# RAPE/NURSING CARE OF VICTIMS

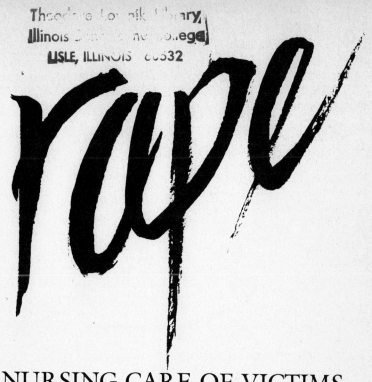

# NURSING CARE OF VICTIMS

## Theresa S. Foley, R.N., C.S., Ph.D.

School of Nursing,
Psychiatric–Mental Health Nursing Program,
The University of Michigan,
Ann Arbor, Michigan

## Marilyn A. Davies, M.N., R.N.

Clinical Administrator,
Western Psychiatric Institute and Clinic,
University of Pittsburgh,
Pittsburgh, Pennsylvania

WITH 23 ILLUSTRATIONS

## THE C. V. MOSBY COMPANY

ST. LOUIS • TORONTO • LONDON  1983

**MOSBY**

A TRADITION OF PUBLISHING EXCELLENCE

*Editor:* Alison Miller
*Assistant editor:* Susan R. Epstein
*Manuscript editor:* Carlotta Seely
*Design:* Kay M. Kramer
*Production:* Barbara Merritt, Mary Stueck

Printed in the United States of America

The C.V. Mosby Company
11830 Westline Industrial Drive, St. Louis, Missouri 63141

**Library of Congress Cataloging in Publication Data**

Foley, Theresa S.
  Rape—nursing care of victims.

  Bibliography: p.
  Includes index.
  1. Gynecologic nursing. 2. Rape victims—
Medical care. 3. Rape victims—Counseling.
4. Rape—Psychological aspects. I. Davies,
Marilyn A. II. Title.
RA1141.F64    1983        362.8'83       82-18764
ISBN 0-8016-1620-4

TS/TS/VH   9  8  7  6  5  4  3  2  1        01/A/071

TO OUR PARENTS

Thelma E. Carmichael Foley and James B. Foley

*TSF*

Florence C. Brickner and Harry A. Brickner

*MAD*

# Preface

One of the most prominent reasons for writing this book has been our experience with victims of abuse and violence and their significant others. Thus we have tried to provide information we consider essential to providing compassionate, comprehensive, and professional nursing care to victims and their significant others.

Statistics on the incidence of abuse and violence are staggering, and projections of future trends suggest that the occurrence of such crimes is likely to increase. It is important, therefore, that nurses be prepared to provide professional care to victims and their significant others. As a social issue, rape and sexual abuse are not just crimes between one man and one woman or child; the crimes reflect an increasing incidence of abuse and violence in Western society. Experts in victimology generally believe that Western culture and socialization processes sanction abuse and violence as a way of life, particularly as a learned response to stressors in daily living. Since women are most frequently the target of oppressive sexual abuse and violence, it is important to address the problem as an issue that directly or indirectly touches one's personal life and reflects socialization processes in need of change.

Teaching others about the problem of violence and abuse and, most importantly, ways to provide nursing care to victims is critical in a time so replete with such maladaptive behaviors. With the increasing specialization and integration of content in nursing curricula, it is important that nurses have available a book that exceeds what can be offered in a single lecture. Nurses not only provide care to victims but also are potential or actual victims of abuse and violence as well. Nurses see victims in every field of practice, not just in an emergency department or medical care unit. For example, nurses see victims as clients seeking care in obstetrical and gynecological clinics, as patients undergoing surgery that can reactivate a rape or sexual abuse trauma, in counseling as psychiatric–mental health nurse therapists, and as children and families in pediatrics. Nurses come in contact with victims as school nurses responsible for assessing stress reactions and the health of children, as community health nurses in the homes of families, as administrators responsible for developing programs and policies related to health and social issues, and as researchers investigating the nature of abuse and violence and the effectiveness of treatment interventions. The importance of content on victimology being included in nursing curricula is evident from the endorsement of the American Nurses' Association Council of Specialists in Psychiatric and Mental Health Nursing of a "Resolution on Victimology," which is reprinted in Appendix V.

Rape and child sexual abuse are problems that have great national, local, and personal concerns for many people. As crimes, rape and sexual abuse have far-reaching effects on the victim's psychological, physical, and social well-being and that of her* significant others. Often the victim becomes involved with multiple care-givers in a variety of social systems that are insensitive to her needs. Professional nurses concerned about rape and sexual abuse victims are asking important questions, such as "How can professional nursing effect change so that better and more sensitive care is provided to victims and their significant others?"

This text was written to facilitate change in three areas: (1) the education of professional nurses so that they are prepared to provide sensitive and competent care to rape and child sexual abuse victims and their significant others; (2) the awareness and sensitivity of health care delivery systems and social systems that provide services to rape and child sexual abuse victims; and (3) support for research on the nature of rape and child sexual abuse, the care of victims and their significant others, and the evaluation of intervention strategies.

The subject matter of this book is arranged in sequential chapters to facilitate a cumulative learning process. Each chapter presumes that the reader has integrated the knowledge and values from each preceding chapter. While completing the text, readers should experience an active learning process that results in a total synthesis of subject matter, application of theory to nursing practice, and a personal growth experience.

At the end of each chapter are learning activities designed to augment the text and to facilitate the learning process. Completion of the exercises is therefore recommended. Annotated suggested readings are also included for those readers who wish to pursue further information on a specific subject.

We believe that professional nursing practice is grounded in a theoretical framework. Stress adaptation theory was selected as a major theoretical framework for this text. As crimes, rape and child sexual abuse not only are maladaptive acts influenced by life stressors, they also require of the victim and her significant others an adaptation process to the acts themselves as stressors. While stress adaptation theory is emphasized, other theoretical frameworks, including general systems theory, social network theory, developmental theory, and crisis intervention theory are also incorporated into the text. We believe that a synthesis of the basic principles of these theories, through the cumulative learning experience provided in the text, provides professional nurses with a firm knowledge base from which to provide quality care to rape and child sexual abuse victims. As a well-designed course of instruction, the book is adaptable to service settings and existing curricula in schools of nursing regardless of their theoretical frameworks. The flexibility of the text is intended to allow options for use of the chapters within existing graduate and undergraduate curricula and service settings.

---

*The authors acknowledge that males are nurses and victims of rape and child sexual abuse. In this text, to facilitate writing style, the authors generally refer to victims and nurses as females.

Part I of this book presents factual information related to rape. We believe that nurses are sometimes confused and uninformed about facts related to rape. Part I consists of two chapters that present an initial learning experience to help the reader sort through relevant data, descriptive information, and research findings to discover these facts. In Chapter 1, Myths and Facts about Rape, we focus on factual information such as: Who is the victim? What is the victim like? Who is the rapist? What are specific facts surrounding the crime of rape? Specific characteristics around the rape itself and the offender are presented to provide important facts that must be addressed before the nurse can provide competent care to rape victims. Special situations that arouse curiosity and are often left unaddressed are also presented in this chapter, such as gang rape, homosexual rape, and repeat rape.

Chapter 2, Men Who Rape, discusses the rapist in more detail. Many myths about the rapist and the victim stem from misperceptions of rape as a sexually motivated act. Two major myths about the rapist are (1) that he is an all-American boy who has tremendous sexual prowess and cannot restrain his sexual urges, or (2) that he is a black, lower-class male who derives demented pleasure from ravishing women. Included in the discussion is a description of the multiple motives for rape, since the victim's response corresponds to the type of offender that she encounters. Although the rapist is not the major focus of attention of the text, we believe it is necessary to discuss treatment programs for offenders to emphasize that they are treatable and, if untreated, they repeat rape and abuse with increasing severity and violence in subsequent offenses.

Part II of the book consists of three chapters that address specific responses to rape. After discovering facts about rape, nurses need to work through their own feelings. Once nurses accept and understand their own responses, they are better prepared to understand the responses of victims, families, and society.

Chapter 3, Nurse Response to Rape, begins with an active learning process by which nurses who work with rape victims assess which factors influence their responses to rape victims. Nurses are asked to explore their own developmental stage of life and life events as well as current social roles, family relationships, and social systems, as these all influence their response to rape victims. We firmly believe that working with rape victims can be a positive growth experience. Rape victims elicit many feelings within the nurse, such as anger, doubt, and anxiety. These feelings can be understood through a process of self-awareness and value clarification. Unless a nurse knows and understands herself, she cannot adequately care for rape victims. The end of this chapter explores expanded roles in nursing, such as advocacy, education, consultation, and research, which offer nurses exciting opportunities to synthesize knowledge and skills into more active professional contributions to victim care.

Chapter 4, Victim Response to Rape, answers the question, "How do victims respond to rape?" Rape victims are not "typical." Their reactions to the violence and abuse experienced during rape vary widely. Depending on individual vulnerability, rape victims experience a stressful response pattern characterized by specific phases, both acute and long-term. Rape is seen as a life-threatening experience that elicits adaptive responses from the victim. Nurses are instrumental in supporting rape victims through this stress adaptation process.

In Chapter 5, Family Response to Rape, family responses are understood as an adaptation to the rape of someone emotionally close to them. Sometimes a major time commitment of nurses has to be in active intervention with family members. In this chapter, using social network theory, we emphasize that nurses need to assess who is the most important emotionally supportive person to the rape victim. Such persons as family members, mates, friends, and children of victims influence a rape victim's responses. It is important that nurses recognize that those persons who are closest to a victim are not necessarily those who can best understand and support the victim. When family members are themselves in crisis, they cannot be expected to adequately support a rape victim. In understanding a family's response to rape, nurses first need to have a basic understanding of how to assess healthy family functioning. Families have acute and long-term stress-adaptation responses to a rape experience that are similar to victim response patterns. Nurses have unique opportunities to help families adapt to the rape experience. Nursing intervention is particularly critical at this time since rape victims typically turn to family members or significant others for support, and the response of these persons can impede or facilitate the victim's resolution of the rape.

Part III consists of five chapters specifically designed to prepare professional nurses to provide competent nursing care to rape and child sexual abuse victims and their families. Advanced nursing skills include physical and psychological assessment, goal-directed nursing interventions, and provision of adequate follow-up care. Although the adult victim is emphasized throughout the book, a special chapter is devoted to the sexual abuse of children.

Chapter 6, Hospital Care of the Rape Victim, presents operational guidelines for the rape examination. We stress the importance of sensitivity to the victim's psychological needs in a discussion of technical and interpersonal nursing care guidelines before and throughout the rape examination. The rape examination emphasizes a procedure that focuses on the victim's physical needs and evidence collection that ensures legal admissibility in court. Examination of the accused rapist and male rape victims is also discussed. The chapter concludes with a discussion of the victim's follow-up care needs. Nurses who are particularly familiar with rape victimology may choose to proceed directly to this chapter for medical management information.

Chapter 7, Basic Counseling and Crisis Intervention, focuses specifically on crisis intervention and counseling of rape victims. In both traditional and expanded roles, professional nurses help rape victims by applying crisis intervention techniques. Nurses assist rape victims to reorder perceptions, learn adaptive coping mechanisms, and organize their support systems. The major emphasis in short- and longer-term counseling is the development of an empathic relationship between the nurse and the rape victim. Within the context of the nurse-victim relationship, concerns and fears of rape victims are worked through and the victim's self-esteem and self-confidence are increased. The creative listening model that emphasizes accurate empathy, nonpossessive warmth, and respect of rape victims is presented. Three phases of a counseling relationship in helping rape victims are also discussed. These phases consist of self-exploration, self-understanding, and action.

Chapter 8, Rape Victim Advocacy, discusses the concept of advocacy as it relates to meeting the rape victim's needs. In this chapter we make a distinction between principles of nursing advocacy and the role and functions of volunteer advocates in rape victim care. Professional nurses who understand the role of volunteer advocates can facilitate utilization of this resource as a secondary support for rape victims. In their professional role, nurses are particularly effective as advocates for rape victims. Nurses implement principles of advocacy in providing care to rape victims and their significant others whether that be in hospital emergency departments or community settings such as rape crisis centers and community mental health centers. This chapter discusses the legal system, including police investigation of the rape and criminal prosecution of the rapist. The role of nurses as mediators in ensuring rape victims sensitive and competent care in the emergency department is presented. Another important role of nurses, discussed in this chapter, is that of an expert witness in criminal proceedings. Nurses must be adequately prepared for this important task.

Chapter 9, Counseling Victims Through the Court Process, is particularly designed for nurses who counsel victims who decide to prosecute their assailants. The court process can be a threatening situation, and nurses need to recognize that rape victims need support in preparing for hearings, coping with concerns that arise during the trial, and adapting to a verdict. For rape victims who need longer-term counseling, we have found a cognitive-behavioral strategy to be most effective and have presented one such model in this chapter.

The major emphasis of this text is on the nursing care of the adult rape victim. However, we do recognize the critical problem of child sexual abuse. Many rapists have a history of child sexual, physical, and psychological abuse. Chapter 10, Child Sexual Abuse, presents information relevant to child sexual abuse and focuses on nursing interventions with child victims and their families. The medical management of the child and the psychological management of the child's parents are emphasized. Several approaches to the prevention of child sexual abuse are also presented.

The appendixes of the book provide the reader with rich resources. Some content contained in the appendixes is referred to in the text of the book. Reference is made, for example, to forms to be completed during a rape examination or a child sexual abuse examination, guidelines for interviewing a child victim, and films as teaching aids. The appendixes also contain a useful list of rape prevention strategies.

We hope that nurses will find the content helpful in developing nursing care plans and in applying the American Nurses' Association Standards of Practice in the nursing care of rape victims and their significant others. Finally, we hope that as a result of this endeavor, victims of rape and child sexual abuse receive compassionate, comprehensive, and professional nursing care, and that more nurses become actively involved in the field of victimology. As Brownmiller aptly said in *Against Our Will: Men, Women and Rape:*

> Fighting back. On a multiplicity of levels, that is the activity we must engage in, together, if we—women—are to redress the imbalance and rid ourselves and men of the ideology of rape.

*Theresa S. Foley*
*Marilyn A. Davies*

# Acknowledgments

Kahlil Gibran said in *The Prophet,* "You give little when you give of your possessions, it is when you give of yourself that you truly give." We gratefully acknowledge those who gave of themselves during the writing of this book and enhanced its quality. The length and scope of the book have resulted in indebtedness to many individuals. Our expression of gratitude will never adequately convey the value we place on their contributions. Foremost, we wish to express indebtedness to the many victims of rape and child sexual abuse who have so openly shared their trauma and suffering and cooperated in efforts to improve the quality of care received by victims within institutions.

An abiding gratitude and special thanks are due to Dr. Aaron Beck, Dr. Ann Burgess, Dr. Ellen Frank, and Dr. A. Nicholas Groth for their consultation, colleagueship, and encouragement in the completion of this work. Without reports of their research and clinical practice much of this text could never have been written. Directors and staff of community agencies providing services for victims and families have been invaluable resources. These include the Assault Crisis Center of Ann Arbor, Michigan; the Center for Victims of Violent Crimes in Pittsburgh; Children's Hospital of Pittsburgh; the Harrisburg Area Rape Crisis Center of Pennsylvania; the Interagency Task Force on Rape-Related Services of Pittsburgh; the Pennsylvania Coalition Against Rape; Pittsburgh Action Against Rape; the Rape Crisis Center of Syracuse, New York; Parents United/Parents Anonymous of Pittsburgh; and the Sexual Assault Center, Harborview Medical Center in Seattle, Washington. Selections from *Stinky: The Berkeley Rapist* have been reprinted by permission of The Sterling Lord Agency, Inc.; copyright 1978 by Lacey Fosburgh.

We also appreciate the dedicated efforts of students and colleagues who reviewed and contributed constructive criticism that enhanced the quality of this work: Patricia Bartone, Dr. Carolyn Carter, Marcia Glass, Dr. Lyn Ramik Finneran, Patty Hayes, Professor Erma Meyerson, Doris Mikel, Nancy Noel, and Priscilla Tait. Special thanks are due to persons providing technical assistance for their competence, dependability, interest, and hard work that enabled completion of this book: Florence C. Brickner, Marsha Comans, and Rita Faigen.

Finally, we wish to express our deepest gratitude to our extended families and to Carl and Bill for their love, understanding, and encouragement, which made this work possible. Hopefully, the care that victims and their families receive will be better for sacrifices that these persons made during the writing of this book.

*Theresa S. Foley*
*Marilyn A. Davies*

# Contents

# PART I

# Facts
# about Rape

## CHAPTER 1

# Myths and facts about rape

RAPE. The word insults our sensitivity. The sound of it leaves us feeling vulnerable and threatened. The act, of course, is worse. . . . The need to control and prevent rape is universal. All of us face the possibility of rape.

From Heath, M., and Mercardante, M., editors: *A handbook for victims,* 1979.

## CHAPTER OUTLINE

## LEARNING OBJECTIVES

After reading this chapter the student will be able to:

1  Define rape within social and legal perspectives
2  List and define five terms that describe sexual assaults other than rape
3  Differentiate between myths about rape and facts about rape
4  State eight rape myths and their results on victims and society
5  Identify high-risk characteristics of rape victims that relate to age, race, sex, occupation, socioeconomic status, and prior psychiatric illness
6  Describe literature findings related to styles of attack and motives for rape
7  Identify and explain five variables that characterize a rape situation
8  Select four rape myths and refute them with facts about rape

In researching the topic of rape for the first time, the uninformed nurse will find that many questions arise. What is rape? Is rape a sex crime? Who is the typical victim? Are most victims promiscuous? What are the chances of rape happening to me? What happens during the assault?

This chapter presents an overview of current issues related to defining rape. These include (1) social criteria that define an act as rape, (2) legal evidence that proves a rape has transpired, and (3) how rape differs from other sexual assaults. The chapter stresses the need for nurses to acquire a specialized knowledge of the subject matter. By defining the term *rape*, it helps the nurse understand the concept of rape from both social and legal perspectives. This discussion also explores the myths and facts about rape.

Myths are false beliefs. Myths about rape arise from the ways in which men and women in our society are socialized; their net effect has been for the victim to blame herself for the assailant's behavior. Facts consist of findings from descriptive and empirical research. In this chapter, rape myths are presented and discussed. Next, facts about rape, based on collected data and research findings, are presented to refute rape myths and provide nurses with the necessary knowledge base for providing care to rape victims.

## DEFINITIONS OF RAPE

The term *rape* is derived from the Latin word *rapere*, which means to steal, seize, or carry away. Rape involves "stealing" sexual relations from another person. For this book, we define rape as *the use of threat, physical force, or intimidation in obtaining sexual relations with another person against his or her will*. The intent of rape is to humiliate and degrade the victim by using sex as a weapon to express violence, power, and aggression.

Rape is considered a violent crime that falls between the acts of assault and robbery: "It is, in one act, both a blow to the body and a blow to the mind, and a "taking" of sex through the use of threat."[10] For a woman, rape implies total loss of self. The woman is treated as a function and an object rather than as a person. For these reasons, women live in fear of rape.

## Social definitions

Social definitions of rape occur when society labels certain behaviors as rape. Such labeling is used for an act that is a deviation from the behavioral norms of a society. For example, in primitive tribal societies a man actually seized or stole whatever woman he wanted for a wife. After raping her, the man would bring the woman into his tribe as his mate. Such behavior was an acceptable tribal ritual. In contemporary Western society this type of behavior would be considered deviant and labeled as rape.

Over the years social definitions of rape have reflected social values related to sex roles and socialization of men and women. Traditionally women have been raised to competitively seek men's attention and affiliation, to barter their sexuality as a prize to trade in winning men. Men have been raised to be aggressors in initiating sexual relationships. "Scoring" or "making a mark" has defined their masculinity, adequacy, and identity. Historically the prosecution of rapists has reflected the social concept of rape in the context of male power and dominance through ownership and the assertion of male dominance (manhood) through the defilement and reduction of another man's property value.

> Society's view of rape was purely a matter of economics—of assets and liabilities. When a married woman was raped, her husband was wronged, not her. If she was unmarried, her father suffered since his investment depreciated. It was the monetary value of a woman which determined the gravity of the crime. Because she had no personal rights under the law, her own emotions simply didn't matter.[5]

Today the issue of male ownership and abuse of another man's property continues to be reflected by the social belief that a father safeguards his virgin daughter, a husband protects his "faithful" wife, whereas no one claims a prostitute. Thus if an assailant attacked all three women in the same way, he could be accused of raping the first two women but not the prostitute.

Society often misperceives rape as a *sexual crime* in which women are viewed as objects for the man's release of sexual tension. This attitude is based on the belief that the victim is simply irresistible and that the rapist acts impulsively and injudiciously in giving vent to sexual passion. It is exemplified by Arizona legislators who, in amending the statutes on sexual assault, perceived the essential issue as "sex and in the same old terms: women 'own' it, men crave it."[2]

Social definitions of rape ignore a wide range of offensive and serious sexual assaults such as date rape or acquaintance rape. The date rape consists of a social relationship in which sexual intercourse was not expected or agreed to, but, under duress or threat of force, it is insisted upon and forced upon an unconsenting woman. Date rapes have their origin in the learned socialization patterns of men and women. Marital rape is even more difficult to prove than date rape because of society's values and attitudes toward a husband's rights to sex within the marriage contract.

## Legal definitions

Today courts of law in the United States recognize three elements as comprising an act of rape: (1) the use of threat, duress, physical force, intimidation, or deception; (2) sexual relations or vaginal penetration, however slight; and (3) nonconsent of the victim. Thus an American court of law has defined rape as

> the penetration or an act of sexual intercourse with a female, not one's wife [in most states], against her will and consent whether her will is overcome by force or fear resulting from the threat of force, or by drugs or intoxicants; or when, because of mental deficiency, she is incapable of exercising rational judgement; or when she is below an arbitrary "age of consent."[3]

Although oral and anal intercourse is considered by many victims to be more traumatic and humiliating than penile-vaginal attacks, many states do not consider this form of assault as an act of rape. However, some states are changing their laws to include oral and anal rape in the legal definition of rape. Some states are also making it possible for a wife to charge her husband with rape.

The underlying element in legally defining rape, both for the victim and for those who corroborate her decision to prosecute, is the *element of consent*. This issue becomes clear in the victim's description of the act as

> sexual invasion of the body by force; an incursion into the private, personal inner space without consent—an internal assault from one of several avenues and by one of several methods [which] constitutes a deliberate violation of emotional, physical, and rational integrity and is a hostile, degrading act of violence that deserves the name of rape.[3]

Rape is characterized according to the element of consent as follows:

1. *Rape.* Sex without consent.
2. *Accessory to sex.* Inability to consent or not consent to sex because of the victim's stage of personality or cognitive development.
3. *Sex-stress situation.* Initial consent to sex followed by something going drastically wrong in the situation; usually the male has exploited the initial agreement.[3]

### CLINICAL EXAMPLE

Heather is a 19-year-old, white, college student who has been living in the dormitory on campus. One weekend she was alone while her roommate was away to see friends. Heather and her boyfriend, Patrick, decided to have a good time. They got a bit intoxicated and danced to some records, then decided to get high on marijuana and watch the late show on TV in the dorm lounge. Patrick escorted Heather back to her room and forced his way in after her. She protested but he insisted he just wanted to stay a minute and hold her a bit. She said dorm regulations cut off visiting hours after 1:00 AM and he had better leave.

Patrick became angry and threw her on the bed saying he wanted to have sex with her. Heather tried to force him off but was not strong enough to move him; his fury frightened and perplexed her. She started to scream but he twisted her arms and put a pillow over her head threatening to smother her if she resisted. She cried, saying she wanted to save herself for marriage and yelled vulgarities at him but that only excited him further. Patrick ripped

Heather's clothes off. Anytime she tried to resist, it just seemed to incite his anger. At one point he grabbed a perfume bottle, smashed it, and used the glass to cut up her breasts, forcing a pillow over her face to muffle her cries. He then forced sexual relations on Heather vaginally, flipped her over, and held her face down. He told her she was a bitch for teasing and leading him on; certainly she should know that "after you've dated a man for awhile sex is expected," so it was her fault that he was upset. He continued telling her she was "not such hot stuff after all," . . . that her hips were too fat and her chest was too small, and "no guy really wants to settle for that." After a period of berating Heather, he then raped her anally, biting parts of her body and pulling her hair as he shoved her about. Before leaving he told her not to tell anyone or he would take revenge. He reminded her that no one would believe her anyway as they had been dating and they would think she had provoked him. Then he left and sneaked down the back stairwell.

The preceding clinical example demonstrates social and legal definitions of rape. The offender (Patrick) reflects the social concept of rape by asserting male dominance through the use of physical force to obtain sexual relations. His attitude is expressed through offensive and dehumanizing statements that reflect his view of his girlfriend as an object for the release of tension. Legally the elements that comprise an act of rape are present: (1) use of threat and physical force, (2) vaginal penetration, and (3) nonconsent of the victim.

## Other sexual assaults

Definitions of rape, as used by researchers, have included impairing the morals of a minor, oral and anal sex, indecent assault, manual contact with the victim's genitals, incest, seduction, child molestation, and other forms of sexual assault. Other terminology that may arise in the course of caring for rape victims includes the following:[6]

*Attempted rape.* In this type of assault substantial steps must be taken by the assailant toward the completion of an act of rape; that is, the assailant must have been exposed and been attempting to subdue and penetrate the victim but for some reason (e.g., interrupted by police) was unable to do so.

*Statutory rape.* Statutory rape is sexual intercourse between a person 18 years of age or older with another person less than 14 years of age who is not his spouse. This definition specifies age but not force. Therefore statutory rape can be a sexual relationship by mutual consent that violates parental consent or standards.

*Incest.* Incest involves sexual intercourse, marriage, or cohabitation with a blood relative without regard to the legitimacy of such acts. It includes a sexual relationship between adopted children and their parents.

*Indecent assault.* This type of assault includes any touching of the "private parts" of the body (the genital area, breasts, or buttocks) of another, except spouse, under circumstances in which the assailant knows such conduct is likely to cause alarm.

*Simple assault.* In simple assault a person attempts to cause bodily harm or injury to another or puts that person in imminent fear of such injury.

*Aggravated assault.* In aggravated assault a person causes or attempts to cause serious bodily harm to another individual with full knowledge of the seriousness of the act or behaves in a reckless manner manifesting extreme indifference to the value of human life.

*Involuntary deviate sexual intercourse.* This is forcible oral or anal intercourse with another person without his or her consent either by threat of force or when such person is unconscious, mentally deranged, or under the age of 14. It could, for example, consist of the assailant forcing the victim to perform fellatio (have her mouth on his genitals) or submit to cunnilingus (forcing his mouth onto the victim's genitals). Many victims do not understand these technical terms, but they will verify acts if the nurse gives an explicit description of them.

*Child sexual abuse.* This type of assault is the forcing of sexual contact onto a child by another person. (See Chapter 10 for a complete discussion of this subject).

## MYTHS ABOUT RAPE

Misconceptions surrounding the crime of rape are both numerous and as old as the human race, with some accounts dating back to biblical times. Currently rape myths can be categorized in two ways: (1) myths related to victims and (2) myths related to men who rape. Table 1-1 presents the more predominant rape myths that exist today.

Many people agree with the rape myths that suggest that rape victims provoke their assault in conscious or unconscious ways. For example, people believe that many women are "asking for it" by dressing provocatively or by acting seductively. These women are construed as presenting themselves in a manner that is "irresistible" to any

**Table 1-1. Rape myths**

| Myths related to victims | Myths related to men who rape |
|---|---|
| Rape is provoked by the victim. Victims are responsible for their victimization either consciously or by default. All women really want to be raped. | Rape is an impulsive, uncontrollable act of sexual gratification (i.e., a sexually frustrated man sees an attractive young woman and "just can't control himself"). |
| Only young, beautiful women in miniskirts are raped. It can't happen to me; only other types of women get raped. Only "bad girls" get raped. Rape reflects a demographic strain caused by sex-marital status imbalance in the community. Only promiscuous women get raped. | Rapists are abnormal perverts or men with an unsatisfied sex drive. Only "sick" or "insane" men rape women. The primary motive for rape is sexual. The rapist is a sexually starved psychopath. |
| Women are raped when they are out alone at night, primarily in dark alleys. If women stay at home, they will be safe. | Most rapes involve black men and white women. Blacks are more likely to attack white women than black women. All rapes are interracial. |
| Any woman could prevent rape if she really wanted to. No woman can be raped against her will. Victims generally do not resist their attackers. Any woman who resists her attacker will be killed. | Rapists will flee if the woman resists. |

From Foley, T.S.: Counseling the victim of rape. In Stuart, G., and Sundeen, S.: Principles and practice of psychiatric nursing, St. Louis, 1983, The C.V. Mosby Co.

man's natural sexual drives. Any blame for the sexual assault is directed totally toward the rape victim.

Other people believe that women place themselves in situations or places that make them a higher risk for sexual assault. These people are also attributing blame to the rape victim. For example, a woman who is walking down a dark alley or goes out alone at night "should know better" because she is increasing her risk of an assault. Likewise a hitchhiker or a woman who allows herself to "be picked up" at a bar or party is also judged to be soliciting or encouraging a sexual assault.

Other women are viewed as secretly desiring sexual encounters, but, when violence occurs, the women are accused of seeking revenge or attempting to avoid societal disapproval by "crying rape." Many people believe that "only bad women are raped" and that women can truly resist an attacker.

Many people subscribe to the myth that rape is a crime of passion, an impulsive act of sexual gratification. They believe that men who rape are sexually frustrated and "can't control themselves." These myths condone the rape as expressing a legitimate sexual need or urge.

Other myths related to men who rape describe offenders as special, identifiable characters. For example, "dirty old man," or "black men against white women," or "perverted" are descriptions used for rapists. Many people do not believe that a normal-appearing and normal-acting man could commit rape.

In general, rape myths reflect positions, values, or feelings determined by society. Rape myths are not founded in facts. Many of the rape myths arise and are perpetuated by socialization processes that specify sex-role behaviors and attitudes toward women. If women are raped, it is because they have failed to heed the dictates of society. Society conveys to rape victims that they are responsible for the assault. This results in ignoring the multifaceted nature of the problem, blaming the rape victim, and reinforcing her guilt and shame.

## FACTS ABOUT RAPE

*Uniform Crime Report* statistics show that reported forcible rape is rising faster than assault, homicide, or any other violent crime in the United States. Rape *increased* 5% during the first 6 months of 1976, while all other violent crimes *decreased* by 5% nationally. According to the FBI, 1979 data show that 75,789 women reported forcible rapes, assaults, or attempts to commit rape by actual or threatened force. In 1979 the number of reported forcible rapes was up 13% over 1978 and up 35% over 1975. The actual scope of the problem is underestimated because many rapes go unreported. Even if better reporting has resulted in higher statistics, researchers estimate the ratio of unreported to reported rapes as ranging anywhere from 2 to 1 up to 20 to 1. For example, for 75,789 reported rapes in 1979, approximately 757,890 (10 to 1) to 1,515,780 (20 to 1) rapes actually occurred. In the United States a rape is reported every 7 minutes.

Crime rates are based on reported cases, and rape is believed to be the most unreported violent crime because of the victim's fear of the assailant, embarrassment over the crime, and societal reactions to rape. The crime rate is the number of crimes for every 100,000 vulnerable people. A crime is, thus, a victim risk rate. The victim risk rate for a woman being raped in her lifetime has been reported as 1 in 10.[11]

## Characteristics of the victim

Although all women face the possibility of rape, according to reported statistics some people are more at risk than others. This section will identify and describe the characteristics associated with the high risk of becoming a rape victim. Factors to be considered include age, race, marital status, sex, occupation, and socioeconomic status. Table 1-2 summarizes the data discussed below.

*Age.* Despite the popular myth that rape happens only to the young, in actuality it happens to persons of all ages. In the literature the youngest rape victim is reported to be 5 months old and the oldest one 91 years old. In a synthesis of research findings, Katz and Mazur[8] report that the high-risk age groups are teenagers (13-17) and young adults (18-24). (These age groups carry high risk for *all* serious violent crimes.) The most frequently cited rape victims are 14 years old.

*Race.* Regardless of age, black females report more rape than any other racial group. Some authors report the rates for rape of adolescent black females to be 20 times higher than those of white women of the same age. Contrary to popular myth, most rapes are *intraracial*. Nationally 3% of rapes are between black men and white women, 4% involve black women and white men. Some studies have found that the percentage of victims by race approximated the average racial population of the area; that is, the percentage of black, Chicano, or Anglo victims reporting rape reflected the racial balance of the city. It should also be noted that many nonwhites tend to use formal systems such as the police or hospital emergency room more frequently than do wealthier, white, middle-class victims who can afford private care. Thus statistics regarding race reflect the general socioeconomic characteristics of persons seeking care in health care systems and are not specific to rape. When interracial rapes do occur, they tend to be more violent, particularly when a white offender and a nonwhite victim are involved.

*Marital status.* Statistics indicate that the majority of rape victims are unmarried at the time of the assault. This fact is understandable in view of the peak age (14 years old) and the high-risk age groups (between 13 and 24) for the crime. The majority of victims live with one or both parents, or with another person.

*Sex.* Although most victims are females and most rape literature defines rape in terms of the female, male rape has been reported. Because of the ways in which men are socialized, they tend not to report the crime or they express embarrassment and rage when they do report it. Estimates of male rape in sexually heterogenous samples have been reported as 4% to 5%, and vulnerability among male college students is reported as 30% in contrast to a 50% vulnerability rate for females.

**Table 1-2. Characteristics of victims**

| Characteristics | High-risk factors |
| --- | --- |
| Age | 13-24 |
| Race | Black |
| Marital status | Single |
| Sex | Female |
| Occupation | Student |
| Socioeconomic status (SES) | Lower |

*Occupation.* Because most victims are young, the majority are also students. Women in certain professions are particularly easy targets: waitresses, cleaning ladies, clerks, and nurses. Many of these women work late hours, travel alone, and have a pattern of entry to and exit from work that facilitates the offender's efforts to plan the attack. In addition, a wide range of other occupations, from nuns to prostitutes, is reported in the literature.

*Socioeconomic status.* Statistics on reported rape indicate that upper- and middle-class females are *less* at risk of rape than women of lower socioeconomic status. However, it has been suggested that the percentage of upper-class victims may be greater than statistics reflect because these women do not use established reporting mechanisms; instead they seek care from private physicians. In general, lower socioeconomic status is characteristic of the black female, who is more vulnerable to all serious crimes.[8]

CLINICAL EXAMPLE

Anne is a 19-year-old, black, single college student attending a community college near her urban home. As she returned to her home after class one evening, two men asked her for directions and then in a surprise attack proceeded to drag her behind a campus building where they raped her. They threatened to kill her if she did not comply with their demands and later to take revenge if she reported to the police. Anne said she did not want her parents to know about the rape.

The victim in this example has many characteristics that place her at high risk for rape: age (young adult), race (black), marital status (single), sex (female), and occupation (student). As a woman who walks home alone in a specific pattern, she is a target for offenders who plan their attack.

*Repeat rape victims. Repeat rape* is defined as going through or experiencing a rape again. Data on the occurrence of repeat rape (also called *victim recidivism*) deserve examination from health professionals. Although preliminary data on repeat rape are quite limited, a few pilot studies have collected data from victim data forms that are filled out at the time of entrance into a health care system and from unstructured interviews related to victim response to rape.

According to preliminary data, the average age of repeat rape victims is not significantly different from the age of other rape victims (generally called first-time victims). Educational levels are also quite similar. However, early research findings indicate the following differences in characteristics of repeat rape victims.

1. Repeat rape victims are lower in socioeconomic status than first-time victims and are either unemployed or on public assistance.
2. Repeat rape victims have a higher frequency of seeking professional help for emotional problems than first-time rape victims.
3. A notable feature of repeat rape victims is transiency, defined as rootlessness or passing through a place with only a brief stay. This feature is not predominant with first-time rape victims.[9]

Recent work in the field of victimology has led to a closer look at victim recidivism. One national survey of victims of violent crimes revealed that 28% were prior victims of violent crimes. Unfortunately, data on rape victims were not included in this survey. A more recent study, reporting data collected from rape victims, revealed that 24%

were repeat rape victims. On interview, repeat rape victims revealed that the prior assault often involved incest. Because repeat rape has received little research attention, only limited facts can be related to this type of assault. Repeat rape, therefore, deserves further examination and well-designed research studies.

### Characteristics of the rapist

The demographic characteristics of the rapist are closely related to those of the victim. Factors to be considered include age, race, marital status, intelligence, and socioeconomic status. Table 1-3 depicts a profile of the rapist; a discussion of the variables cited in the table follows below.

*Age.* The rapist is usually a young man in the age group of 15 to 24. This is not surprising because adolescent and young adulthood years are a time of psychologic distress for men as they attempt to establish their sexual identity, power status, and adequacy as a "man." Thus rape is a symptom of the offender's internal psychologic developmental crisis, arising at a time when many demands are being placed upon him for managing his life and when he has insufficient resources to cope with successive pressures; or rape is a symptom of a crisis state in which the man is temporarily overwhelmed by stresses that he ordinarily has sufficient resources to cope with.[4]

*Race.* Most reported rapes are committed by black men against black women. However, one must question whether the crime rate and incidence of rape among blacks is really higher than among whites, or whether the statistics are not, in fact, a reflection of general discriminatory practices within American culture. It is known, for example, that more blacks are convicted of crimes and receive more severe sentences (death, life imprisonment) than whites.

*Marital status.* Many rapists are married, have girlfriends and families. All rapists report readily available sexual partners for gratification of sexual needs. Data on marital status for convicted rapists show most to be married. Rapists who are not convicted tend to be single.

*Intelligence.* The rapist is of *average intelligence* but falls below his educational and vocational or career potential. His ability to be successful and master the demands of school and work are a direct result of his inability to tolerate and channel frustration.

*Socioeconomic status.* It is characteristic of the rapist to come from a *lower socioeconomic background*, which some experts believe to be characterized by physical aggression and sexuality or culturally sanctioned modes of proving one's masculinity and sense of identity that foster rape.

**Table 1-3. Profile of the rapist**

| Variable | Characteristic |
| --- | --- |
| Sex | Male |
| Age | 15-24 |
| Race | Black |
| Marital status | Single (nonconvicted) |
| Intelligence | Average |
| Socioeconomic status (SES) | Lower |

### Rape situation variables

This section describes literature findings that report facts related to the rape situation. The "facts" are derived from reported rape cases, so the reader is cautioned that these statistics must be considered within this limitation. Table 1-4 summarizes current information related to rape situation variables. As demonstrated in the table, specific variables include style of attack; motives for rape; relationship between victim and offender; where and when the rape occurs; use of force, violence, or weapons; and victim precipitation.

*Style of attack.* Two styles of attack characterize rape situations. One is a *confidence rape* in which the assailant obtains sex under false pretenses by first gaining the victim's trust and then betraying the trust by deceit or violence. The second type is a *blitz rape* in which victims and offender lack prior interaction. It is "out of the blue" and a sudden, unexpected attack.[4] In the clinical examples discussed earlier in this chapter, Heather was a victim of a confidence rape by a date, whereas Anne was a victim of a blitz rape by strangers.

*Motives for rape.* The intent of rape is to humiliate and degrade, not merely to "take" the victim's most intimate parts; power and control, violence and aggression, and sadism are the motives of the rapist. The penis is merely the weapon used to achieve the rapist's motives; sexual gratification is rarely the intent, and where it does exist rapists report it to be both combined with aggressive aims and an unsatisfying experience failing to meet fantasized expectations.[4] The rapist attempts to demonstrate his masculinity by contempt for anything feminine. This is done by acts such as (1) urinating, defecating, or ejaculating on the victim's face; (2) forcing the victim

**Table 1-4. Rape situation variables**

| Variables | Characteristics of situation |
|---|---|
| Style of attack | Confidence rape <br> Blitz rape |
| Motives for rape | Power/control <br> Violence/aggression <br> Sadism |
| Relationship between victim and offender | Stranger (adult) <br> Acquaintance (adolescent) |
| Where rape occurs | Residence of victim or offender <br> Lower socioeconomic neighborhoods <br> Western metropolitan city |
| When rape occurs <br> Time of day <br> Day of week <br> Season | Nights: 8:00 PM to 4:00 AM <br> Weekends <br> Summer months |
| Use of force, violence, or weapons | Knife or gun <br> Physical and verbal abuse |
| Victim precipitation | Two thirds of assaults are planned |

into bizarre acts such as rubbing her face or tongue into urine, feces, or vomit; (3) ridiculing and humiliating the victim by forced sexual acts such as fellatio and cunnilingus; (4) putting her in a degrading, helpless position at his mercy and command with a terrifying fear for her life; and (5) frequently a final act of force by inserting objects such as bottles and broomsticks into her vagina. For a more detailed discussion of the motives for rape, see Chapter 3.

Two types of rape that reflect particular motivational aspects are the gang rape and the homosexual rape. *Gang rape* is defined as rape by multiple offenders. *Homosexual rape* is defined as rape by a member of one's own sex.

CLINICAL EXAMPLE

I had gone grocery shopping. It was midnight and I took advantage of the stores being open to get stuff done that I can't do when I'm working all day. When I came out my front tire was flat. There were a couple of young guys who offered to give me a lift to the gas station up the street two blocks. It was so cold out in the snow so I took them up on it. How could I be so stupid? They stopped up the street and forced a blindfold on me, then took me to a part of town I don't know to an apartment where a couple of guys met them. They took turns raping me all night and seeing who could perform the most feats. When morning came they took me back to my car and left me like discarded garbage. I feel so filthy dirty, so embarrassed for being so stupid . . . so hurt.

This clinical example demonstrates gang rape—a type of rape that is more common than most people believe and particularly frequent among adolescents. Generally gang rapes last for several hours and show no seasonal specificity. They are usually planned in advance and tend to be associated with high levels of violence and sexual coercion as one male in the group "outdoes" the preceding offender in demonstrating his "adequacy" as a male. Often gang rapes are committed by young males who have been out drinking. According to Katz and Mazur,[8] the youths pick as targets adolescent females from their own neighborhood. These females are often those who have a reputation for being sexually promiscuous or who have achieved some meritorious recognition (e.g., honor student or homecoming queen) that sets them apart from their peers. Black women and Spanish-American women are reported as 10 times more susceptible to this form of assault than white women. It is difficult to collect accurate data on gang rapes because research data vary with definitions of gang rape in terms of the offenders and the victims.

Most homosexual rapes are committed by men who equate their actions with those that they believe to characterized heterosexual, aggressive males. Herman[7] found that among prison rapists the typical sexual aggressor does not consider himself a homosexual or even to have engaged in homosexual acts. This attitude seems to be based upon the offender's startlingly primitive view of sexual relationships, one that defines as "male" whichever partner is aggressive and as "homosexual" which ever partner is passive. In this study the aggressors used such language as "fight or fuck" and "we're gonna make a girl out of you." It is also noteworthy that prison inmates often perceive homosexual offenders as asserting their masculinity through sexual dominance and control, degradation, and conquest of the victim, all of which are characteristic of the rape of women.

Thus, regardless of the victim's sexual identity, motives for homosexual rape remain the same as for other rapes (power/control, violence/aggression, and sadism). Only the available object, the victim, differs.

*Relationship between victim and offender.* The stereotype of the rapist being a stranger to the victim is a fact in well over half of reported rape cases. The majority of adult victims are raped by strangers, whereas the majority of adolescents and children are raped by persons known to them.

The definition of *stranger* varies in the rape literature and thus limits the strength with which conclusions can be made. For example, Amir[1] found 42% of his sample assaulted by a stranger, defined as one with whom "no previous contact existed, and no acquaintanceship established before the offense," and another 10% in the category of "stranger but general knowledge . . . offender is only known visually to the victim without any other contact between them" (52% of total). Other authors report the percentage of "stranger" victim-offender relationships ranging from 33% to 60%. The frequency of acquaintance between victim and offender as reported in the literature is affected by diverse definitions of stranger on a continuum from a "pick-up" to a "casual acquaintance." Furthermore, statistical data are not definitive because a large number of rapes are unreported when the victim and the offender know one another, as is often the case with the adolescent, the young college woman, or the date rape. Many rapists tell their victims that no one will believe them since the victim knows, has dated, or is otherwise acquainted with the offender. This threat holds some weight since (1) the general populace believes many rape myths; (2) studies have shown that less than 50% of situations in which the victim and the offender are acquainted are judged not to be a case of rape or do not receive a conviction; and (3) convicted rapists report 13 nonconvicted rapes for every convicted offense. The fact that adolescent victims and adolescent offenders tend to be acquainted is not surprising in light of the victim's age range, which is characterized by a high level of social activity and dating.

The notion of the "stranger rapist" is believed by most women and lulls them into a false sense of security with men they know. Rapists known to the victim include same-age mates; friends; dates; boyfriends; incestuous offenders such as fathers, uncles, brothers, cousins; and men from all paths of life.

*Where rape occurs.* The 1976 *Uniform Crime Report* statistics indicate that 42% of all rapes continue to occur in metropolitan regions with a population of 250,000 or more. Women residing in metropolises of over 250,000 are three times more likely to be raped than women residing in suburbs; they are four times more likely to be raped than women residing in rural areas. However, there appears to be a change in the direction of rape from major urban locations to suburban areas. In 1976, forcible rape increased 3% in suburban areas bordering large cities and decreased 1% in large cities. This distribution of the incidence of rape could reflect better reporting, an increase in the crime, perceived respectability by the victim, or improved services to the victims.

It appears that some areas of the country are less safe to live in than others. Women in the north central states are less at risk (43 rapes per 100,000) than women residing in the southern states (46 rapes per 100,000) or western states (69 rapes per 100,000). According to the *Uniform Crime Report* for 1976, the safest place to reside to avoid rape is the northeastern United States (37 rapes per 100,000).

Like all violent crimes, most rapes take place in *lower socioeconomic neighborhoods* and in the victim's or the offender's *residence*. Because of social activity styles, adolescents are more likely to be assaulted in the rapist's home or that of a third party. For example, many adolescent and young adult rape victims have been taken into the assailant's confidence as an acquaintance or at a social gathering. They may accept an invitation for a ride home, to see the assailant's apartment, or go with him to another party only to have their confidence betrayed. However, staying at home is no guarantee that women can avoid being raped. Women are also raped in their own residences by men who claim to be friends or pose in such roles as repairmen or census takers. Rape in one's residence is particularly common for adult women more often than for adolescents.

*When rape occurs.* Because since most social activities take place outside ordinary working hours and days, it is not surprising that most rapes occur on *weekends* and during the *night* from 8 PM to 4 AM, particularly if the assailant is a stranger. The night and weekend characteristic of rape is comparable to the evidence of other violent crimes. In warm-weather areas rape is distributed over the 12 months, but in cold-weather areas the national picture reflects a pattern of greater frequency in the summer months. The increased incidence of reported rape in summer months may reflect the increased numbers of persons who are participating in outdoor activities.

*Use of force, violence, or weapons.* Although rape-murders rarely occur, they usually receive the greatest media exposure. Despite the fact that murder rarely accompanies rape, *force and violence are the rule* rather than the exception in rape. Rape generally resembles aggravated assault, in which the weapon most commonly used by the assailant is a knife or, secondly, a gun. According to Katz and Mazur,[8] the following seven situations are associated with increased degrees of violence: (1) adult victims and victims older than the offender are subjected to greater physical force; (2) group rape involves more violence than single-assailant rape; (3) if the offender has been drinking but the victim has not, there is more violence; (4) black offenders are more violent than white offenders (thus black women have endured more abuse than white victims); (5) violence increases when the offender experiences sexual impotence at the time of the assault; (6) a distant victim-offender relationship results in more violence; and (7) more violence occurs if the rape takes place outdoors, as the offender tries to subdue the victim.

*Victim precipitation.* The National Commission on the Causes and Prevention of Violence defines victim precipitation in forcible rape as "when the victim agreed to sexual relations but retracted before the act or when she clearly invited sexual relations through language, gestures, etc."[3] The commission found that rape victims were responsible for less precipitant behavior (as defined) when compared to other violent crimes, as shown in Table 1-5.

In an effort to develop rape prevention programs, researchers are now beginning to investigate the behavior of women in pre-rape situations and within the actual act of rape. Because this behavior merits and needs further study, the National Center for the Prevention and Control of Rape has funded research studies on the subject; it has also attempted to alert adolescents to the misunderstandings and mixed messages often communicated by males and females during dating and erotic play through an educational film about the date rape.

**Table 1-5. Precipitant behavior of victims in rape and other violent crimes**

| | |
|---|---|
| Homicide | 22.0% |
| Assault | 14.4% |
| Armed robbery | 10.7% |
| Unarmed robbery | 6.1% |
| Rape | 4.4% |

From Brownmiller, S.: Against our will: men, women and rape, New York, 1975, Simon & Schuster; Mulvulhil, J.D., and others: Crimes of violence, vol. 3, staff report to the National Commission on the Causes and Prevention of Violence, Washington, D.C., 1969, U.S. Government Printing Office.

For many individuals there is a fine line of discrimination between a woman's invitation for sexual relations (by which she is held accountable for rape) and an act of rape (in which nonconsent is explicit). However, the fact that more than two thirds of all rapes are *planned* and premeditated refutes the myths related to victim precipitation. For example, a woman attacked in her home by a stranger or by a man who betrays her confidence in him is not responsible for precipitating the assault.

### CLINICAL EXAMPLE

Marjorie, age 20, had been dating a young man who she met at a fraternity party at the local college campus near her home. The couple dated on several occasions, and the young man invited Marjorie to his fraternity formal. Marjorie was very excited about the invitation and looked forward to the social evening. After thoroughly enjoying the formal, the couple returned to the young man's fraternity house. Marjorie began to notice that her date was drinking quite heavily and politely asked him to take her home. Marjorie's date disagreed and told Marjorie that he would take her home shortly. After several hours of continued drinking, Marjorie's date passed out on a living room couch. Marjorie was frightened to go home alone and accepted a ride home from another fraternity brother. As they were leaving, the fraternity brother pulled a knife, grabbed Marjorie, and dragged her beside the fraternity house. Marjorie was too frightened to scream but tried to resist the man's sexual assault. The man warned Marjorie to stop struggling and he proceeded to beat her about the face until she was semiconscious. Another couple leaving the fraternity party found Marjorie approximately one-half hour after her assault. The couple helped Marjorie to an emergency room where she received immediate medical attention and a rape examination. Marjorie was admitted to the hospital for overnight observation.

An analysis of the preceding clinical example points out specific variables related to the rape situation:

*Motive.* Sexual gratification was not the offender's intent because he used violence to control the victim. By beating the victim to a semiconscious state, the rapist assaulted her and used her as an object of his aggression.

*Relationship.* The victim was lulled into a false sense of security by assuming that an acquaintance (a fraternity brother of her date) was a safe person to accept a ride from.

*Where and when.* Following a social activity (fraternity party), the assault occurred outdoors and late at night. These characteristics are comparable to many other violent crimes.

*Force and violence.* The assault resembles aggravated assault because the rapist caused serious bodily injury. The use of a weapon (knife) further substantiated a violent intent.

*Victim precipitation.* In this example it is clear that the victim did not invite sexual relations and did not consent to the assault.

## SUMMARY

As direct care providers to rape victims, nurses have a responsibility to become knowledgeable about the multifaceted nature of rape. Rape is a painful, violent experience in which sexual intercourse is forced on a rape victim (usually female) by a rapist (usually male). Systematic data support associations between rape and certain high-risk characteristics in rape victim profiles. In addition, variables in the rape situation contribute to a victim's risk of being involved in a violent, dehumanizing experience.

When necessary, nurses present relevant information to victims, families, and members of society in order to refute rape myths. They intervene in processes that reinforce a victim's guilt and shame. Professional nurses do not convey to rape victims that they are responsible for the assault. Instead, knowledgeable nurses separate rape myths from rape facts and assess their impact on rape victims, persons closest to rape victims, and others in society.

## Learning activities

### EXERCISE 1. Rape myth-fact test

*Directions:* Check your response on the following true or false statements. Respond to every item. Then check your responses with the answer key at the end of the Learning Activities for this chapter.

| True | False | |
| --- | --- | --- |
| ___ | ___ | 1. Rape is a minor crime affecting only a few women. |
| ___ | ___ | 2. Victims are responsible for their victimization either consciously or be default. |
| ___ | ___ | 3. Nationally, rape is a warm-weather crime. |
| ___ | ___ | 4. Only promiscuous women get raped. |
| ___ | ___ | 5. Forcible rape is the highest rising violent crime in our nation today. |
| ___ | ___ | 6. Any woman can prevent rape if she wants to. |
| ___ | ___ | 7. Violence accompanies all cases of rape. |
| ___ | ___ | 8. There is a low rate of false report in cases of rape. |
| ___ | ___ | 9. Today in most states a woman cannot prosecute her husband for rape. |
| ___ | ___ | 10. Most reported rapes are interracial. |

|  True | False |     |
|-------|-------|-----|
| ____  | ____  | 11. No woman's dress gives a man the right to rape her. |
| ____  | ____  | 12. It is not easy to prosecute a rapist and secure a conviction. |
| ____  | ____  | 13. Rape is an impulsive, uncontrollable act of sexual gratification. |
| ____  | ____  | 14. Most reported rapes have a higher incidence in rural settings. |
| ____  | ____  | 15. If a woman does not resist or struggle, she literally has not been raped. |
| ____  | ____  | 16. Women are raped when they are out alone at night, primarily in dark alleys. |
| ____  | ____  | 17. No woman's behavior gives a man the right to rape her. |
| ____  | ____  | 18. Sexual assault occurs only among total strangers. |
| ____  | ____  | 19. Most rape victims precipitate the crime. |
| ____  | ____  | 20. Rape is a violent attack in which sex is the weapon and the primary motive is aggression or power. |
| ____  | ____  | 21. A woman is more apt to report rape by a friend or relative than by a stranger. |
| ____  | ____  | 22. Any woman can be a victim of rape regardless of social or economic class, age, or race. |
| ____  | ____  | 23. Rapists tend to be attracted only to pretty women. |
| ____  | ____  | 24. Any woman can be a victim of rape regardless of her place of residence. |
| ____  | ____  | 25. A victim's demographic and social variables do not bias juries in determining if a situation or act is a case of rape. |

## EXERCISE 2. The nurse's definitions of rape

*Directions:* The following eight items describe cases involving varying degrees of sexual assault. Evaluate whether you think rape has occurred by marking the response that corresponds best to your opinion:

A. Strongly agree
B. Agree mildly
C. Disagree mildly
D. Strongly disagree

The answer key is located at the end of the Learning Activities for this chapter.

A B C D 1. An 80-year-old, black, widowed woman lives alone. She answers the doorbell and finds a man who says he is there to check and replace her water meter as ordered by city regulations. The woman lets him in, whereupon the man shoves her into the bedroom, beats her brutally, and forces sexual relations on her.

A B C D 2. A 24-year-old, white, married woman agrees to work overtime for her boss one evening to complete a project on time. During a break the two smoke marijuana, and the boss has a few beers. Just before quitting work he threatens to fire her unless she complies with his sexual advances. (In the past the woman has always refused the boss's sexual advances.) He forces sexual relations on her and, with an apology for his intoxication, slips $10 in her pocket on the way out.

A B C D 3. A 23-year-old, white, single woman who has been living with her parents initiates more of a social life for herself. She attends a singles club and meets a young man who asks her out for the evening. The man drives about town, suggesting they "make love," to which she ambivalently objects. Finally he drives to a motel and rents a room. There the woman acquiesces to his continued sexual advances.

A B C D 4. An 18-year-old, black, single female has a date with an acquaintance for the second time. She agrees to a double date for a party. Once at the party it becomes obvious that she and her friend are the only two females there. Although uncomfortable about the situation, the woman decides not to worry since she knows her date. Later she engages in heavy petting and necking with the man. The man's friends enter the room where they are and force oral and anal sexual relations on the woman without her consent. After that her date takes her home.

A B C D 5. A 34-year-old white nurse meets some of her colleagues after work for a drink in a bar. There she meets a man and spends several hours talking and dancing with him. The man offers to take her home since she is slightly intoxicated. The woman invites him in for a "nightcap," and he takes advantage of the opportunity by having sexual intercourse with her.

A B C D   6. A 48-year-old, white, single woman who teaches at a university is struggling with the loss of her youth and beauty. At a faculty party she meets a bachelor who bestows compliments on her and raises her spirits. The man convinces her to take a tour of the house and in a back bedroom seduces her into "making love." Embarrassed at her lack of control, the woman tells him she feels she has been raped. He tells her she's "all wet" and that she ought to "grow up."

A B C D   7. An 18-year-old black divorcee escorts her child to a visitation with his father. When she arrives at the apartment, the man invites her in for a beer and to meet his new fiance. To be polite she agrees to meet the woman. After several beers she suddenly finds herself thrown to the floor and restrained by the woman while her former husband forces sexual relations on her.

A B C D   8. A 20-year-old, white, single female is living with her boyfriend and his family. Following an argument with him, the woman goes to a bar for several drinks. On the way home she secures a ride from a taxi driver. The driver picks up a man and drops the two off at the man's home despite the woman's protests. The man forces sexual relations on the woman, threatening to kill her if she does not comply or if she reports the incident to anyone. He has a sawed-off shotgun with him. In the morning the man calls a taxi and lets the woman go.

## EXERCISE 3. Victim profile characteristics and rape situation variables

Review the situations in Exercise 2 and determine, when possible, the risk of rape based on the victim profile characteristics and the rape situation variables listed below.

Victim profile characteristics:

Age
Race
Marital status
Sex
Occupation
Socioeconomic status

Rape situation variables:

    Motive
    Relationship between victim and offender
    Where rape occurs
    When rape occurs
    Use of force or violence
    Victim precipitation

**Answer key to Exercise 1. Rape myth-fact test**

| | | |
|---|---|---|
| 1. F | 9. T | 17. T |
| 2. F | 10. F | 18. F |
| 3. T | 11. T | 19. F |
| 4. F | 12. T | 20. T |
| 5. T | 13. F | 21. F |
| 6. F | 14. F | 22. T |
| 7. F | 15. F | 23. F |
| 8. T | 16. F | 24. T |
| | | 25. F |

**Answer key to Exercise 2. The nurse's definitions of rape**

| | |
|---|---|
| 1. A | 5. D |
| 2. A | 6. D |
| 3. D | 7. A |
| 4. A | 8. A |

## REFERENCES

1. Amir, M.: Patterns in forcible rape, Chicago, 1971, University of Chicago Press.
2. Ben-Horion, D.: Is rape a sex crime? The Nation, p. 115, Aug. 16, 1975.
3. Brownmiller, S.: Against our will: men, women and rape, New York, 1975, Simon & Schuster.
4. Groth, A.N., with Birnbaum, H.J.: Men who rape: the psychology of the offender, New York, 1979, Plenum Press.
5. Haros, C.V.: Rape, New Cannon, Conn. 1974, Tobey Publishing Co., Inc.
6. Harrisburg Area Rape Crisis Center: Focus: volunteer training, Harrisburg, Pa., 1977, the Center.
7. Herman, D.: Rape culture. In Freeman, J., editor: Women: a feminist perspective, Palo Alto, Calif., 1975, Mayfield Publishing Co.
8. Katz, S., and Mazur, M.A.: Understanding the rape victim: a synthesis of research findings, New York, 1979, John Wiley & Sons, Inc.
9. LeGrand, C.E.: Rape and rape laws: sexism in society and law, Calif. Law Rev. **61**(3):927, 1973.
10. Medea, A., and Thompson, K.: Against rape, New York, 1974, Farrar, Straus & Giroux, Inc.
11. U.S. Department of Justice: Uniform crime report for the United States, 1973, 1974, 1976, 1978, 1981, Washington, D.C. U.S. Government Printing Office.

## ADDITIONAL REFERENCES

Biancinti, T.A., and Tjaden, C.: The crime of rape in Denver, Denver, 1971, Denver Anti-Crime Council.

Burgess, A.W., and Holmstrom, L.L.: Rape: victims of crisis, Bowie, Md., 1974, Robert J. Brady Co.

Chapman, T., and Gates, M., editors: The victimization of women, vol. 3, Sage yearbooks in women's policy studies, Beverly Hills, Calif., Sage Publications, 1978.

Cohen, M. Garofalo, R., and Seghorn, R.: The psychology of the rapist, Seminars in Psychiatry 3:307-327, 1971.

Frank, E.: Psychological response to rape: an analysis of response patterns, doctoral dissertation, Pittsburgh, Pa., University of Pittsburgh, 1979.

Heath, M., and Mercardante, M., editors: A handbook for victims, Pittsburgh, Pa., 1979, Interagency Task Force on Rape-Related Services.

Holmstrom, L.L., and Burgess, A.W.: The victim of rape: institutional reactions, Lexington, Mass., 1978, John Wiley & Sons.

Keller, E.: Training manual, St. Paul, Minn., 1979, Minnesota Program for Victims of Sexual Assault.

Klemmack, S., and Klemmack, D.: The social definition of rape. In Walker, M.J., and Brodsky, S.L.: Sexual assault, Lexington, Mass., 1976, D.C. Heath & Co.

MacDonald, J.M.: Rape: offenders and their victims, Springfield, Ill., 1971, Charles C Thomas, Publisher.

MacLean, J.: Rape: what's being done to stop it? In These times: a special report, Chicago, 1975, New Majority Publishing Co.

Metzger, D.: It's always the woman who is raped, Am. J. Psychiatry 133:405-406, April 1976.

Miller, J., et al.: Recidivism among sex assault victims, Am. J. Psychiatry 135:1103-1104, Sept. 1978.

Mulvihil, D.J., et al.: Crimes of violence, Vol. III, A staff report to the National Commission on the Causes and Prevention of Violence, Washington, D.C., 1969, U.S. Government Printing Office.

Pittsburgh Action Against Rape: Training manual, Pittsburgh, Pa., 1979.

Shore, B.: An examination of critical process and outcome factors in rape, Pittsburgh, Pa., 1979, University of Pittsburgh School of Social Work.

Tobac, S.: The effects of a rape crisis center's training program on volunteers' rape myth-fact awareness and their attitudes toward women: review of literature, master's thesis, Pittsburgh, Pa., 1979, University of Pittsburgh.

Travis, M.: The most common myths concerning rape—and the facts, Brainerd (Minn.) Daily Dispatch, May 1976.

Warner, C.: Rape and sexual assault, management and intervention, Germantown, Md., 1980, Aspen Systems Corp.

Women and the criminal law: the victim in a forcible rape case: a feminist view, Am. Criminal Law Rev. 2:347, Winter, 1973.

## ANNOTATED SUGGESTED READINGS

Brownmiller, S.: Against our will: men, women and rape, New York, 1974, Simon & Schuster, Inc.

The history of rape is presented in a well-documented manner with a careful scrutiny of the central issues. The author utilizes a historical perspective to disclose rape as an act embedded in and supported by our culture. Challenged are the myths, attitudes, and assumptions that surround rape so as to obscure its nature and perpetuate the crime. While some generalizations without qualifications are occasionally made, the book remains a classic for anyone attempting to understand the problem and work on any aspect of its eradication.

Burgess, A.W., and Holstrom, L.L.: Rape: crisis and recovery, Bowie, Md., 1979, Robert J. Brady Co.

The authors report the findings of longitudinal work with rape victims, including (1) crisis responses of rape victims, (2) counseling approaches effective in helping victims, and (3) recovery issues identified by rape victims. The text includes a number of articles reprinted from journals that emphasize treatment approaches in victim care. The book is useful across a wide variety of disciplines concerned with human services, particularly for those persons most likely to see the victim in the immediate aftermath of the rape assault.

Chappel, D., Geis, R., and Geis, G., editors: Forcible rape: the crime, the victim, and the offender, New York, 1977, Columbia University Press.

This book is a collection of some of the most important writings on heterosexual forcible rape. It reflects the authors' belief that social action, scientific inquiry, and reflection must go hand in hand. The authors suggest that they and the reader may disagree with some of the readings; however, the articles serve a necessary function in stimulating the reader's attention, discussion, rebuttal, and refinement of the issues. Particularly useful is the introduction, which provides an overview of current literature in a framework that draws a parallel to developments in the feminist movement, the behavioral sciences, and legal reform concerning forcible rape. A carefully selected bibliography is included.

Evans, L.J.: Sexual harassment: women's hidden occupational hazard. In Chapman, J.R., and Gates, M., editors: The victimization of women, vol. 3, Beverly Hills, Calif. 1978, Sage Publications, Inc., Yearbooks in Women's Policy Studies.

This article discusses sexual harassment as an expression of the prevailing male view of women and its use to remind working women of their "proper role" as wife, mother, or sex partner. The author identifies the scope of the problem and the myths associated with it (e.g., women enjoy sexual harassment); discusses related public policy and the courts, citing evidence of Title VII not being upheld and women being blamed for men's behavior (comparable to rape); and refutes notions of reverse discrimination with respect to sexual harassment.

Gager, N., and Schurr, C.: Sexual assault: confronting rape in America, New York, 1976, Grosset & Dunlap, Inc.

The authors present multiple dimensions of the crime of rape in an informative, insightful, and thought-provoking manner. Legal, medical, and psychologic aspects of rape are considered. The "politics of rape" are given attention with a discussion of ways society effectively predisposes men to rape and women to become victimized. The reader is given significant practical information and a comprehensive consciousness-raising introduction to rape as a problem. The book does not address counseling or self-help approaches in assisting victims with resolution of the rape crisis.

Griffin, S.: Rape: the all-American crime. In Chappell, D., and others, editors: Forcible rape: the crime, the victim, and the offender, New York, 1977, Columbia University Press.

This article is a precursor of the feminist literature on the crime of rape and male-female relations, as reflected in the power structure of American social systems. Culturally rooted rape myths are discussed in the context of females dominated by males mirroring our social system. To end rape the author proposes dissolving patriarchal systems.

Kjervik, D.K.: The stress of sexism on the mental health of women. In Kjervik, D., and Martinson, I.M., editors: Women in stress: a nursing perspective, New York, 1979, Appleton-Century-Crofts.

This chapter discusses the socialization processes of our society that affect the mental health of women, particularly those that teach women to believe they are inferior to men. The author describes the stages of growth women pass through in overturning and confronting the effects of sexism to become more assertive and autonomous individuals. The chapter presents approaches for a therapist to implement in feminist-oriented counseling to facilitate this process. It closes with a discussion of implications for education and research.

Parsons, J.: Cognitive developmental theories of sex-role socialization. In Frieze, I., and others: Women and sex roles: a social psychological perspective, New York, 1978, W.W. Norton & Co., Inc.

This chapter examines the major differences between cognitive-developmental theory, Freudian-identification theories, and social learning theories. It presents cognitive-developmental theories of sex-role acquisition stemming from the works of Piaget and Kohlberg. The author suggests that this model provides the best framework for analyzing sex-role acquisition; and for discussing differential valuing of the male and female role, the emergence of prejudices regarding individual behaviors and capabilities, and the basis from which to eliminate prejudices.

Schultz, L.G., editor: Rape victimology, Springfield, Ill., 1975, Charles C Thomas, Publisher.

Lectures and essays from social work nursing, medicine, law, sociology, and the feminist movement are collected in this book, as well as victims speaking to various dimensions of rape as a problem. The social aspects of rape and the child as a sexual assault victim are given special focus. The anthology is wide in scope and provides a good introduction to rape, touching on areas neglected in similar collected works.

Walker, M.J., and Brodsky, S.L., editors: Sexual assault, Lexington, Mass., 1976, Lexington Books.

This book presents a comprehensive compilation of scientific research, informed observations, and knowledge of professionals from recent addresses, essays, or lectures on a variety of aspects of rape as a problem. The editors describe their purpose as being to "raise the complex issues of causes and prevention of rape and to offer some preliminary answers to show the range of current developments in dealing with the victim and understanding rape through a readable and scientifically sound text."

Weis, K., and Borges, S.: Victimology and rape: the case of the legitimate victim. In Schultz, L.G.: Rape victimology, Springfield, Ill., 1975, Charles C Thomas, Publisher.

This article discusses ways in which women are socialized to become victims and men to become offenders. It gives attention to ways in which socio-cultural attitudes and roles are perpetuated and exploit both males and females, particularly in the dating situation. The origin of the "legitimate" victim, victimology, and rape are explored.

## CHAPTER 2

# Men who rape

Rape became not only a male prerogative, but man's basic weapon for force against woman, the principal agent of his will and her fear . . . his victorious conquest over her being, the ultimate test of his superior strength, the triumph of his manhood. . . .

From Brownmiller, S.: *Against our will: men, women and rape,* 1975.

## CHAPTER OUTLINE

## LEARNING OBJECTIVES

At the conclusion of this chapter the student will be able to:

1  List six myths about the rapist, describing the effects of belief in the myths, and their corresponding facts

2  Differentiate between anger rape, power rape, and sadistic rape

3  Describe interactions between rapists and victims during three phases of a rape experience

4  Explain three types of sexual dysfunctions in rapists during the assault

5  Identify three areas of emotional conflict for the offender

6  List nine areas of psychologic assessment in the diagnostic evaluation of an offender

7  Describe four treatment modalities that are used in treating rapists

There are as many myths about the rapist as there are about the victim. These myths reflect the socialization processes in Western society, including the many taboos associated with a sexual offense. By all appearances the rapist is no different from the accepted norm of other men in our society, a fact which greatly complicates the problem of rape for women and the understanding of it by both men and women. Because rape, a sexual offense, is popularly misbelieved to be a sexually motivated crime or a crime of passion, the victim is often held accountable for having seduced the offender. A result of this simplistic explanation is to minimize or overlook conflicts within the offender.

Exploring facts about offenders raises a number of questions: Who is the rapist? Is every man a potential rapist? What motivates a man to rape? Can a rapist be cured? Is the rapist insane or mentally retarded? Can women prevent a rapist from carrying out a rape? Many of these questions were discussed in Chapter 1. A fuller discussion of facts about the rapist is presented in this chapter, including (1) myths about the rapist, (2) motives for rape, (3) interaction between rapist and victim, (4) sexual dysfunction of the rapist, (5) criminal characteristics of the rapist, and (6) mental status of the rapist. Thus an understanding of the offender is a multidimensional phenomenon.

## MYTHS ABOUT THE RAPIST

The first serious study of the psychologic nature of a rapist is less than four decades old, yet men have been raping women since the beginning of history. Generally our knowledge about the psychology of the offender is incomplete. Many nonreported and nonconvicted offenders escape attention and treatment. Because it is characteristic of the offender to "act out" his conflict rather than to seek professional help, he comes to public attention through the legal system only when convicted of an offense. As prison and treatment facilities are mandated by law to guarantee "sexually dangerous" persons safe for release into the community, more scientific investigations into the nature of the offender's conflicts and treatment have emerged.

Because many women are raised to "capture" a man as proof of feminine adequacy and attractiveness, it is a direct threat to the security and self-esteem of the rapist's wife or girlfriend to think of "her man" having sex with another woman. Rapists are husbands, brothers, sons, friends, and neighbors next door. It is hard to believe that someone loved or known to us would violently assault another person, and the harshness of this reality is often coped with by the general populace through myths about the rapist.

Table 2-1. Myths about rapists, results of the myths, and facts

| Myths | Results | Facts |
|---|---|---|
| Rapists are sex fiends releasing pent-up impulses. | Belief in this myth excuses the offender for behavior misperceived as a crime of passion. Normal behaviors (e.g., sleeping nude) are labeled as provocation or precipitation even when the victim is attacked by surprise in her own home. Rapists are not brought to trial nor charged with offenses. | All rapists report readily available sexual partners. In no case has sexual provocation on the victim's part been found. Rapists report sexual dysfunction (e.g., impotency, retarded ejaculation) during the assault but not with consenting sexual partners. |
| Rapists would not rape if prostitution were legalized or if castration were the punishment for such acts. | This myth perpetuates notions of rape as a sexual crime rather than a violent one. | Motives for rape are power, anger, and sadism; therefore castration and legalized prostitution do not treat the underlying conflict that perpetuates the behavior. |
| Rapists will flee if the woman resists. | One who believes this myth subcribes to a blame-the-victim model and perpetuates notions of the crime as an act of passion. | Force (e.g., verbal threats or physical force) is used to subdue the victim in all rapes. Lack of resistance does not imply consent or provocation; it reflects women's socialization to be passive and submissive, to feel fear and terror when faced with aggression, to defer to men rather than fight back. Women aim to survive by whatever means seems appropriate, given the assailant encountered. Resistance by the victim is essential for some offenders to become sexually aroused and may cause more harm rather than the expected release to safety. |

Table 2-1 presents myths about the rapist, the results of believing these myths, and the relevant facts that dispel them. As demonstrated in the table, myths about the offender serve to protect rapists and give women and society a false sense of security by blaming the victim for the assault. Myths about the rapist excuse and minimize the offender's behavior by describing rape as a crime of passion. Many people believe rape would not exist if prostitution were legalized; others believe that women invite rape.

Facts about the rapist are collected from research and clinical studies of offenders as well as from data collected by agencies and bureaus that work with or treat offenders.

**Table 2-1. Myths about rapists, results of the myths, and facts—cont'd**

| Myths | Results | Facts |
|---|---|---|
| Rapists are "dirty old men" or just young boys "sowing wild oats." | This myth minimizes the violation of a woman's rights, the situational crisis imposed on the victim, and the long-term resolution process. | Rapists are most often between the ages of 15 to 24 years; almost none are found over the age of 45. |
| Raping is a one-time act reflecting a momentary lapse of judgment; it is not a serious offense. | Belief in this myth fails to acknowledge the offender's inadequacy in interpersonal relationships, gender identity, impulse management, and chronic immaturity. | Raping is a repetitive offense; convicted offenders report 13 rapes for every convicted offense.<br>Even in the majority of reported rapes, no suspect is apprehended and convictions are rare. |
| Rapists are mentally ill or mentally retarded and not responsible for their acts. | Society does not consider rape abnormal unless it is extremely brutal and the victim has physical proof of that brutality.<br>One who believes this myth excuses the offender for his behavior. | Rapists exhibit defects in their personality structure, including denial of their behavior and projection of responsibility for their acts. These defects in psychologic functioning do not exonerate them from their behavior; to do so would corrupt their treatment and rehabilitative therapy.<br>Alcohol and drug abuse are common secondary diagnoses that reflect the offender's difficulty with impulse management, his dependency, and his demands for immediate gratification.<br>There are more descriptive similarities than differences between rapists and nonrapists: married or previously married, moderate to heavy drinking, skilled and semiskilled trades, and not provoked by the victim. |

*Continued.*

**Table 2-1. Myths about rapists, results of the myths, and facts—cont'd**

| Myths | Results | Facts |
|---|---|---|
| All rapists have similar characteristics. | Belief in this myth results in applying a treatment approach that may be contraindicated and fails to meet the offender's individualized needs. | Equalizing all rapists objectifies their personhood and fails to recognize the uniqueness of different human beings. Definitions of the rapist's characteristics depend on the source—popular literature, the rapist, researchers. Men rape for different reasons: power, anger, sadism. Personality structure is unique to the offender. |
| Rapists are not treatable. | One who believes this myth supports outdated laws that lead to incarcerating the offender and function solely as preventive detention, not treatment. With the underlying conflict for rape untreated, the incarcerated offender continues to rape while in prison and when released. | Current research suggests that rapists can benefit from some form of specialized treatment based on a comprehensive assessment and a wide selection of approaches that meet individualized needs. The effectiveness of any given treatment approach, including measurement of recidivism, has yet to be established. Most rapists are "treated" in maximum security prisons, an environment not conducive to meaningful psychologic change. |

The next sections of this chapter present facts about the rapist, including motives for rape, sexual dysfunction during rape, criminal characteristics of the rapist, and treatment programs for rapists.

## MOTIVES: WHY DO MEN RAPE?

Popular belief views rape as an act motivated primarily by a need for sexual gratification. Factual data suggest that rape is a violent crime performed by a rapist to express and address issues of anger, power, and sadism. As such, it is a pseudosexual act (more accurately viewed as a sexual deviation and sexual offense) that has a complex and multidetermined etiology.

Rape is *always* characterized by the motivational components of anger, power, or sadism—with one of the motives *predominant* in a given rape situation (where sexual behavior is used to meet nonsexual needs). In many ways the power rapist and the anger rapist are similar—for example, both have past and current conflictual relationships with women. However, it is the predominant manner in which the conflict is acted out that differs—for example, through degradation of the victim or physical brutality. The following discussion, based largely on the work of Groth,[9] is a synthesis of clinical and research findings about motives of the rapist. It begins by presenting three clinical examples that illustrate the differences between the three motivational conflicts acted out by different rapists.

### CLINICAL EXAMPLE: POWER RAPE

All my life I felt I was being controlled, particularly by my parents, that people used me without any regard for my feelings, for my needs, and in my rapes *the important part* was not the sexual part, but *putting someone else in the position in which they were totally helpless.* I bound and gagged and tied up my victims and made them do something they didn't want to do, which was exactly the way I felt in my life. I felt helpless, very helpless in that I couldn't do anything about the satisfaction I wanted. Well, I decided, I'm going to put them in a position where they can't do anything about what I want to do. They can't refuse me. They can't reject me. They're going to have no say in the matter. *I'm in charge now* [emphasis added].[9]

### CLINICAL EXAMPLE: ANGER RAPE

I was *enraged* when I started out. I *lost control* and *struck out with violence.* After the assault I felt relieved. I felt I had gotten even. There was no sexual satisfaction; in fact, I felt a little disgusted. I felt relieved of the tension and anger for a while, but then it would start to build up again, little things, but I couldn't shake them off [emphasis added][9].

### CLINICAL EXAMPLE: SADISTIC RAPE

I needed to find a victim . . . . She was thumbing a ride . . . . I told her to get into the back seat and attach the seat belt. I sped away looking for a place to turn off. I found a side road . . . and before she could think to undo the seat belt, I had the gun pointing at her head and said, "Don't!" I told her to clasp her hands together and to hold them out in front of her. I handcuffed her wrists . . . . The next move was to open the passenger side door, still pointing the gun at her, put handcuffs on her ankles, and then take a cord and draw her legs and arms closer together—by the way, as I recount this, I find I'm getting an erection—then . . . assault her . . . . I have no memory of ever having a legitimate, consenting sexual fantasy. Originally, the fantasy associated with my offense was that sexual intercourse itself would be painful to the victim . . . . I never found the fantasy to be convincing in reality . . . . I suspect a good deal of it was finding a scapegoat for my anger—anger at everybody and everything . . . . It came out in the fantasy, the power to hurt, taking out an awful lot of hate that I am unable to show otherwise, a combination of hostility and sexual tension. The picture in my mind was one of torturing the victim with everything from matches and cigarette butts to a propane torch, electrical stimulation, needles, and so forth.[9]

### Power rape (55-65%)

Power rape is characterized by *unresolved life issues over power and mastery* that are the dominant forces motivating the offender. Typically this offender presents himself as a shy, quiet, "good boy," with a lack of assertiveness in approaching life tasks. His occupational history is often far below his aptitude and potential abilities, reflecting his low level of aspiration and low self-esteem. He may withdraw from school or show poor scholastic performance along with inadequate social skills.

The power rapist tends to have a very low self-esteem with pervasive feelings of worthlessness, vulnerability, and inadequacy. His sense of inadequacy is particularly acute in the sexual arena, where his masculine identity is most severely called into question and where he feels a need to prove himself as a desirable, potent, strong, and competent man. He thus has a rich fantasy life about his sexual conquests of women who initially resist his advances but eventually succumb to his sexual prowess, becoming sexually aroused and receptive to his approach. It is not unusual for this type of offender to believe, despite the victim's resistance, that she is enjoying every minute of the assault and to tell her, "You're really liking it, aren't you? You're really hot for me. I'll bet this is the best loving you've ever had!" and to ask her for a date when he finally lets her go. This astounds most victims, who find such arrogance and distorted self-perception hard to believe. In the feminist literature, MacKellar[16], commenting on the rapist's insecurity, states: "The man who rapes does so because he lacks a better means for making the point, 'I am a man.'"

As illustrated in the preceding clinical example, the rapist who acts on power motives has usually felt under the control of women, whether they be his mother, wife, or girlfriend. By capturing a woman he places her in the position he has felt and despised. He forces her to experience what he despises about himself: being weak, helpless, submissive. Because the rapist is out to prove his adequacy, any *force* or physical aggression is used primarily to *subdue* rather than to harm the victim. It is not unusual for him to keep the victim captive for hours and repeatedly assault her and for her to cooperate with his demands in order to survive, all of which adds to her sense of degradation and is further used to discredit her in court.

In fantasy the power rapist obsessionally plans the assault in minute detail and then stalks his victim (usually a stranger), like the predatory criminal, to make certain that his conquest is accomplished. In planning the rape this type of offender reports feelings of anxiety, excitement, anticipated pleasure, and erotic arousal. However, in reality the rape falls short of his fantasies and he finds little sexual satisfaction. Because sexual relations were not negotiated, he is not reassured by his own performance or the victim's response to him. He tends to blame the victim for her lack of response or to find something the matter with her rather than confront his own sense of inadequacy; he *needs* to believe that the victim wanted and enjoyed the assault as well as to rationalize the fact that she did not match his sexual fantasies. Otherwise his fantasied self-image would be threatened. For the power rapist the act of raping is a counterphobic behavior that puts to rest fears about his sense of manhood and heterosexuality or any disturbing thoughts about homosexuality. His defenses for coping (denial, inhibition, avoidance, projection) make psychotherapeutic treatment an extended intervention ranging from 4 to 6 years.

### Anger rape (35-40%)

Anger rape is always characterized by *physical brutality* and more *force or intimidation* than would be necessary to subdue the victim if the sole intent were to overpower and penetrate the victim. The rapist may use either a blitz or confidence style of attack, but more frequently he gains the victim's confidence by misrepresenting himself, for example, as a repairman or a census taker. In his attempt to batter, hurt, and debase the woman, the assailant views rape as the ultimate offense and expression of his rage. The dominant effect is one of *rage, hated, anger, and contempt* toward the victim, which is expressed by profanity, insults, and forced sexual acts that are degrading for the victim. Stressing the anger in rape, feminist Pauline Bart[3] points out: "Psychiatrists say a gun is a substitute phallus . . . . I find the reverse to be true. When it comes to rape, a phallus is a substitute gun. Rape is a power trip, not a passion trip. The rapist is more likely to rape in cold blood, with contempt and righteousness, than with passion."

As demonstrated in the preceding clinical example, a rapist with anger as his motive derives a sense of relief, rather than sexual gratification, from the discharge of anger. The release of anger is cyclic, so when rage builds up again the offender seeks a release for it through rape, which has become a maladaptive learned behavior to reduce stress. The tension he feels is generally not identified as a precursor to premeditated rape but as a sense that "something is about to happen." Because the rapist does not recognize this tension as a cue to his behavior, in most cases he does not seek help that would prevent his explosive and exploitive act. Frequently he neutralizes his response to his own behavior or dissociates himself from the assault while it is in progress, as if he were an observer to his own action.

Typically the assault by a rapist with an anger motive is precipitated by an upsetting event, such as a dispute with his girlfriend or wife, that he reacts to intensely. The rape becomes a symbolic expression of his rage and revenge toward significant women in his life. The anger rapist commonly feels mistreated or put down by women. Even if his feelings are actually distortions, he holds them to be true, and the rape serves to discharge the anger he feels about the perceived mistreatment. Because it takes time for frustrations to reach an explosive point, the aggressive rapist acts on a sporadic and infrequent basis.

The anger rapist's relationships with significant others in his life are characterized by conflict, irritation, and aggravation, which he displaces onto the victim. The victim may be a stranger who is a symbolic substitute for the target of his wrath; in other cases she is the actual person with whom he is angry. A direct result of displacing his hostility is to never work through difficulties in heterosexual relationships that arise during adolescence. For this offender adolescence represents a developmental crisis. In some cases he uses excessive defenses to resolve his heterosexual identity. He may exaggerate masculinity through activities such as aggressive sports and high-speed driving. Frequently he overidealizes his own mother, alternately perceives real women as depriving or untrustworthy, and carries this split perception into ambivalent relationships with women which he fails to resolve.

Because the aggressive rapist inflicts considerable physical trauma on the victim, which provides corroborating social and legal evidence, it is believed that more of these offenders receive convictions than do other types of rapists. This results in a misrepresentation of the actual number of anger rapists in the general population. It is the opinion of researchers that the power rapist is far more common than the anger rapist, yet statistics do not reflect this fact.

Finally, since anger rape is an explosive incident, it can be understood as a temporary decompensation of psychotic proportions that occurs in men who have been unable to resolve their intense rage with women. Compared to other types of offenders, anger rapists are most amenable to treatment. This is partially related to the fact that they have higher social and occupational levels of adjustment and fairly mature relationships with both sexes, although less so with women.

### Sadistic rape (5%)

A third pattern of rape, sadistic rape, is characterized by a fusion of sexual and aggressive needs into a single psychologic experience. Aggression itself becomes eroticized; without some degree of violence the sadistic rapist does not experience sexual excitation. He sees the victim's struggle, torment, anguish, and protestation as her sexual excitation rather than as a refusal, even when she is fighting for her life. Frequently this offender is impotent until he elicits resistance from the victim. The more she struggles, the more sexually aroused and aggressive he becomes, with the aggression subsiding after intercourse. A self-perpetuating cycle of increasing intensity results: the more aggression aroused, the more powerful the rapist feels; the more powerful he feels, the more excited he becomes—to the extent that he may, in a frenzy, commit a "lust murder."

As illustrated in the preceding clinical example, the sadistic assault may involve bondage and torture or bizarre ritualistic acts; it is usually committed without a display of anger. The *intent* of the sadistic rapist is to inflict pain, torture, and abuse on his victim; it is not sexual gratification. The offender aims to punish, degrade, humiliate, and destroy his prey. He thrives on a sense of omnipotence. His masturbatory fantasies focus on sadistic themes; he is fond of collecting mementos of his victims and sadomasochistic pornography. His *victim* is usually a *stranger* who symbolizes something he wants to destroy, for example, promiscuous women or prostitutes. His assaults are both premeditated and carefully planned to avoid discovery; they are sporadic and repetitive, with each successive assault showing an increase in the degree of violence. The sadistic quality of the rapist's assaults generalizes to his other relationships, both consenting sexual relationships and other less dramatic criminal offenses.

Although the sadistic offender is usually married, he reports poor sexual adjustment in his marriage. It is not uncommon for him to engage in extramarital affairs or to be involved in a series of divorces. In many ways he is similar to an anti-social personality or psychopathic character. However, he differs from these personality types in that his aggression tends to be diffused, unorganized, sexualized, and not used for adaptive purposes. The sadistic rapist tends to view the world as a hostile place and to mistrust every human contact with an overriding sense of paranoia that interferes with any satisfying sense of interpersonal mutuality. These developmental difficulties arise during the childhood years prior to adolescence, and the hostile view of the world and aggressive self-defense become sexualized with the onset of puberty.

The sadistic rapist is the least amenable to treatment because the onset of his interpersonal difficulties occurred in childhood. Although sadistic rape is the least common type of rape, it captures the fascination of the general public and is widely publicized in the media (as seen in Jack the Ripper or the west coast Hillside Strangler). The most grotesque assaults perhaps epitomize the public's worst fears about rape and reflect the most flagrant stereotypic notions about rape.

## MULTIPLE MOTIVES FOR RAPE

Although clinical observations of offenders tend to identify predominant types of rapists according to their motives, every case of rape has certain common features. All rapes occur in the sexual arena where men feel acutely vulnerable and inadequate in their relationships with women. These men are dependent on women for sexual gratification and resent them for their ability to refuse or reject them. Rape enacts the man's revenge and retaliation for perceived victimization; or it represents capture and control of the woman, thereby making her refusal impossible. The rapist attempts to discharge his hostility and contempt for women, to deny his sexual anxieties and doubts, to compensate for his helplessness by exploiting and controlling a woman in a desperate misguided attempt to assert his competency and manhood.

> Rape is equivalent to symptom formation in that it serves to defend against anxiety, to express a conflict, and to gratify an impulse. It is symptomatic of personality dysfunction, associated more with conflict and stress than with pleasure and satisfaction.[9]

Through rape young men may try to defend against homosexual impulses and retain status among their peers, particularly in gang rapes.

The ways in which the victim responds to the assault depend on the type of offender encountered. Table 2-2 depicts the victim's response based on the rapist's motive. As noted in the table, the victim who encounters a power rapist usually has little evidence of physical trauma because she has cooperated with his demands in order to survive. The victim's survival behavior results in feelings of guilt over compliance with demands, and she is likely to receive little to no support from significant others. Also, the victim fears the assailant's return and retaliation. Therefore she may

**Table 2-2. Victim response according to type of rapist motive**

| Type of rapist motive | Victim response |
| --- | --- |
| **Power rape** | |
| Minimal force | Little or no evidence of physical trauma |
| Acquainted, same age as victim "Confidence rape" common | No support from significant others: submission viewed as provocation; cooperation viewed as consent |
| | Guilt over sexual act |
| | Anger at self |
| | Self-blame for victimization |
| Sexual inadaquacy/dysfunction | Reassures assailant of potency and sexual adequacy |
| | Cooperates for survival |
| Captures victim for hours | Feels powerless and helpless |
| | Will not try to escape |
| | Hopes for release by complying |
| | Will not risk antagonizing assailant |
| | Fears harm if escape efforts unsuccessful |
| Threats or termination Continue power/control | Fears assailant's return |
| | Fears assailant's retaliation |
| | Lacks sense of self-determination and personal control |
| | Confusion, indecision, doubting |

*Continued.*

**Table 2-2. Victim response according to type of rapist motive—cont'd**

| Type of rapist motive | Victim response |
|---|---|
| **Anger rape** | |
| Use of force<br>　Physically brutal and violent<br>　Aggression blatant | Physical trauma to multiple body areas<br>Aims to survive the assault<br>Less guilt over sexual act |
| Victim not recognized<br>　Stranger or "blind with rage"<br>　Symbolic substitute object | Support and comfort from significant others, police, hospital<br>　personnel, and others in the general populace<br>Less doubt about provocation<br>Less self-blame for victimization |
| "Blitz" style of attack common | Increased awareness of vulnerability<br>Heightened sense of being at risk<br>Realistically assesses high-risk situations subsequently<br>Develops strategies to reduce risk of vulnerability and<br>　accessibility<br>Fears future assaults from assailant<br>Needs to understand assailant's motives and dynamics |
| **Sadistic rape (5%)** | |
| Use of force<br>　Bondage, mutilation, use of<br>　　objects<br>　Sexual organs are focus of<br>　　injury | May not survive the assault |
| Victim a stranger | Futility felt in efforts to establish relationship or<br>　meaningfulness with assailant |
| Premeditated act<br>　Captures victim<br>　Works self into excitement<br>　Repetitive act | Crisis state develops<br>Difficulty resolving crisis state, may need longer-term<br>　counseling<br>Terror and horror |
| Fused sexuality and aggression<br>　Abuses and tortures the victim<br>　Inflicts pain prior to sexual<br>　　assault<br>　Sense of power correlated to<br>　　degree of aggression | Fear of "going crazy"<br>Fear of never recovering<br>Severe depression in some cases<br>Risk of suicide in some cases<br>Reminded of assault by permanent injury—retards recovery |
| Sadomasochistic interests<br>　Bizarre sexual acts<br>　Acts out sadomasochistic<br>　　pornography | Ritualistic behavior to undo the trauma or regain mastery of<br>　self and environment |

From Groth, A.N., with Birnbaum, H.J.: Men who rape: the psychology of the offender, New York, 1979, Plenum Press.

experience confusion and doubt when faced with decisions that need to be made in self-care after the rape. In contrast, victims of anger rape are primarily concerned with having survived the assault and are often in a state of psychologic shock, realizing their close call with death. These victims are much more likely to receive support from significant others and to feel less guilty over their behavior during the rape experience.

Victims of a sadistic rapist may experience extreme terror and sometimes fear they will never recover from the rape. These victims may need longer-term counseling to resolve the rape and to learn adaptive ways of coping (other than posttraumatic responses such as ritualistic behaviors).

## INTERACTION OF RAPIST AND VICTIM

Almost all research has investigated the formal relationship between the victim and the rapist—for example, the stranger-acquaintance status or an age comparison. A few studies have investigated the attitude of the offender toward his victim, but there is a dearth of research on the interaction between the rapist and the victim during the assault itself. If women are to be helped to avoid rape and prepared to cope with it when it cannot be avoided, each of the stages of the assault must be studied further.

In Webster's dictionary *interaction* is defined as "a mutual or reciprocal action or influence." According to this definition, it would be accurate to say that there is no interaction between victim and rapist. The victim is an object, symbol, or tool upon which the rapist acts out his motives. The rapist does not relate to the victim. In fact, he both depersonalizes himself from what he is doing to her and neutralizes his feelings about the assault. Thus the victim's reaction falls upon deaf ears. Because the victim is an object or function for satisfying her assailant's needs, there is no mutuality in the act of rape. In interviewing men who did not complete the rape act, Ben-David[2] found that these men were unable to rape the woman if she had been able to elicit in them some emotional feelings for her; in such cases she had become a real person to the rapist, no longer an object. Brodsky[4] also found rapists to report the development of an interpersonal relationship between victim and offender as an effective deterrent to the crime. In light of these facts, the following section presents findings in the literature on the interaction of the victim and the rapist. It is divided into three stages: (1) prior to the rape, (2) during the rape, and (3) terminating the rape. Elements of one stage of the rape interaction often overlap into other stages. For example, the rapist may both *test and threaten* the victim at the same time in an effort to subdue her.

### Prior to the rape
#### Selecting the victim

The potential rapist first seeks out a woman who seems (to him) vulnerable. Typical victims include women intoxicated from drugs or alcohol; divorced, widowed, separated, or single-parent women, who may be less alert to cues because of the stress of their crisis; any woman sleeping alone; women returning home alone late at night and feeling tired from a day's work; or mentally-ill or retarded women. Although the rapist usually claims that he seeks out the "ideal American woman," the actual victim does not fit any set of ideal characteristics. The rapist bases his selection on whoever seems *most available, least able to defend herself,* or is *least alert*. The style of attack may be either blitz or confidence rape.

The rapist selects an environment that he thinks will allow easy entry—a first-floor apartment, an empty laundromat, a basement, a poor neighborhood with buildings in disrepair—and where he is not likely to be interrupted. Selkin[19] comments that unsuspecting women—such as nurses, teachers, and volunteers—who are friendly and like to help others unknowingly court the danger of being raped. The woman who *denies* that rape can happen to her, as most women do, is particularly vulnerable at the selection stage because she ignores the cues of danger, which often seem like simple social amenities. In the acquaintance or date rape the victim's confusion is even greater.

### Testing the victim

At this point the rapist wants to know if the potential victim can be intimidated; if so, he then threatens her into submission. Because women are generally socialized to be nonassertive and nonaggressive, the testing phase of the rape sequence is the focus of self-defense training for women. However, because aggression excites rather than deters some offenders, clinical researchers caution that a swift self-defense is not a fail-safe answer to prevention. The woman must assess the type of offender she has encountered, and in many cases the time this takes is sufficient for him to subdue her. According to Groth and Cohen,[14] the testing point of interaction is important to the rapist because he may lose his opportunity to rape if he guesses wrong, or he may be convicted and sentenced to prison if caught.

Usually the rapist's modus operandi is verbal. He may use insinuating remarks and admonitions such as "Don't scream!" or "Take your pants off!" He may test the victim's response to inappropriate caresses and grabbing. (In the work setting feminists call caresses and grabbing "petty rape.") Some rapists try to terrorize the victim by hitting, scratching, or throwing her down. Many women resist a brutal style of attack and the offender is scared off. However, with Western society's emphasis on physical attractiveness or beauty, many women are frightened of being disfigured or maimed. Insecure about their body image, women may readily submit to a rapist's demands, especially if they fear that they will be killed (although sadistic rape-murder is rare) or if the rapist uses a weapon. Robbing the victim is another way some rapists test the victim's willingness to submit to him, as in the case of the Berkeley Rapist.

CLINICAL EXAMPLE

"Shut up, you bitch, or I'll kill you," a man's voice said . . . . He blindfolded her with a pillowcase and said he wanted money. She was relieved, but after he left to get her purse in the living room, she heard him moving about for too long. Then, he came back closer, she heard the sound of denim falling as he stepped out of his pants. She knew she would be raped . . . . [8]

The clinical example above describes the rapist who intimidates his potential victim through verbal abuse. The robbery tests the woman's submissiveness, and helps to assure the rapist of the woman's compliance.

### Intimidating and threatening the victim

After testing the victim, the rapist suggests that he will engage in illegal behavior if necessary to gain her compliance. He may tell her he has a prison record, that he would not hesitate to murder her or hurt her loved ones if she refuses to cooperate. He makes clear a penalty if she refuses to cooperate with him and the reward she will receive (for example, no bodily harm) if she complies with his demands. Selkin[19] refers to the intimidation process as a "carrot and stick" stage in which the rapist calms the hysterical, frightened victim. He reassures the victim that everything will be just fine if she cooperates, and he may express concern for her health or future relationships with men. This is clearly a stage of negotiation whereby the rapist attempts to secure orderly and controlled behavior from the victim; if he does not subdue her, he faces intolerable anxiety from not being in control of the situation. At this point some victims will bargain by agreeing to certain demands—for example, oral but not anal intercourse. However, the victim's power to negotiate has been lost by the fact that she has acceded to any form of intimidation, and the rapist will then proceed to do as he wills with her. This stage of the rape is the *turning point* on which the remaining sequence of events are balanced.

In an effort to study deterrance of rape by potential victims, Brodsky examined the verbal interactions between the potential victim and the assailant by using a combination of film vignettes and verbal responses from interviews with convicted rapists. Depending on the nature of the rapist, the most successful deterrants included a successful interpersonal contact or ability to relate to the assailant (removal of self from object status), arousal of sympathy, and verbal attack or discouragement. Based on preliminary findings, Brodsky suggests the following strategy:

> If the rapist approaches with great verbal or suggested physical aggression or antagonism, then crying, signs of weakness, protests about body difficulties and open exhibition of great personal distress may be useful. For these men there is much lower success likelihood for active, verbal resistance. On the other hand, for the men who are highly tentative, relatively more polite, and who have preceded the actual rape threat with a number of preliminary conversations and tentative judgements about the woman, then the woman may be well advised to try active rejection and verbal or physical attack.[4]

Brodsky notes that these results are consistent with Selkin's findings[19] that communicating explicit unavailability to the assailant is an effective method of preventing rape. However, even tactics rated with the greatest success are valid only in specific situations. Other factors that are important in deterring a rapist include the woman's tone of voice, her posture and gait, the amount of confidence she conveys, and other similar nonverbal messages. Knowledge of this most important stage of the rape interaction remains very limited. More research needs to be done to validate when certain prevention tactics work, when they do not, and with what type of offender.

### CLINICAL EXAMPLE

> I didn't want a beer but I thought if I drank it he would be a little more likely to take me home like I had asked. But, he just kept driving around and before I knew it we were in the middle of the woods on the edge of the park. He parked the car and put his arms around me. I told him I wanted to go home and he said he'd take me home in just a little but he just wanted to talk with me some and get to know me. So we talked about a lot of stuff. Then, all of a sudden, bam! He unlocked the front seat in the jeep and the next thing I knew I was flat on my back with him on top of me. I fought like hell but I couldn't move with his weight on top of me.

## During the rape
### Sexual transaction

The sexual aspects of an assault are the ones people are most curious about, partly because the act is misperceived as a sexually motivated encounter and also because the most private side of one's life is exposed. Telling the events of a sexual transaction to the police, the medical personnel, the district attorney, the judge, and the public (including one's family and friends) can make many victims feel as though they are being raped a second time. Contrary to popular myth, the rapist is not a ravishing lover. In most cases he exhibits some type of sexual dysfunction (discussed later), and intercourse occurs in less than half of the rapes that are reported. It is the rule, rather than the exception, for the rapist to force oral and anal sex on his victim. The more he views these acts as sexually deviant or degrading to his victim, the more likely he is to insist on these modes of sexual transaction. It is during the sexual transaction that the rapist's fantasy life comes to the fore and his unique personality is imprinted on the victim. (For this reason, when the police investigate this aspect of the assault, they are not only assessing the question of the victim's consent but also determining the rapist's modus operandi. The nurse can explain this rationale to the victim and perhaps make the painful retelling of the incident more tolerable.) Although in reality the rapist may feel inadequate, he will insist that the victim confirm his fantasied desirability. For example, in confronting both power issues and his need for reassurance, he may ask the victim about her sexual life and interests as well as give her orders or commands.

CLINICAL EXAMPLE

I undressed her and told her to undress me. I began fondling her and asked her if she enjoyed sex with me. Then I told her to go down on me and when I got hard I entered her. I noticed she was wearing a wedding ring, and I asked her if I was as good as her husband.[10]

The clinical example above demonstrates the rapist testing notions of his sexual prowess and adequacy by asking the victim if she enjoyed sex with him and if he was "as good as her husband."

The rapist is confronted with a parodox: He cannot reveal his true identity or he will be reported and caught; thus he is unable to obtain the intimacy essential to satisfaction from a sexual experience. The sexual transaction falls short of his fantasies as the rapist struggles with the conflicts inherent in the assault:

1. Need for intimacy versus need for concealment
2. Need for control versus need for affection
3. Need for sexual gratification versus hatred and contempt felt for the victim[19]

The assault reveals the precise conflicts that the rapist tries to gratify with his behavior and the ones that characterize the offender according to his motives: power, anger, or sadism. It is during the sexual transaction that motivational conflicts are enacted.

### Meaninglessness of the victim to the rapist

From interviews with imprisoned sex offenders, Ben-David[2] found that regardless of the motive for the assault (power, anger, or sadism), the victim is not a partner of equal standing, as in normal personal interactions. The victim is not perceived as a person having equal rights, unique characteristics, and a unique personality. The victim becomes meaningless to the rapist through two techniques: neutralization and depersonalization.

*Neutralization technique.* Rape is a transgression of the accepted moral code of even criminal society because it causes harm to another person. Harming another person violates the rapist's self-concept, creating pressure to reestablish a sense of psychologic equity. Thus the rapist felt psychologic distress by denying he harmed his victim and usually reports, instead, feeling victimized by the woman, circumstances, and society. A reversal in thinking allows the rapist to feel that he has not violated the moral code or his self-concept, and psychologic equity is reestablished.

*Depersonalization process.* In a depersonalization process the victim has the role of object or symbol to the rapist. The rapist behaves as if the victim is entirely unknown to him, even if the two have been acquainted for a long time. The victim is disrobed of her person and personality during the rape and left with only a sexual role. The symbolic role that the rapist gives her has meaning only to him. During court hearings the rapist may report being unable to remember what happened or that the victim's description was not of him; he may plead insanity or claim a Jekyll and Hyde personality.

As a result of the rapist's neturalization and depersonalization processes, "the victim plays a role in a complicated play, unaware of the type of play or the role she has been cast in. The role was forced on her and at the same time it removes her human and social role."[2] Ben-David's findings are consistent with those of others who have conducted clinical research with sex offenders.

> From a practical-preventive point, one may advise women that, in an attempted rape situation they have to behave in an "unexpected" way, for example, not to defend themselves or to surrender, but try to raise in the rapist personal feelings for them. They have to behave in such a way that the rapist will be unable to relate to them in an impersonal way; they have to behave in a way that stirs in the rapist human feelings for them.[2]

## Terminating the rape

Selkin[19] states that the manner in which the rapist departs from the victim can be viewed as a diagnostic signature. For the rapist the central issue in terminating the rape is to prevent, or delay, the victim from reporting the assault so that he will not be caught. At this point his motivational conflicts reemerge through themes such as guilt, fear of retaliation, omnipotence, or anger, which are enacted in his unique style of departure. Some rapists try to confuse the victim about the precise moment when they are leaving.

CLINICAL EXAMPLE

When he was about to leave, he tied her wrists behind her back and put her face down on the bed. Then he picked up the lamp beside the bed and balanced it on her naked back. He turned the bulb on. He told Sarah not to move. "He said when I heard the front door shut I could get up . . . . I heard him open the door, but I didn't hear it shut." Sarah Hughes stayed in that position, the lamp balanced on her back for close to an hour. She was afraid Stinky was waiting and watching, ready to kill her if she moved.[8]

Some rapists threaten to harm the victim if she reports the incident to the police. A rapist may instill fear by reminding the victim that he knows where to find her, that no one will believe her anyway, or that he knows the "ropes of the system" and can get off the charges with a good lawyer. Other rapists feel guilty and apologize for their behavior; they may plead with the victim not to call the police.

CLINICAL EXAMPLE

He said he was sorry for doing it, something just came over him. He asked me to forgive him. Then he tried to get me to stop for something to eat with him, he wanted to take me out like on a date. I told him I just wanted to get home so he drove me to my house. Then he asked if he could call me for a date. I was scared and just wanted to get away from him so I said, "Sure, call me later." But it made me sick to my stomach.

According to Selkin,[19] the themes that the offender expresses in his style of terminating the rape are diagnostic for his personality pattern. Here he expresses the same conflict that he enacted throughout the rape transaction.

## SEXUAL DYSFUNCTION DURING RAPE

It is artificial to separate a discussion of the rapist's sexual functioning during the rape from his motivational conflicts for the act or the interaction stages with his victim. However, the public tends to focus on this aspect of the assault, and the courts use evidence of the sexual transaction to determine the rapist's guilt or innocence. According to Groth and others,[13] in reality, rape is a pseudosexual behavior in which sex is used as a weapon to express issues of power and aggression and sex is used to meet nonsexual needs of the offender. Selkin[19] found that vaginal intercourse occurred in less than half of reported rapes, whereas anal and oral intercourse were common. None of the offenders studied by Groth and Burgess[12] reported sexual dysfunction in any of their consenting sexual relationships; the dysfunction was specific to the rape situation. And in *no* case has the offender reported needing to rape for the purpose of sexual gratification.[11] That fact corroborates the position that the intent of rape is power and aggression, not sexual gratification.

In a sample of 170 convicted offenders, Groth and Burgess[12] found that one third of the men reported some type of sexual dysfunction at some point during the assault. This was regarded as a conservative estimate since 11% of the men reported being interrupted or deterred and a higher frequency of sexual dysfunction is expected under such circumstances. The *most frequent* type of dysfunction was impotence, and the *least common* type was premature ejaculation. The following clinical examples illustrate types of sexual dysfunction during rape as reported by convicted rapists.

CLINICAL EXAMPLE: RAPIST'S IMPOTENCE DURING RAPE

When he lost his erection, he'd get mad and scream, "Act like you want it you bitch . . . Act like you like it." His face was up next to mine, kissing me, and that was just awful, a nasty, awful, sloppy kiss, and he was angry the whole time. He didn't like women. He couldn't. I thought he was punishing me, he was so rough and hurtful. I told him it really hurt. I was all dry and tight, but he didn't care at all.[8]

## CLINICAL EXAMPLE: RAPIST'S RETARDED EJACULATION DURING RAPE

He had an erection and he just went back and forth, for hours. He had no interesting moves or variety. I could have been a board. A couple of times he speeded up, and I thought he was going to come. But he didn't.[8]

## CLINICAL EXAMPLE: RAPIST'S PREMATURE EJACULATION DURING RAPE

At first she was real friendly, and I got turned on. When I started taking the initiative, she got turned off, and I wasn't prepared for that. She started struggling with me, and I overpowered her, but I had some problems getting into her. I had only half a hard-on, because I already shot my load. I came off during the struggle.[9]

In rape with a power motive the offender is likely to be handicapped by impotence, retarded ejaculation, or premature ejaculation. *Impotence* (erective inadequacy) consists of partial or complete failure to achieve and sustain an erection. Some offenders force the victim to stimulate them manually or orally to overcome this condition. Other offenders overcome this condition only when the victim struggles or resists; this is characteristic of rape with an anger motive, in which eroticization of aggression is a condition essential to completion of the act.[12] Groth and Birnbaum[9] found impotency the most common sexual dysfunction, comprising 46% of all cases, and that 16% of offenders reported some degree of impotency, usually occurring in the initial stage of the assault. In a power rape the offender tries to reassure himself of his sexual adequacy, competence, and identity. He expects the woman to eventually succumb to his sexual abilities with wild abandon. In reality, he finds little sexual satisfaction in the rape because of either his handicapped performance or because of the victim's response.

The second most common type of dysfunction among rapists is *retarded ejaculation* (ejaculatory incompetence). Retarded ejaculation consists of a failure to ejaculate during intercourse even after 30 to 60 minutes of steady intravaginal penetration. According to Masters and Johnson[17] retarded ejaculation is an infrequent complaint in the general population. However, this condition ranks second among rapists and comprises 45% of the incidence of their sexual dysfunction. This rate of occurrence is a dramatic departure from that of the general population. Retarded ejaculation is particularly hurtful for the victim, who is not sexually aroused or lubricated and as a result suffers a high incidence of genital trauma.

In rape with an anger motive the offender attempts to discharge his rage on the victim rather than obtain satisfaction from sexual gratification. He tends to view sex as dirty and degrading, and he casts women in roles as "whores and bitches." The sexual act is satisfying only to the extent that it enables him to hurt the victim. However, he is faced with a dilemma in that he frequently reports difficulty in achieving an erection or ejaculation during the assault; and since sex is his weapon he is handicapped in discharging his rage. When he is impotent or cannot ejaculate, this further incites his rage toward the woman; and it is his eroticized aggression that generally enables him to have an erection but does not guarantee that he will ejaculate.

The least common type of sexual dysfunction reported by rapists is premature ejaculation. *Premature ejaculation* consists of ejaculation at the moment of penetration or immediately before intromission. Only 9% of offenders cited this dysfunction occurring during the assault. Some offenders report spontaneous ejaculation during the assault without ever penetrating the victim. Since these reports rely completely on subjective self-reports, it is possible that this dysfunction also accounts for those rapes in which the offender does not attempt to penetrate the victim. In addition, many women are in a state of shock during the assault and are unaware of whether or not the man has ejaculated.

It would be erroneous to assume that the rapist experiences only one type of sexual dysfunction during a given assault. For example, he may experience initial erective impotency and overcome this, but then he may need to contend with retarded ejaculation. The rapist's *sexual dysfunctioning is symptomatic of his psychodynamic conflict* in which he experiences inadequacy, anxiety, and rage. It is the impact of his psychologic conflicts on his physiologic functioning that accounts for his sexual dysfunctioning and the absence of sperm when evidence is collected.[9] Groth and Burgess found evidence of sperm in *less than half* of their study sample of 92 rape victims and a high incidence of physical trauma in these cases. They concluded that "the absence of sperm does not mean that a woman was not raped."[12] This proves to be an important finding because of the crucial role that the medical record serves in supporting the victim's allegation of rape. In collecting evidence many physicians overstep their role by indicating on the medical record that the victim was not raped because no sperm was found; and attorneys may attempt to impeach a victim's character and credibility on the same account. It is important, therefore, to educate the public, who serve as jurors in rape cases, about these findings to ensure that the medical examination is not unduly emphasized in court proceedings and to help guarantee appropriate prosecution of offenders in the absence of positive physical and laboratory results.

## CRIMINAL CHARACTERISTICS OF THE RAPIST

One of the myths surrounding the crime of rape is that it is not a serious offense, rather merely a case of harmless youth "sowing a few wild oats." However, research findings refute that claim. Rape is a repetitive, compulsive act in which the offender is more violent and aggressive with each succeeding assault as he attempts to achieve a fantasied experience that continues to escape him.[13] Convicted rapists report that for every convicted rape offense they have committed 13 nonconvicted rape offenses.[10] This suggests that the incidence of the crime is higher than reported statistics reflect. In a study of 239 individuals charged with rape offenses, Henn and others[15] found that defendants charged with rape typically had a history of antisocial behavior that included other types of violence. This is consistent with other research findings. Amir[1] found that almost half (49%) of those charged with rape offenses had a previous arrest record, although most were for antisocial behavior such as crime against property. Svalastoga[20] found that 67% of rapists taken to court had a previous criminal background, and Mohr[18] reported 57.9% with a prior criminal record. Such findings make it clear that rape is more than child's play, and the repetitive quality of the offense suggests that it is a serious problem—more serious than most of society acknowledges.

## MENTAL ILLNESS OR SYMPTOM FORMATION

Another popular myth is that the rapist is mentally ill. This myth represents an effort to rationally explain an act that does not make sense. To date, research evidence does not indicate that the rapist is mentally ill. Rape is not listed as a mental illness in the 1980 diagnostic manual of the American Psychiatric Association (the DSM III). The strongest suggestion that rape may be a mental aberration stems from the work of Groth and Burgess, who assert that the offender's behavior is a sexual deviation, a psychosexual developmental crisis. Yet a crisis is not considered sufficient in itself as a basis for diagnosing a person as being mentally ill. However, research regarding the rapist's motives and diagnostic assessments indicates that severe borderline psychotic states and various types of personality disorders have been found[5] and in that respect the rapist's behavior constitutes a mental disorder.

Basing their categories on the rapist's motive, Cohen and others[6] suggest three types of personality disturbance: (1) explosive personality—rape: aggressive aim; (2) inadequate personality—rape: sexual aim; and (3) antisocial personality—rape: sex-aggression diffusion. Cohen's categories reflect a belief that rape is sexually motivated and that the rapist uses force to gain access to the victim. Clearly he differs from other researchers. Most researchers and clinicians are aware of the limitations that diagnostic labels impose and the narrowed perceptions and misunderstandings they create. Therefore they have found it more useful in understanding the offender and planning treatment programs to identify the most apparent defects in his personality and their severity.

The core areas of emotional conflict for the offender center are (1) impulse management, (2) gender identity, and (3) interpersonal relationships. First, the rapist has poor impulse management, which is characterized by explosive anger and an inability to delay gratification and tolerate frustration. It is as though he is propelled into action rather than being able to harness that energy and adaptively channel it toward goal-directed ends. Although some offenders are unable to recognize their frustrations, others have a defective awareness of, and ability to cope with, the demands of life. Second, the offender lacks a solid gender identity and an adequate sense of masculinity. He has not been successful in managing his life effectively, even in nonsexual areas such as academic pursuits and employment, because of his inability to channel his impulses for adaptive outcomes. Therefore he does not feel good about himself. The offender copes by denying his deeply rooted low self-esteem, lest it shatter an already weak masculine self-image. Thus the concrete signs of masculine mastery and competency heralded by the values of our society—physical aggression and sexuality—become prime targets in the offender's efforts to gain a sense of adequacy.

The offender's efforts to achieve a masculine self-image are hampered by his impaired ability to negotiate interpersonal relationships, the third area of conflict. While growing up, the offender did not learn to be sensitive to the needs of others, to their feelings or concerns; people were simply obstacles to his gratification. His demanding, self-centered personality structure precluded the formation of meaningful relationships; and women, therefore, came to be viewed as objects for his gratification or for venting his impulses. Here lies the core of interaction between rapist and victim during the sexual assault: there is no meaningful interaction because the offender detaches himself from the woman's personhood and depersonalizes and neutralizes his own responses. The rapist subsequently rationalizes and minimizes his behavior and projects responsibility for his acts onto the woman (or others), thereby maintaining a stance that the world is a hostile environment. This approach to life characterizes all his interpersonal relationships, not just the sexual assault. Therefore the offender's distorted view of morality and interpersonal relationships becomes a focus in treatment. Burgess and Lazare[5] concluded that "whether the act of rape is symptomatic of a long-standing and serious personality disorder or of a temporary regression under unusual stress, it is *always* symptomatic of some psychological defect." Stated differently, Groth[9] concluded that "rape is not a symptom of mental illness but of personality dysfunction. It is the result of defects in human development." The question then becomes, What does one do to treat and rehabilitate the offender?

## TREATMENT PROGRAMS FOR RAPISTS

Because the focus of this book is the nursing care of rape victims, the following discussion of treatment programs for offenders is intentionally brief. It is limited to an overview of the multiple approaches used in treating the core areas of conflict that the offender experiences. To date, there is insufficient objective, systematic research to determine the long-term effectiveness of any given approach. However, as various treatment modalities are used with offenders, understanding of the rapist is expanded; this, in turn, facilitates a better understanding of the victim's response and increases the probability of designing effective prevention programs in our society. The first task in designing a treatment program is a diagnostic assessment of the offender. The second task in treating the offender is designing an individualized treatment program specific to his needs.

### Clinical assessment of the offender

Since effective treatment and rehabilitation of the offender is based on a careful assessment of his conflict, the importance of a comprehensive diagnostic evaluation and dynamic formulation cannot be overemphasized. Groth cites two key questions to be answered in relation to *each* phase or facet of the offender's development and functioning:

1. How competent is he in managing this life task (the power issue)?
2. How frustrated or dissatisfied is he with this aspect of his life (the anger issue)?[9]

A diagnostic evaluation of the offender follows a format similar to that used in completing a psychiatric assessment of clients; it enables the interviewer to identify target areas of concern and the clinical significance of each category of information explored. The interviewer obtains information in the following areas: (1) identifying information; (2) family background; (3) medical history; (4) educational development; (5) military history; (6) interpersonal development including social, sexual, and marital history; (7) occupational history; (8) recreational interests; and (9) criminal history.[9] Since the offender tends to deny his conflicts and project responsibility for his acts onto others, multiple collateral sources must be sought to obtain a comprehensive evaluation. Collateral resources include the following: (1) observation of the offender's behavior and interaction with others; (2) clinical interviews that obtain historical data and impressions about his values, feelings, attitudes, and thought processes; (3) field investigations that may involve a home visit or interviews with the offender's significant others; (4) a medical examination to determine his health status and any possible relationship to his criminal sexual activity; (5) documents containing data from the records and files of formal agencies that he has had contact with; (6) standard psychometric tests; (7) physiologic measurements to record his reactions during interviews and treatment sessions; and (8) referrals that report all aspects of his ability to manage his life.[9]

These data are then compiled in a formulation that reflects a holistic picture of the offender and his offense

> against the background of the offender's developmental history, the social-environmental context of this development, the environmental-situational context of the crime, the current psychological and emotional life of the offender, and the social-environmental features of the life situation that the offender would reenter if released.[14]

From a comprehensive diagnostic evaluation and profile of the offender, an individualized treatment program is designed with the intent to reduce, inhibit, or eliminate his sexually assaultive behavior. Often the selection of available treatment programs is determined by the setting in which the offender is found. A treatment program may encompass a combination of any of three modalities: (1) incapacitation, (2) psychotherapy, (3) programs in psychosocial development.

## Incapacitation
### Incarceration

Imprisonment is the most obvious method of preventing the offender from harming members of the community. However, this approach is simplistic because it does not treat the dynamic conflict of the offender that triggers his assaultive behavior. As discussed earlier, the object of the rapist's assault is often substituted in the prison setting, where he engages in homosexual rape. Furthermore, although a 20-year prison sentence can be leveled for rape, the actual sentence delivered is often closer to 24 months, followed by an early probation. Contrary to current practice, a period of confinement of about 5 years and a gradual release into the community have been found to be an effective treatment.

### Chemical or surgical castration

The notion of castration is an expression of the sense of outrage experienced by the community toward the rapist and is often viewed by the layman as punishment rather than treatment for the offense. In chemical castration an antiandrogen hormone, medroxyprogesterone acetate (Depo-Provera), is administered to lower the offender's level of sexual arousal or responsiveness. The theory behind this method is that a decreased libido or potency will enable the offender to benefit from other treatment approaches that focus on his core conflict areas. Surgical castration has the same net effect; however, it is not a reversible procedure and may exacerbate an already prevailing sense of sexual inadequacy, which may further enrage the offender. Both chemical and surgical castration inhibit sexual drive, but to be effective they must be used in conjunction with other treatment modalities that rehabilitate the offender.

### Psychotherapy
#### Individual psychotherapy

The aim of individual psychotherapy is to facilitate the offender's awareness of his conflict areas, gain insight into the forces that trigger his behavior, experience again the emotional relatedness he could not handle adaptively, mature emotionally, and learn better ways to cope with his conflicts. Prognostic criteria for a successful course of individual psychotherapy for the offender are usually based on the following:

1. A circumscribed chief complaint
2. A history of a "meaningful" relationship with another person during his early life
3. An ability to interact flexibly with the evaluator and have access to his feelings during the evaluation interview
4. An above-average psychologic sophistication and intelligence
5. A motivation for change[7]

Because few offenders meet all these criteria, the use of this treatment modality is restricted. Furthermore, the effectiveness of individual psychotherapy on a long-term basis in resolving the offender's conflicts remains to be tested. However, this method is employed as a treatment approach with selected offenders, and in these cases the following pattern usually occurs.

In the *initial phase* of treatment the offender denies responsibility for his behavior, and his conflicts with authority figures surface. He does not trust those responsible for his therapy or confinement and views himself as a victim of the system. Through clinical skillfulness this initial *resistance* is overcome, and the offender engages in a *middle phase* of therapy. At this time he uncovers his nuclear conflict, which is characterized by a dichotomization of men and women based on perceptions of his relationship with his parents in childhood. His rage with a controlling, rejecting, and often seductive mother is recognized as being displaced onto substitute women, whom he dichotomizes as whores or madonnas. His relationship with either a weak and ineffectual father figure or a harsh and brutal one is acknowledged. It is this early triangular relationship that the offender comes to recognize as the source of his sense of helplessness, worthlessness, and rage. The uncovering phase is critical in breaking through the offender's defensive process of projection and helping him begin to *admit* and examine his own responsibility for failure to master life's tasks. The process of self-admission surfaces the offender's core conflict, which then becomes the focus of therapy.[9] Groth and Cohen note:

> The dilemma of on the one hand wanting to turn over the responsibilities of his life management to others (since he feels incapable of self-mastery) and assume a passive-dependent position on the other hand fearing that to do so would be tantamount to self-destruction since there is no one who would or could be capable, concerned, or caring enough to assume such responsibility (since he feels incapable of being loved) constitutes the core conflict operating within this type of patient. . . . It is this combination of self-hatred, hurt, and depression that lies at the base of the sexual psychopathy.[14]

As the offender comes to grips with his personality, he experiences depression and sometimes entertains suicidal thoughts. Careful clinical intervention assures the offender that the therapist has not abandoned him and that the offender *can* learn to manage his life and impulses, thereby stimulating a sense of self-esteem. Gradually the offender comes to identify with the therapist and expresses an interest in making restitution for his behavior or participating in prevention programs in the community. At this time he learns adaptive behaviors and tests their effectiveness; he acquires new skills in interpersonal relationships, skills that give him a sense of mastery and self-esteem. The offender is no longer a victim of himself. The major clue to his recovery is his ability to empathically recognize the needs and feelings of others, to no longer dichotomize people as good and bad but to differentiate among them, and to recognize his own needs and feelings apart from others. Successful treatment requires that each phase of individual psychotherapy be manifested.

### Group psychotherapy

Individual psychotherapy is often complemented by group psychotherapy. Through the group mode, the offender experiences both a sense of responsibility to the members as well as a feeling of being cared for by them.

Where conflict with authority figures becomes tumultuous when dealt with on an individual basis, the offender's psychotherapy peers will confront him with his inability to establish effective interpersonal relationships and with his nonadaptive defensive maneuvers of denial, projection, and rationalization. It is in this way that the offender acquires the peer-group experiences that have been lacking in his developmental history. He learns competition, cooperation, and collaboration with his peers; he learns to give and take; and in the process he learns the social skills necessary to establish satisfying interpersonal relationships. The offender gains insight into the provocative behavior that has caused others to reject him, discovers that he cannot blame others for his behavior, and begins to learn healthier ways of relating to people. It is this new insight that enables him to become the "captain of his ship." With this knowledge and a healthier set of behaviors acquired through group psychotherapy, the offender can attain an adequate sense of masculinity both intraphysically and in relation to his peers.

### Programs in psychosocial development

One approach in rehabilitating the offender is through programs that teach him the skills he lacks so that he can better manage his life's tasks. Although there is a wide range of educational courses in human development, the following programs represent a potpourri from which an individualized treatment program for an offender can be planned.[9,14]

*Recreational programs* offer the offender an opportunity to release energy in a healthy, adaptive manner and to learn interdependency skills through team effort in sports. *Vocational programs* teach trade skills that can enable the offender to become self-sufficient and master life's demands upon release from treatment or incarceration. *Sex education programs* give the offender basic information on human sexuality, which he is often lacking, and an opportunity to explore his attitudes through counseling and therapy directed at specific problems. *Social skills training programs* address the offender's deficiencies in interacting and communicating, enabling him to become more effective at establishing and maintaining close interpersonal relationships. Parent-effectiveness training teaches him the skills he needs to function and cope as a parent. In some settings nurse clinicians have worked in expanded nursing roles in these programs to facilitate the offender's social rehabilitation. *Empathic skills training programs* develop the offender's ability to recognize and be sensitive to the needs and feelings of others in opposition to his narcissistic, self-centered focus. Empathy training is accomplished through group methods such as encounter groups or consciousness-raising groups. *Emotional regulation* is learned through programs that teach the offender how to recognize and express anxiety, frustration, and anger in constructive ways. Programs directed toward emotional regulation include assertiveness training, relaxation exercises, and biofeedback strategies. *Religious counseling* facilitates the offender's development of a moral sense, self-respect for others, a sense of hopefulness, and an avenue for restitution for his behavior coupled with a decreased sense of isolation through the experience of a Judeo-Christian brotherhood.

The advantages of psychosocial development courses lie in the fact that they are clearly goal directed and concretized in a manner that enables the offender to perceive his accomplishments and to feel a sense of mastery and pleasure. As such they foster internalization of self-reinforcing activities and behaviors that are healthy and adaptive. The time-limited nature of such programs allows the treatment team to scale a number of such programs from basic to advanced levels, teaching the offender skills he lacked in his earlier development. The design of psychosocial rehabilitation programs can be arranged so that a combination of treatment approaches facilitates an intrapsychic synthesis of new behaviors, attitudes, and styles of coping. The effectiveness of these programs on a long-term basis, alone or in combination with other treatment modalities, remains to be tested.

### Behavior modification

Another approach in rehabilitating the offender is the application of behavior modification techniques in decreasing or eliminating the offender's sexual response to rape. It should be remembered that the offender consistently underestimates his sexual arousal to rape cues on self-report inventories. Thus physiologic measurements that record his reactions during the treatment sessions should always be used as a measure of the effectiveness of the treatment. The behavior modification approaches most commonly employed include (1) aversive conditioning, (2) covert sensitization, (3) hypnotherapy, (4) fading, and (5) systematic desensitization. The application of behavior modification in treating sexual offenders is a fairly recent approach, and its long-term effectiveness is only beginning to be evaluated. More commonly it is applied in conjunction with one of the other available treatment modalities.

## SUMMARY

This chapter has examined the nature of the man who rapes. Raping behavior is repetitive, with each successive offense being a more violent assault. Motives for the offender's sexual assault include power, anger, and sadism. Rape is understood as a symptom of the offender's psychologic dysfunction resulting from impairments in various aspects of his human development. The rapist tends to view women as very powerful by virtue of their womanhood. The woman is put on a pedestal, admired, courted, and seen as giving or controlling favors. Thus the rapist feels that the way to countercontrol a woman is through aggression or making her do exactly as he wills. The man who rapes feels the same before the act as the man who murders or robs, only the expression of the motive is different. Frequently the offender rapes with impunity because conviction rates are low. Sentencing often indicates that it is considered a lesser offense to murder than to rape, and so offenders are encouraged to rape *and* murder to obtain lighter sentences. As yet there is no known cure in rehabilitating the rapist. However, inroads have been made into understanding the offender and treatment modalities have been developed. Treatment approaches designed to rehabilitate the offender include (1) incapacitation in the form of incarceration and/or chemical or surgical castration, (2) individual psychotherapy, (3) group psychotherapy, and (4) programs in psychosocial development. The seriousness of the problem of rape and its many dimensions has been aptly summarized by Groth:

> A solution to this problem will require making basic changes in our society. Rape is more than a clinical issue, it is a social, economic, legal, cultural, and political issue that requires multidisciplinary and interagency cooperation. There is no room for professional conceit or territorial possessiveness if we expect to combat sexual assault successfully.[9]

## Learning activities

### EXERCISE 1. I learned statements*

*Directions:* The following is a list of unfinished sentences to complete. Divide your notepaper into two columns. In the left-hand column write a response to the unfinished sentence; the intent here is to focus on content learned from reading the chapter. In the right-hand column write your personal feelings as they correspond to each item in the left-hand column; the focus here is on your feelings and personal values. Allow 10 to 15 minutes for this exercise. Next, break into groups of three for discussion and share the completed responses with your classmates. This portion of the exercise is *optional*. It could also be done with colleagues at work or roommates.

| Statements | Feelings |
|---|---|
| 1. I discovered that the rapist is . . . | _____ |
| 2. Rape is a pseudosexual act because . . . | _____ |
| 3. Sexual gratification as a motive for rape is . . . | _____ |

---

*Adapted from Smith, M.: A practical guide to value clarification, La Jolla, Calif., 1977, University Associates, Inc., pp. 64-65.

|  | Statements | Feelings |
|---|---|---|

4. The primary motive for rape is . . .  _____

5. Anger rape is characterized by . . .  _____

6. Core areas of conflict common to all rapists are . . .  _____

7. Rapists humiliate and degrade victims because . . .  _____

8. Violence as a condition for sexual excitation characterizes . . .  _____

9. Lust-murder is . . .  _____

10. Rape is equivalent to symptom formation in that . . .  _____

11. The rapist's interaction with the victim is . . .  _____

12. Meaning of the victim to the rapist is . . .  _____

13. In the past I have unknowingly courted the danger of rape by . . .  _____

14. I would be intimidated by a rapist if he . . .  _____

15. The critical turning point for completing the act of rape is . . .  _____

16. To stir human feelings in the rapist I would . . .  _____

17. Sexual prowess of the rapist is . . .  _____

18. Rapists report sexual dysfunction only . . .  _____

19. The criminal record of the rapist suggests . . .  _____

20. Absence of sperm on evidence collection means . . .  _____

21. Personality dysfunction of the offender consists of . . .  _____

22. Rape as a form of mental illness is . . .  _____

23. In my judgment, the best treatment program for a rapist is . . .  _____

24. I want to learn more about . . .  _____

## EXERCISE 2. Rape prevention*

*Directions:* Match the type of assailant in the right-hand column with the most successful method of deterrence described in the left-hand column.

| Method of deterrence | Type of assailant |
|---|---|
| 1. ____ Forceful physical resistance. | A. Dominant, aggressive, antagonistic, assaultive. |
| 2. ____ Crying and passivity. | B. Highly tentative, relatively polite, preliminary conversations and judgments about potential victim. |
| 3. ____ Aggressive, forceful refusal; unequivocal, flat no. | |
| 4. ____ Open exhibition of great personal distress. | C. None of the above; explain your answer. |
| 5. ____ Protests about bodily difficulties. | |
| 6. ____ Verbal attacks, shouting, screaming, cursing. | |
| 7. ____ Signs of weakness, arousal of sympathy. | |
| 8. ____ Interpersonal liaison or contact. | |

*Adapted from Brodsky, S.L.: Prevention of rape: deterrence by the potential victim. In Walker, M.J., and Brodsky, S.L., editors: Sexual assault, Lexington, Mass., 1976, Lexington Books.

## EXERCISE 3. Psychology of the offender

*Directions:* Answer all questions with reference to content from the chapter. Place a check in the appropriate column to show your response to each true-false statement. Answers can be found at the end of the Learning Activities.

| True | False | |
|---|---|---|
| ____ | ____ | 1. Rape is a crime of violence. |
| ____ | ____ | 2. Males are never subject to rape. |
| ____ | ____ | 3. The rapist selects an attractive young woman to assault. |
| ____ | ____ | 4. All rapists have similar characteristics. |
| ____ | ____ | 5. Rape happens after careful planning. |
| ____ | ____ | 6. Rapists are sex fiends seeking sexual gratification. |

| True | False | |
|------|-------|--|
| ____ | ____ | 7. The rape victim is usually a stranger to the rapist. |
| ____ | ____ | 8. Rapists cannot be treated or rehabilitated. |
| ____ | ____ | 9. Rape is an expression of intrapsychic dysfunction. |
| ____ | ____ | 10. Legalizing prostitution would eliminate rape. |
| ____ | ____ | 11. Some rapists require victim resistance to become aroused. |
| ____ | ____ | 12. Lack of victim resistance does not imply consent to rape. |
| ____ | ____ | 13. Rapists are not mentally insane. |
| ____ | ____ | 14. Raping fulfills the sexual fantasies of the rapist. |
| ____ | ____ | 15. The anger rapist is least amenable to treatment. |
| ____ | ____ | 16. Fighting is always the best deterrence to rape. |
| ____ | ____ | 17. Rape is equivalent to symptom formation. |
| ____ | ____ | 18. Oral and anal intercourse usually occur in rape. |
| ____ | ____ | 19. The rapist successfully obtains intimacy in the sexual experience. |
| ____ | ____ | 20. The victim is meaningless to the rapist. |

## DISCUSSION QUESTIONS*

1. Why do you think women vomit, burn their clothes, even commit suicide after being sexually assaulted?
2. Why do you think a victim would not report an assault against her by a friend or relative?
3. Why do you think relatives of a person who has been sexually assaulted find it hard to cope with what has happened?
4. Do you think you should consider the possibility of your being sexually assaulted or should you just dismiss it as being "something not nice"?
5. How can you best safeguard your home against entry by a possible assailant?
6. Why do you think the FBI ranks sexual assault with murder and aggravated assault as a "violent crime"?

---

*Reprinted with permission from Discussion Guide for the program "A Crime of Violence, Rape and Sexual Assault, Current Affairs Division, Key Productions, Inc., p. 6.

### Answer key to Exercise 2. Rape prevention

| Method of deterrence | Rationale for answer selection |
|---|---|
| 1. B | a. The dominant, aggressive rapist tends to be deterred by crying, signs of great personal distress, weakness, passivity, and interpersonal liaison or contact (Brodsky, p. 88). |
| 2. A | |
| 3. B | |
| 4. A | |
| 5. A | b. The highly tentative, preliminary assessing rapist tends to be deterred by forceful and aggressive resistance, verbal attacks, and explicit refusals (Brodsky, p. 88). |
| 6. B | |
| 7. A | |
| 8. A | |

### Answer key to Exercise 3. Psychology of the offender

| | | |
|---|---|---|
| 1. T | 8. F | 15. F |
| 2. F | 9. T | 16. F |
| 3. F | 10. F | 17. T |
| 4. F | 11. T | 18. T |
| 5. T | 12. T | 19. F |
| 6. F | 13. T | 20. T |
| 7. T | 14. F | |

## REFERENCES

1. Amir, M.: Patterns in forcible rape, Chicago, 1971, University of Chicago Press.
2. Ben-David, S.: Rapist-victim interaction during rape, paper presented at the Third International Symposium on Victimology, Germany, 1979; Department of Criminology, Bar Ilan University, Ramat Gan, Israel, Mimeographed.
3. Bart, P.: Rape doesn't end with a kiss, Viva, **2:**40, 1975.
4. Brodsky, S.: Prevention of rape: deterrence by the potential victim. In Walker, M.J., and Brodsky, S.L., editors: Sexual assault, Lexington, Mass., 1976, D.C. Heath & Co.
5. Burgess, A.W., and Lazare, A.: Community mental health: target populations, Englewood Cliffs, N.J., 1976, Prentice-Hall, Inc.
6. Cohen, M.L., Garofalo, M.A., Boucher, R., and Seghorn, T.: The psychology of the rapist, Sem. in Psychiatry **3:**307, 1971.
7. Davanloo, H., editor: Basic principles and techniques in short-term dynamic psychotherapy, New York, 1978, SP Medical & Scientific Books.
8. Fosburgh, L.: The Berkeley rapist, New Times, **5:**28, May 15, 1978.
9. Groth, A.N., with Birnbaum, H.J.: Men who rape: the psychology of the offender, New York, 1979, Plenum Press.
10. Groth, A.N.: Personal communication, Conference on the Sexually Abused Child, Pittsburgh, Pa., December 1979, Pittsburgh Action Against Rape.
11. Groth, A.N., and Burgess, A.W.: Rape: a sexual deviation, Am. J. Orthopsychiatry **7:**400, July 1977.

12. Groth, A.N., and Burgess, A.W.: Sexual dysfunction during rape, New Engl. J. Med. **297**(14):764, Oct. 1977.
13. Groth, A.N., Burgess, A.W., and Holmstrom, L.L.: Rape: power, anger, and sexuality, Am. J. Psychiatry **134**(11):1239, Nov. 1977.
14. Groth, A.N., and Cohen, M.L.: Aggressive sexual offenders: diagnosis and treatment. In Burgess, A.W., and Lazare, A., editors: Community mental health: target populations, Englewood Cliffs, N.J., 1976, Prentice-Hall, Inc.
15. Henn, F.A., Herjanic, M., and Vanderpearl, R.H.: Forensic psychiatry: profiles of two types of sex offenders, Am. J. Psychiatry **133**(6):694, June 1976.
16. MacKellar, J.: Rape: the bait and the trap, New York, 1975, Crown Publishers, Inc.
17. Masters, W.H., and Johnson, V.E.: Human sexual inadequacy, Boston, 1970, Little, Brown & Co.
18. Mohr, J.W.: Rape and attempted rape. In Sexual behavior and the criminal law, Part III, a preliminary report, Oct. 1965, Mimeographed. Forensic Clinic, Toronto Psychiatric Hospital.
19. Selkin, J.: Rape, Psychol. Today **8**:71, Aug. 1975.
20. Svalastoga, K.: Rape and social structure, Pacific Sociol. Rev. **2**:48, Spring 1962.

## ADDITIONAL REFERENCES

Abel, G.G., Blanchard, E.B. and Becker, J.V.: An integrated treatment program for rapists. In Rada, R.T., editor: Clinical aspects of the rapist, New York, 1978, Grune & Stratton.

Abel, G.G., Blanchard, E.B., and Becker, J.V.: Psychological treatment of rapists. In Walker, M.J., and Brodsky, S.L., editors: Sexual assault, Lexington, Mass., 1976, Lexington Books.

Barlow, D.H., and Agras, W.S.: Fading to increase heterosexual arousal in homosexuals, J. Applied Beh. Anal. **6**:355-366, 1973.

Herman, S.H., Barlow, D.H., and Agras, W.S.: An experimental analysis of exposure to "explicit" heterosexual stimuli as an effective variable in changing arousal patterns of homosexuals, Beh. Research and Therapy, pp. 335-345, December, 1974.

Katz, S., and Mazur, M.A.: Understanding the rape victim: a synthesis of research findings, New York, 1979, John Wiley & Sons.

MacDonald, J.: Rape: offenders and their victims, Springfield, Ill., 1971, Charles C Thomas, Publisher.

Pacht, A.R.: The rapist in treatment: professional myths and psychological realities. In Walker, M.J., and Brodsky, S.L., editors: Sexual assault, Lexington, Mass., 1976, Lexington Books.

Resnik, H.L., and Wolfgang, M.E.: New directions in the treatment of sex deviance. In Resnik, H.L., and Wolfgang, M.E., editors: Sexual behavior: social, clinical and legal aspects, Boston, 1972, Little, Brown & Co.

Skyes, G.M., and Matza, D.: Techniques in neutralization: a theory of delinquency, Am. Sociol. Rev. **7**:664-670, 1957.

## ANNOTATED SUGGESTED READINGS

Bart, P.: A study of women who both were raped and avoided rape, J. Soc. Issues **37**:4, 1981.

The researcher interviewed 13 women who were both raped and avoided being raped. The women avoided rape when: they were attacked by strangers; they used multiple prevention strategies, such as screaming and physical struggle; the assault occurred outside; and the primary concern was not being raped. The same women were raped when: they were attacked by men they knew, particularly if a prior sexual relationship existed with the man; only talking or pleading was used as a preventive strategy; the assault occurred in their homes; their primary concern was not being killed or mutilated; and force was threatened. Readers will find this issue of the journal useful because the contents are focused entirely on matters related to rape victimology.

Brodsky, S.L.: Sexual assault: perspectives on prevention and assailants. In Walker, M.J., and Brodsky, S.L., editors: Sexual assault, Lexington, Mass., 1976, D.C. Heath & Co.

The author describes models of blame and prevention strategies that relate to each model according to the manner in which one's pervasive, consistent assumptions about the nature and causes of rape are formulated: (1) victim blame and prevention, (2) offender blame and prevention, (3) societal blame and prevention, and (4) situation blame and prevention. Finally, the author discusses unconventional proposals for rape prevention which are creative and innovative.

Brodsky, S.L.: Prevention of rape: deterrence by the potential victim. In Walker, M.J., and Brodsky, S.L., editors: Sexual assault, Lexington, Mass., 1976, D.C. Heath & Co.

The author reports an investigation conducted in four sequential steps to study the verbal interactions between potential victim and assailant for use in deterrence of rapists. The author investigated what it was successful rape resisters did, if these actions could be identified, validated and disseminated so that other women confronted with sexual assault, and unable to flee or resist, could benefit. He describes two types of assailants and interactional patterns identified as potentially successful deterrents to rape.

Burgess, A.W., and Lazare, A.: Community mental health: target populations, Englewood Cliffs, N.J., 1976, Prentice-Hall, Inc.

The first part of the book explores ways in which biologic, psychologic, social and behavioral models can be employed to fully understand multiple dimensions of a clinical problem. The attitudes and concepts are then applied to the management of specific problems. Of particular usefulness is Chapter 12, by Groth and Cohen, "Aggressive Sexual Offenders: Diagnosis and Treatment," and Chapter 11, "Victims of Violence."

Chapman, J.R., and Gates, M., editors: The victimization of women, vol. 3, Beverly Hills, Calif., 1978, Sage Publications, Inc., Yearbooks in Women's Policy Studies.

Chapter 1 examines rape as a perversity that is a natural result of a sexist social order. The author discusses sex-role socialization within the framework of three concepts: the morality of submissiveness, the morality of chivalry, and the morality of justice. Chapter 2 focuses on male victimization of women by (1) reviewing theories and research in the area of human violence and aggressions, (2) examining the differential effect on males and females from exposure to violence, (3) discussing rape as a prototype of female victimization, and (4) describing one treatment program for sexually aggressive men.

Conroy, M., and Ritvo, E.R.: Common self-defense: a practical manual for students and teachers, St. Louis, 1976, The C.V. Mosby Co.

This book offers women a course in self-defense designed to facilitate awareness of dangers and equip oneself to live securely and comfortably in the face of threats that exist. The curriculum overcomes the need for atheletic skills often required for martial arts defense courses and the psychologic roadblocks to learning (anxiety, fear, discomfort) experienced by women in the face of threats to personal safety. It is organized around three strategies: (1) eliminating potential dangers in one's life, (2) recognizing and avoiding dangers through forethought and common sense rather than physical techniques, and (3) physical techniques that all women can master and that do not require constant conditioning.

Feshbach, S., and Malamuth, N.: Sex and aggression: proving the link, Psychol. Today **11**:111, 1978.

The UCLA researchers' results suggest that men who view pornography in which sex and violence are fused, such as *Playboy* and *Penthouse*, tend to be more stimulated (than control groups) by the idea of rape and less sympathetic to victims. The authors report research studies investigating the link between sex and aggression by which they arrived at their conclusion. The article may stimulate ideas regarding community and media projects that nurses can implement. It closes with recommended preventive measures.

Geis, G.: Forcible rape: an introduction. In Chappel, D., and others, editors: Forcible rape: the crime, the victim, and the offender, New York, 1977, Columbia University Press.

The first chapter of this book provides the novice reader in the field of rape literature with an objective critique of ideological concerns and empirical questions. The first section critiques the work of the feminist writers, including Brownmiller, Griffin and Grear, Medea and Thompson, Gager and Schurr, and Russell. The second section critiques the interrelated aspects of behavioral science investigations of rape, including studies on seasonal rape rates, general correlates of reported rape, victim-related research, the rapist, crosscultural work, and legal matters.

Groth, A.N., with Birnbaum, H.J.: Men who rape: the psychology of the offender, New York, 1979, Plenum Press.

This book is written in nontechnical language and easy-to-read style. It should be required reading for nurses working with victims or offenders. The book is based on the authors' experience with over 500 offenders over a 15-year period. It examines the psychologic and emotional factors that predispose the man to rape and to react to situational and life events by sexually assaulting women. It offers a framework for understanding the offender's developmental history, life-style, and motivations for raping and gives guidelines for identification, diagnostic assessment, and treatment of offenders.

Medea, A., and Thompson, K.: Against rape, New York, 1974, Farrar, Straus & Giroux.

The authors have one brief passage on "The Little Rapes" which brings the reader's attention to the many ways in which women are verbally harrassed on the streets and social situations. The authors draw attention to the social amenities involved, the woman's fear of being assertive (labeled rude), and her inclination to feel guilty if she defines her personal space.

National Center for the Prevention and Control of Rape: Rape and older women: a guide to prevention and protection, Rockville, Md., 1979.

The guide attempts to help older women prevent rape and reduce the emotional stress created by fear of rape that influences a woman's social activities, independence, and overall quality of life. Specific avoidance behaviors to reduce the risk of victimization in high-crime, low-income residence areas and the use of people as "security systems" to deter crime are presented. Although the guide is designed specifically for the elderly, the content is also suitable for younger age groups and men in educational programs that teach crime prevention strategies.

Pickering, M.: Women on the defense: basic self-defense for women runners, Runners World **10:**108, 1979.

As more women are running, the incidence of attacks upon them has increased. This article describes ways the woman runner can short-circuit potential threats by taking precautions in advance of running and by knowing what she can do if an attack occurs. The author describes ways (specific to the woman runner) to avoid confrontations, physical and mental preparation for potential assaults, nonphysical responses women have used to repulse attackers, and physical responses. Particularly useful are two tables summarizing (1) 10 Ways to Avoid Attack—Around the Home and When Running, and (2) 10 Ways to Handle Attack.

# PART II

# Responses
# to Rape

## CHAPTER 3

# Nurse response to rape

What you and I really need is a moment of truth and a habit of truth with ourselves. My willingness to be honest with myself . . . will be the decisive factor and the essential condition for growth as a person.

From Powell, John, S.J.: *Why am I afraid to tell you who I am?* © 1969, Argus Communications, Allen, Texas. Used with permission.

## CHAPTER OUTLINE

**Definition of a value**
**Values related to rape and sex roles**
**Value clarification process**
**Phases of nurse response to rape**
  Choosing values
    Denial of rape facts

Cognitive dissonance
Anxiety
Anger
Action
  Data inquiry
  Emergency nursing care
  Counseling

Education
Consultation
Prizing
  Rape crisis center volunteer
  Public education
  Social action
  Research
**Summary**

## LEARNING OBJECTIVES

After reading this chapter the student will be able to:

1 Define a full value

2 List seven criteria for an operational definition of the value clarification process

3 Explain four common behavioral responses of nurses during the choosing-values phase of the growth experience

4 Describe four areas in which nurses direct their anger about rape

5 Explain four behaviors of the action phase of the nurses' growth experience

6 Identify four ways nurses publically demonstrate values about rape

Working with rape victims forces upon nurses the need to assess their own values related to rape and sex-role behaviors. Unless nurses are comfortable with their own values, it will be difficult for them to convey comfort and support to rape victims. Otherwise nurses will focus on their own thoughts and feelings rather than keeping the rape victim's needs in perspective.

This chapter presents value clarification as a framework through which nurses assess their own responses while working with rape victims. We believe that nurses who care for rape victims go through a positive growth experience in clarifying their values about rape. Emphasis is on two major principles: (1) there is no "right" or "wrong" set of values about rape, and (2) nurses who are comfortable with their own values can direct their energies into constructive actions to make the rape experience less anxiety producing for victims. This chapter also presents expanded roles for nurses who have full values related to rape. Structured Learning Activities at the end of the chapter facilitate the value clarification process applied to rape.

## DEFINITION OF A VALUE

There are many definitions of a value. In this text a *value* is defined as a personal belief or attitude about the truth, beauty, or worth of something. One can value concepts, objects, people, or behaviors. Values give meaning and direction to a person's life. A *full value* is defined as a strong, motivating belief or attitude that involves three essential components: (1) thoughts, (2) feelings, and (3) actions. A full value is formed by a dynamic process between the cognitive, affective, and behavioral components of one's personality. It is a guide, a norm, a principle by which a person lives. This principle becomes strong enough to influence behaviors and patterns of living. For example, nurses who fully value rape prevention participate in public speaking about this issue, write articles on the subject, organize safety programs, or develop protocols for nursing care of rape victims in the clinical setting.

A person is not born with values. Rather, a person is born into a culture and a family that together promote, teach, and impart values over a lifetime of experiences. Socially meaningful experiences generally include other persons who become significant to the maturing person throughout the developmental phases of childhood, adolescence, and adulthood.[12,13]

The pattern of value development is unique for each person. Values may be imparted through moralizing from parents, child care helpers, religious leaders, or authority figures. A child may model the values of a significant parent, teacher, or guardian. Often values are acquired through the process of reward for certain values and punishment for others. As cognitive processes develop, a person experiences various value systems through books, movies, television, or school. Friendships and peer relationships begin to take on special meaning and values become shared. Norm values may be established by a peer group.

During adolescence and young adulthood a person begins to explore and question values and to choose ones that are comfortable. The choice is not easy! As certain values come into competition with others, decisions must be made about their priority—the importance of some values relative to other ones. For example, nurses may decide during their medical-surgical experiences that they would like to specialize in cancer nursing. But they cannot act on their values because they must first complete their basic nursing education. Similarly pediatric nurses who show an interest in becoming advocates for abused children do not always have the time to become active in this area. Both types of nurses have values, but neither has developed *full values*.

## VALUES RELATED TO RAPE AND SEX ROLES

Depending on their knowledge about rape, nurses hold certain views and values about this act. The predominant ones, which may differ from facts about rape, include the following:

1. *Rape is a sexual act.* It is perceived as an impulsive act caused by sexual impulses that cannot be controlled. The rapist may overcome an unwilling woman or he may be seduced.
2. *Rape is an insane act.* The rapist is an abnormal, sick man in need of psychiatric care. Society needs to be protected from the assaultive rapist. He should be jailed or hospitalized.
3. *Rape is a culturally determined act with heavy social implications.* What is defined as rape in one society may be socially acceptable in another. It is necessary to explore the social definition of rape rather than the act itself.
4. *Rape is related to sex roles.* Cultural conceptions about the nature of male and female roles influence societal views of rape. Intersexual activities, customs, and the status of men and women need to be examined before one can decide on the issue of rape.
5. *Rape is a violent act.* A humiliation for women, rape is a violent and aggressive act, an expression of hostility by a male.
6. *Rape is an act of oppression.* Rape typifies male dominance of females. It represents a form of male suppression of females.

As nurses provide care to rape victims, their views about sex-role behaviors also emerge. *Sex-role behavior* is defined as that behavior which is culturally expected and acceptable from those who are biologically identified as male or female. Some examples include:

1. Women are passive, submissive, and dependent on men.
2. Women are defenseless and in need of protection by men.
3. Men are aggressive and powerful.
4. Men and women are equal.
5. Women are oppressed by men and need to be liberated.
6. Women should be housewives and mothers; men should be breadwinners.

Nurses may demonstrate sex-role values through statements they make about rape victims; for example, "If she hadn't gone to that singles club, this wouldn't have happened" or "If she had been home with the kids, she wouldn't be in this mess."

In the process of nursing education and practice, professional nurses learn to achieve objectivity in providing care to clients. One framework for achieving such objectivity is value clarification. The next section describes this process as it relates to rape.

## VALUE CLARIFICATION PROCESS

Value clarification is a process by which nurses can discover their values related to rape. Value clarification does *not* provide a "right" or "wrong" set of values or attitudes on rape. No one set of values is appropriate for everyone because each person is a unique personality in a particular set of situations and has been socialized with a different set of values. Value clarification is a means to an end. The value clarification process involves three major steps: (1) choosing values, (2) action, and (3) prizing. Within these three steps are seven criteria:[12,13]

1. Choosing values
   a. A person chooses a value freely.
   b. The value is chosen from alternatives.
   c. The person carefully studies the consequences of each alternative.
2. Action
   d. The value influences a person's behavior.
   e. The value is acted on repeatedly and becomes a pattern of life.
3. Prizing
   f. The value is publically affirmed.
   g. The value is cherished.

Any thought, feeling, or behavior that fulfills all these criteria is considered a full value. If some but not all seven are fulfilled, the thought, feeling, or behavior is not a full value.

Nurses, depending on their particular personalities and life circumstances, have variable responses to rape and to the nursing care of rape victims. Professional nurses need to develop the ability to recognize and assess their own response patterns. In this section nurses are assisted in clarifying feeling and value options before committing themselves to beliefs or values concerning rape. Readers are asked to review the facts and myths about rape and to choose their values freely. Nurses who do not choose values freely become uncomfortable and awkward in their interactions with rape victims. More often, it is the nurses' attitudes and values that are subtly conveyed to rape victims during nursing care. Attitudes and values that are conveyed can help or impede the victim's resolution of the rape: positive experiences with health providers facilitate adaptive responses; negative interactions hinder adaptive responses.

## PHASES OF NURSE RESPONSE TO RAPE

In beginning to explore the subject of nurses' responses to rape, we found, from our own experience and that of colleagues, that many nurses work through predictable phases of a growth experience. Fig. 3-1 depicts the nurse's growth experience within the value clarification framework. As shown in the figure, nurses go through the three major phases of value clarification: (1) choosing values, (2) action, and (3) prizing.

### Choosing values

Nursing actions are influenced by value choices. In their professional training, nurses are exposed to several values or beliefs about rape. They explore the facts and

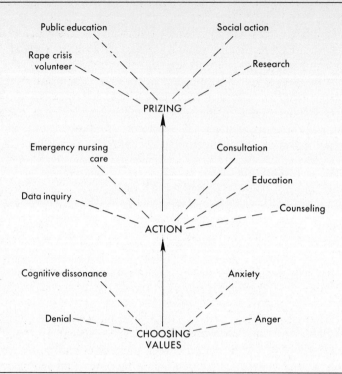

**Fig. 3-1. Positive growth experience of nurses in response to rape.**

myths about rape prior to freely choosing values related to rape. Nurses learn to analyze data before making decisions; value choices about rape and/or nursing actions are made after critical thought and objectivity is achieved. Choosing values related to rape is characterized by four responses: (1) denial of rape facts, (2) cognitive dissonance, (3) anxiety, and (4) anger.

### Denial of rape facts

If nurses choose to believe rape myths, they have difficulty accepting the reality of rape events. Nurses who believe rape myths make comments such as "She was not *really* raped" or "This is not a 'legitimate' rape." Sometimes nurses encounter situations in the emergency room that they consider to stretch the definition of a "legitimate" rape. It is at these times that the nurse's values, reflected in the nurse's social definition of rape and beliefs about appropriate sex-role behavior, conflict with the legal definition of rape. The following example illustrates a situation in which the nurse's personal values could determine whether or not she defines the situation as rape.

#### CLINICAL EXAMPLE

Marian dated Alfred for 6 months. They were at Alfred's apartment where they engaged in kissing and petting. After some period of time Marian stated that she wanted to stop. Alfred continued to pressure for sexual intercourse and, after a struggle, he forced sexual relations on her.

Nurses will have different values about whether the above situation constitutes a case of rape. For example, one nurse may view the victim as culpable because she was not virtuous in her behavior. A second nurse may believe that after such extensive dating the man had a right to sexual intimacies, which the woman could not legitimately refuse. A third nurse may assert that rape could not occur in a close relationship since it is the woman who usually encourages sexual activity or gives mixed messages about refusal. Yet the fact remains that by the legal definition rape did occur in this case because it involved a male forcing intercourse on a nonconsenting female.

The refusal to admit the truth or reality about a rape event is called *denial*. Even though the nurse may "know better" than to doubt the victim, there will be times when the nurse's responses do not match the facts about rape. Sometimes the nurse will overtly or covertly communicate to the victim doubts about the victim's allegation of rape. Other times the nurse communicates doubts about the legitimacy of the victim's allegation of rape to other nurses and colleagues in the presence or absence of the victim.

Nurses who deny rape facts demonstrate *avoidance behaviors* when they do not want to be involved in relating to rape victims. Such behaviors consist of acts of creating a void or departure from an undesirable stimulus or situation. A common example of an avoidance behavior is withdrawal. Nurses who withdraw avoid relating with rape victims in either active or passive manners. *Active withdrawal* is a "pulling away" in which nurses physically put distance between themselves and rape victims. Forms of this behavior occur when (1) nurses who have the time to interact instead leave rape victims alone in examining rooms for extended periods of time; or (2) nurses distance themselves by standing far away from rape victims so that comfortable interaction is impeded. *Passive withdrawal* behaviors are more subtle "pulling away," but they are just as detrimental to helping rape victims. A nonverbal barrier develops between nurses and victims, thus preventing helping relationships from developing. Some examples of less direct withdrawal behaviors occur when (1) nurses act detached and aloof, making if difficult for victims to feel that they are interested or concerned; (2) nurses "forget" rape victims or refuse to talk to them, speaking only when victims ask for specific information or help.

Many rape victims are doubly victimized: once by the rape and again by care providers in the health care system. Often nurses' denial of rape facts is related to values held about rape and rape-related issues such as sexuality and male-female relationships. When nurses entertain the idea that rape myths are indeed myths, they open themselves to cognitive dissonance resulting from new and conflicting data.

### Cognitive dissonance

Initially the nurse believes many of the myths about rape (see Chapter 1). For example, rape is believed to be a sexual act or a crime of passion that only happens to other women who are promiscuous or somehow got their "just desserts." Gradually the nurse's misconceptions about rape are refuted with facts. As the roots of the problem are explored and awareness of one's values about rape are clarified, nurses experience a state of cognitive dissonance. *Cognitive dissonance* is defined in Webster's dictionary as a state that exists when two opposing beliefs exist simultaneously. Such dissonance creates an unpleasant state of tension that the nurse is motivated to resolve.

### CLINICAL EXAMPLE

Cathy is the wife of a minister and is well known for her charitable services in the community. While making a home visit to one of the parishoners, Cathy was raped. The nurse who cares for Cathy views the victim as respectable. However, the nurse has two opposing thoughts: (1) Cathy is a respectable person; and (2) rape only happens to women who ask for it.

To reduce the felt tension from conflicting thoughts, the nurse is motivated to resolve one of the contradictory thoughts. In this situation the nurse has two choices: (1) to believe the myth: People deserve whatever happens to them; or (2) to accept the fact: Rape is a senseless act and respectable people are raped.

Nurses resolve cognitive dissonance in response to rape in one of two ways: (1) denial of rape facts by belief in rape myths, or (2) value clarification regarding rape, sexuality, and male-female relationships. Denying that a situation constitutes a case of rape—even when the rape events meet the legal criteria defining rape—is one way nurses resolve cognitive dissonance in response to rape. Another way is for nurses to clarify their values about rape and rape-related issues.

### Anxiety

As nurses clarify values about rape, the tension from cognitive dissonance is resolved and the facts about rape are usually accepted. If the nurse accepts the facts about rape, *anxiety, shock,* and *fear* are experienced. *Anxiety* is defined by May as a state of "apprehension cued off by a threat to some value which the individual holds essential to his existence as a personality."[9] In contrast, *fear* is a subjective state of feeling that arises from being in danger to life or limb because of a specific stimulus external to the person (e.g., rape, which can be identified).[5] *Shock,* according to Webster's dictionary, is a severe "disturbance in the equilibrium or permanence of something" characterized by feelings of surprise, terror, horror, or disgust.

As a result of an anxiety response, the nurse realizes that human beings are much more similar than different. If raped, the nurse would feel just as awful as the victim. The nurse can no longer assume that rape can happen only to someone else. In realizing that "it could happen to me," the nurse identifies with the victim. Protective emotional distance from the crime is eroded or penetrated by rape facts. Fear, shock, and horror emerge as awareness of rape as a potential personal reality grows.

Variables affecting nurses' feeling responses include personal history, stage of psychologic development, and present life circumstances. For example, it is not uncommon for nurses to experience uncomfortable feelings when they encounter a situation that is very similar to their own. Nurses who have been sexually abused or sexually assaulted feel quite different from those who have never experienced or seen such violent behaviors. Nurses who work with rape victims also need to separate their thoughts about male-female sexual assaults from male-female relationships. They need to understand that a sexual assault is a specific situation that cannot be generalized to all male-female interactions. Sexual intercourse, generally considered the greatest intimacy between two humans, is usually viewed as a pleasurable experience. In contrast, sexual intercourse through sexual assault involves a painful, violent experience. Assessment of similarities to rape victims will help nurses separate their own feelings and reactions from those of rape victims.

Being human, all nurses experience anxiety of varying degrees at some time in their professional careers. During an anxiety response, the nurse engages in some of the following behaviors: checks locks on doors and windows; feels uneasy being alone late at night; and removes a first name from the mailbox. Nurses who work with rape victims feel increased anxiety as they (1) become aware of the violent, aggressive nature of the crime; (2) begin to appreciate the rape victim's helplessness; and (3) experience an urgent need to reduce the victim's pain and suffering by providing high-quality psychologic and physical nursing care.

Since anxiety is not a pleasurable experience, nurses develop various ways of reducing and coping with their anxiety when working with rape victims. In doing so, nurses may behave in overt and covert ways that can be detrimental to the victim's efforts to resolve the rape. Therefore it is important that nurses who work with rape victims recognize such behavioral responses. Examples of common covert behaviors are the physiologic changes of tachycardia, headaches, or sweating. When nurses feel physically uncomfortable, it is more difficult for them to be effective in providing nursing care to patients. Examples of overt behavioral responses to anxiety include:

1. Talking too much
2. Compulsive actions
3. Failure to listen
4. Diagnosing and analyzing
5. Overcompensation by controlling behaviors
6. Advising or giving solutions
7. Ordering, directing, and commanding
8. Moralizing, preaching, and warning[13]

### Anger

The process of realizing that rape is a potential personal reality takes time. It is stimulated by the nurse's gradual awareness of the facts about rape. Covert and overt behaviors used to cope with anxiety, related to the nurse's "rape awareness," become less adaptive and effective, giving rise to an experience of anger. *Anger,* according to Webster's dictionary, is defined as a strong sense of emotional excitement induced by intense displeasure. Arising after the nurse's feelings of anxiety and shock subside, anger is directed in four areas: (1) toward the rapist, (2) toward society, (3) toward the rape victim, and (4) toward the self.

Nurses become angry toward the rapist for inflicting sexual abuse and (if not convicted) for being able to get away with the assault. Nurses often feel that rapists should be punished, either by being jailed or institutionalized. Sometimes nurses find it difficult to provide care to alleged rapists in the emergency room and make comments such as "I hope someone does it to him so he knows what it feels like!"

Nurses also become angry at society for nurturing the conditions that allow rape to occur. Some believe that society should be reformed to ensure that rape does not occur. Such nurses may become interested in prevention-education programs, social action roles to reform society, and the women's movement to establish equal relationships among men and women. Early preventive behaviors, rooted in fear, later generate feelings of anger from an awareness that no person is free of the fear of rape, and the nurse cries out, "Women, men, and children should not *have* to take precautions against rape!"

Blaming the victim is the way nurses sometimes vent their anger and frustration about a rape, especially when there seems to be no outlet for their feelings or when they feel a sense of powerlessness or helplessness. At times the circumstances surrounding a rape are so bizarre or unpleasant that it is more comfortable to blame the victim so that the nurse's anxiety will be decreased. Otherwise the nurse would be confronted with the fact that the rape could have happened to her, and some nurses are unable to even consider rape as a personal possibility. Nurses who have an initial reaction of blaming the rape victim think that the incident could have been prevented if the victim had not provoked the attack or placed herself in a dangerous situation. Angry nurses want to say to rape victims, "How could you be so stupid!" Unfortunately, the impact of blaming rape victims is to increase the victim's sense of guilt and hopelessness.

Nurses also direct anger toward themselves. *Self-directed anger* is expressed in overt and covert behaviors. Overt behaviors include responses such as *helplessness* or *sympathy* toward victims. Covert behaviors include responses such as *guilt, shame,* or statements of *self-blame*.

Nurses feel inadequate when they are unsure of how to help rape victims. Overwhelmed by a rape victim's helplessness and their own feelings of inadequacy, nurses can become ineffective in providing emotional support and physical care. When nurses feel helpless, they lose an objective assessment of their skills and ability to learn what they need to know to become competent practitioners. When nurses feel helpless, they want to reassure the rape victim and diminish the victim's discomfort. Such feelings of helplessness and inadequacy are so unpleasant that the nurse is motivated to act or resolve the feeling state. Nurses also feel sorry for rape victims; this sympathy can be a vehicle for expressing their helplessness. Nurses who sympathize with rape victims can become overinvolved in the crisis situation. They often identify with the emotions of rape victims and may begin to experience the *same* emotions. For example, if the rape victim is anxious, the sympathetic nurse may begin to feel symptoms that characterize an anxiety state (e.g., nausea and trembling). Anxiety is known to be highly contagious in a relationship. Therefore the nurse who feels sympathetic may react to the victim's anxiety level or transmit her own anxiety to the victim, creating a vicious, escalating cycle that is nonproductive in problem-solving or crisis resolution at a time when rational responses are critical.

Nurses direct anger toward themselves when they express a sense of guilt for having believed the myths about rape; they may be very self-incriminating or self-punitive. The nurse may think: "I am *ashamed* that I used to blame and judge the victim as responsible for the crime." "I am embarrassed that I ever thought it was a sex crime." "Something must be the matter with me for being so ignorant." Sometimes nurses are too embarrassed to admit their ignorance to ask the necessary questions to obtain the facts about rape. Other times nurses ask questions in a manner that conceals their ignorance or embarrassment about matters they misperceive to be of a sexual nature.

## Action

The second major step in the value clarification process is action. Nurses make values part of their behaviors and incorporate values into their actions. Values become a consistent and repeated part of nursing performance.

The action phase begins with the development of gentleness and humility toward one's self and the victim. Feelings of incrimination and punitiveness toward self and others are replaced with caring and action. Just as the victim is not at fault for the crime of rape, nurses are able to acknowledge that they are not at fault for earlier states of ignorance. It is not uncommon for nurses to wonder at this time, "Who failed to inform me about rape, and why?" Even though nurses are potential victims, they come to realize that there is a great deal of confusion about the crime and its multidimensional aspects in *all* of society. Nurses realize that as long as their energy is directed toward finding someone to blame, constructive resolution of rape as a problem is impeded.

However, it is necessary to ventilate one's anxiety, anger, dismay, and concern. Giving expression to such feelings facilitates a realistic perception of the event and allows a balance in states of feeling. Thus energy is freed for action. The energy that went into blaming oneself and others is released to investigate the problem of rape and to take constructive action. Action is the phase of growth experience in which the nurse is most vigorous and productive; the nurse is engaged in activity to accomplish specifically valued goals. This phase of the nurse's growth experience is characterized by several behaviors: (1) data inquiry, (2) emergency nursing care, (3) counseling, (4) education, and (5) consultation.

### Data inquiry

In order to determine specific areas or targets for intervention, nurses first must inquire into the etiology of rape. If nurses expect to understand the problem of rape, rape prevention, and how to provide care to victims, they must act to obtain information that meets these objectives.

It is important for nurses to help one another obtain facts about rape and about means of providing empathic, competent care to victims. Once the nurse learns the facts about rape, the net result is the same: the nurse's initial denial is eroded and a set of processes are set in motion. Earlier responses of guilt, shame, self-blame, helplessness, and embarrassment are replaced by constructive behaviors.

### Emergency nursing care

Nurses who work in hospital emergency departments provide direct care to rape victims. Emergency care is directed toward reducing the rape victim's stress state while also meeting physiologic needs. Nurses can help rape victims by providing a supportive environment, by showing concern for the victim's needs, and by demonstrating competent nursing care. One action that professional nurses can implement is to develop a rape exam protocol that meets all the legal criteria for evidence collection yet also remains sensitive to victim needs. (The role of the nurse in hospital emergency departments is thoroughly discussed in Chapter 6.)

### Counseling

Counseling rape victims and their families or significant others is a service offered by rape crisis centers. Nurses function as counselors through these crisis centers and community mental health centers. Counselors must complete a training program at the rape crisis center and maintain consultation regarding those persons seen in counseling. Often nurse counselors have had advanced preparation in a master's program that included supervised experience and education in providing therapy to clients. Counseling on a longer-term basis often is necessary with those victims who decide to prosecute the assailant (see Chapter 9), have a history of psychiatric illness, or have difficulty resolving the rape experience. Counseling the family or significant others of victims is often a short-term intervention (see Chapter 5); cases that require longer-term resolution are likely to be referred to psychiatric-mental health nurses or a professional qualified to provide family therapy.

### Education

Nurses teach facts about rape and the nursing care of rape victims to nursing students and nurses in continuing education courses or workshops. Theory and course content vary between educational settings. Crisis intervention models provide many nurse educators with conceptual frameworks for teaching rape content. Nurses often draw on content taught in prevention-education and training programs at rape crisis centers when teaching nurses about rape and victim care. Since rape is an important knowledge area and nursing care of victims has special significance, nurse educators encourage (1) nursing care of rape victims to be taught as a special entity or course; (2) special emphasis on students' self-awareness and value clarification; and (3) a conceptual framework for teaching students rape content and nursing care of rape victims.

Given the knowledge "explosion" today in scientific and health professions, often nursing educators are limited in the time allotted in a curriculum to teach nursing care of rape victims. Some schools of nursing subsume content on rape under lectures on crisis theory and intervention, use rape as an example of a crisis, and refer students to selected readings. Other curricula provide 2 to 4 hours of lecture time on rape and nursing care of victims; some of these presentations include the use of audiovisual media, such as the rape exam, to complement presentations (see Chapter 6).

The following outline is one model we used for a 2-hour lecture on nursing care of victims of rape:

I. Broad objectives
  A. Gain knowledge to provide the physical and psychologic care to persons who are victims of rape
  B. Develop ability to recognize and assess the responses of persons who are victims of rape and to make appropriate referral when deemed necessary
  C. Identify the interventions indicated in the care of persons who are victims of rape
  D. Develop awareness of the role of the nurse in educating the community regarding issues related to rape

E. Provide an opportunity to review a film on self-protection against rape

II. Class outline
  A. Historical perspectives
    1. Definition of rape
    2. History of rape
    3. Epidemiology
    4. Myths
      a. Social bias
      b. Population vulnerable to rape
  B. Emergency room nursing care
    1. Nurses' role
    2. Medical-legal examination
    3. Examination to obtain evidence
      a. Inspection
      b. Laboratory procedures
    4. Documentation of findings
    5. Treatment
  C. Prevention or alleviation of psychologic trauma
  D. Follow-up care
    1. Somatic reactions
    2. Emotional reactions
    3. Silent rape reactions
  E. Referrals

As more nurse educators act on full values about rape, more content is being developed for use in the education of nurses and others concerned with victim care. Given the extent of violence in our society today—rape, incest, abuse of the elderly, battering of women, psychologic abuse of women, sibling violence, and physical abuse of children—curricula in schools of nursing may expand to reflect the federal government's funding of programs that offer specialized education and training for nurses to work with victims of violence and to develop prevention programs. Finally, rape crisis centers represent an opportunity for nurse educators to impact programs such as victim counseling as well as collaborative relationships with other agencies that provide victim care. Professional input from knowledgeable nurses can influence the quality of training sessions as well as the services offered.

### Consultation

*Consultation* has been defined in a wide variety of ways—including "any professional activity carried out by a specialist," "specialized professional activity between two persons in regard to a third," or "professional activity carried out by a highly trained person"—but without differentiating the consultant's activity of consultation from other functions of the professional's role responsibilities.[1] Caplan defines consultation as

> a process of interaction between two professional persons—the consultant, who is a specialist, and the consultee, who invokes the consultant's help in regard to a current work problem with which he is having some difficulty and which he has decided is within the other's area of specialized competence.[1]

Four types of consultation are recognized by specialists: (1) the management or treatment of one or more cases (client-centered consultation), (2) the management or treatment of a particular client where help is sought to improve handling of the case (consultee-centered case consultation), (3) the development or improvement of a program (program-centered administrative consultation), and (4) the problems of program planning or implementation (consultee-centered administrative consultation). Nurses who function as consultants have preparation at the master's level in programs that provide supervised educational and experiential learning. Often when consultation is sought from nurses in the field of rape work it is in relation to one or more rape victim cases and the management of those cases (client-centered or consultee-centered consultation). It is important to remember that although the nurse consultant offers a professional viewpoint on how to manage a situation, whether it be related to the client or administration, it is the prerogative of the consultee to follow or reject that recommendation.[1]

### Prizing

The final step in the action phase is a deepening awareness of one's feelings—prizing. Nurses cherish values and feelings, are proud of them, and are happy with their choices. Willing to share their values publically, nurses reveal their inner selves and move toward self-acceptance. Once values and feelings are experienced as worthwhile and rewarding, they do not *always* remain full values. Values are never static. Rather they are in a dynamic process that allows change over time. As nurses mature professionally, values change. Encountering situations in which one value may come into competition with another, nurses weigh their values and decide on priorities. Prizing behaviors include (1) rape crisis volunteer, (2) public education, (3) social action, and (4) research.

#### Rape crisis center volunteer

As awareness about the problem of rape and the poor quality of care victims received became more prevalent, rape crisis centers emerged. Gradually more and more professionals have joined these organizations, participated in and contributed to their programs, and applied what they have learned in these settings in their professional work. There are a number of ways in which nurses can participate in the work of rape crisis centers. One of the main services offered by rape crisis centers is *hotline crisis counseling* to rape victims on a 24-hour basis. Nurses who volunteer to work on the hotline do so after completing a training program offered by the rape crisis center. When nurses are "on call," they often provide this service from their residence. When a victim calls the crisis center, the call is forwarded to the nurse at home through an answering service or "telepatch" system, provided by a private agency or telephone company. The nurse provides crisis counseling to the victim, applying the principles of crisis intervention and following the telephone interviewing guidelines with victims of rape (see Chapter 7). The nurse follows the policies and procedures of the rape crisis center by completing the required record forms on all calls received and by reporting the nature of all calls received to the person in charge of hotline volunteers. The role of hotline crisis counselor offers the nurse just beginning to work with rape victims a gradual supervised introduction into this type of work. It allows nurses who work rotating shifts and have demanding responsibilities to contribute to the field of rape work.

Another major service offered by rape crisis centers is that of *advocacy*. Nurses can volunteer to function as nursing or legal advocates for victims of rape. Nursing advocates offer emotional support to rape victims seeking care, act as "watchdogs" to the health care system (e.g., seeing that evidence is properly collected to ensure the victim's rights in prosecuting assailants), and offer assistance with follow-up health care. Legal advocates provide emotional support and information to victims who report to the police and prosecute assailants. Nurses who act as legal advocates also coordinate multiple community systems for victims—for example, medical, police, and court systems or personnel. (Advocacy is discussed in further detail in Chapter 8.) Often nurses' ability to contribute to rape work through advocacy depends on competing professional work commitments, time schedules, and priorities in their personal life.

### Public education

Public education about rape is a major contribution offered by nurses. Most rape crisis centers offer a "speakers training" workshop for volunteers to prepare them for speaking engagements. Nurses who volunteer to do public speaking address a wide variety of audiences such as young school children, teen-agers, parents, church groups, men's and women's groups, and professional groups. Nurses serving as public education speakers will find that faculty in schools of nursing request their services.

A wide variety of educational approaches have been developed by rape crisis centers. Programs focus on primary, secondary, and tertiary prevention. Information on such programs can be obtained by writing to the National Institute of Mental Health, Center for the Prevention and Control of Rape,* which acts as a clearinghouse to identify resource material on rape programs, medical protocols, the criminal justice system, films and videotapes for training, and a wide variety of pamphlets and guides.

The Syracuse Rape Crisis Center in New York has developed a high school program for rape awareness prevention that identifies model content for each level of a prevention-education program as follows:

1. Primary Prevention Education (long-term goal)
   a. Information on why rape occurs, etiology of the problem
   b. Define the nature of rape and child sexual assault
   c. Discuss societal conditions that nurture rape
   d. Explore the myths and facts about rape
   e. Prevalence of rape and child sexual assault
   f. Skills in communicating privacy and the right to say "no" to sexually assaultive or abusive acts
2. Secondary Prevention Education (immediate and personal goal)
   a. Identification of potentially dangerous situations

---

*NIMH, Center for the Prevention and Control of Rape, 5000 Fishers Lane, Parklawn Bldg., C Wing, Rm. 15-99, Rockville, MD 20857.

        b. Communication in dangerous situations to avert assault or seek help
        c. Acquaintance and date-rape situations
     3. Tertiary prevention (preventing long-term psychological trauma)
        a. Imparting information on the psychological impact of rape
        b. Disseminating information on supportive services in the community—crisis and counseling centers, medical and legal services

Prevention-education programs are believed to be important in long-range efforts to eliminate the incidence of rape from society, reduce potential victimization by teaching alternative life-styles and affirming a person's rights to privacy or personal boundaries, and in reducing the psychologic trauma of the crime.[3]

### Social action

Nurses can develop and participate in activities or programs intended to create increased societal awareness of the problem and long-range change in societal conditions that nurture rape. Social action projects are usually of a short-term nature and have a singular objective. Some projects, however, such as revisions within the criminal justice system for interviewing child sexual assault victims, are of a longer duration and require coordinated community and institutional efforts. The following are examples of social action projects:

1. Women committed to eliminating sexist violence in pornography and the media schedule a tour through the local pornography district to increase awareness of society's view of women as sex objects.
2. A group publishes a newsletter challenging attitudes about pornography such as: "Don't some women enjoy pornography?" "Isn't pornography a safety valve or harmless outlet for men who might otherwise commit violent crimes?" "Isn't pornography a trivial issue and where do you draw the line?" The group manages to have the question and answer debate inserted in the newsletters of community organizations.[10]
3. A group of women start a consciousness-raising group composed of men and women. The group selects books to read and discuss regarding incest, the socializing of men and women in our society, sex-role stereotyping, racism and sexism, and rape.
4. A group pickets a local movie theatre that shows films that depict women enjoying sadistic and sexual abuse.
5. A group demonstrates and successfully recalls a judge for an unfavorable decision and prejudicial remarks made in relation to a rape case.
6. A group of women picket and demonstrate in front of a lingerie store that depicts the legs of a mannikin protruding from a garbage can that advertizes "more trash for less." The group writes letters to the editor complaining of the implication that women are "cheap trash."
7. Volunteers in a rape crisis center compile a "rape alert" to circulate in the community. It describes the appearance and modus operandi of rapists that victims have decided not to prosecute (but want to alert other women to).
8. Professional nurse advocates write a local hospital to register a complaint about the refusal of the hospital to treat a rape victim. They seek the backup of com-

munity organizations and top-level officials to enforce the seriousness of the complaint.

*Social action projects* are defined as stopgap measures that bring to a halt practices that are unethical, discriminating, or otherwise objectionable.[14] Confrontation strategies are anxiety producing for nurses who lack experience in this technique for changing a system, particularly for female nurses who have been socialized to be submissive, compliant, and nonassertive. Nurses who express their values about rape through social action projects recognize that change is a *slow* process. For a problem as pervasive as rape, and given the lack of societal awareness about the multiple causes of rape, social action projects have a great impact because of the effort of a group of people addressing the problem. Nurses who are politically aware are beginning to recognize social action roles as an important way of contributing to eradicating the crime of rape and improving services to victims.

### Research

According to Webster's dictionary, *research* is defined as "studious inquiry or examination, especially investigation or experimentation aimed at the discovery and interpretation of facts, revision of accepted theories or laws in the light of new facts, or practical application of such new or revised theories or laws." The mere mention of research is enough to send many nurses to the farthest "closets" of their work settings. Commenting on whether nurses can conduct research within an 8-hour work span, Robb has stated:

> Research is something that nurses, in general, spend a great deal of time busily and guiltily *not doing*. Their reasons are legion and include such frequently identified impediments as lack of time, energy, money, peer and administrative support, expertise, ideas, and tangible rewards.[11]

Current nursing researchers believe that *all* nurses can and should do research. Doing research means that nurses value the practice of nursing sufficiently to investigate their work. According to Diers,[2] the *purpose* of doing nursing research is to modify nursing practice in light of the findings from research studies and ultimately to improve the quality of care provided to patients. Simon[12] states that people *do* what they value and value what they do: nurses who *value* improving the quality of care to patients (in this case, rape victims) *do* research on rape and publish those findings. Nurse researchers are not satisfied with being an expert clinician; they seek scientific verification regarding the effectiveness of clinical interventions and supporting theoretical frameworks. One of the main points emphasized under the action phase of the nurse's response to rape is that the nurse acts on that value system. To date, improved care to rape victims is the direct result of *nursing* research in the field, primarily the work of Ann Burgess and Lynda Holmstrom. Research has refuted many misconceptions about rape and highlighted socializing processes that contribute to the development and belief in rape myths.

Today more nurses are prepared to do research than a decade ago, and more role models are available to inspire and encourage young nurse researchers in their work. Many nurses who have not had the advantage of advanced education in how to write or conduct research still express their value for research by participating in such studies and assisting with data collection. Furthermore, the profession's value of nursing research is evidenced by the availability of funding to conduct research from sources such as the Division of Nursing, the American Nurses' Foundation, and Sigma Theta Tau.* In addition, federal funding for nursing research is available. As a result of intensive lobbying by feminists' groups, the National Center for the Prevention and Control of Rape, mentioned previously, was established within the National Institute of Mental Health and supports research.

The majority of research on rape has asked the questions, What is this? or What is happening here? Problem statements at this level of inquiry include: Why do men rape? What conditions foster or perpetuate rape? How do victims respond to being raped? What are the variables to bring about successful conviction of an offender? How must nurses go about collecting evidence so that it meets criteria to be legally admissable in court proceedings? How does the victim's family respond to the assault? Such problem statements have prompted investigations that resulted in greater understanding of the nature of rape, its roots, ideas about prevention and treatment interventions. Beginning to understand the nature of a problem is the first step of any research process.

After a decade of descriptive studies on rape, researchers are now asking, What will happen if . . . ? or How can I make . . . happen? Research studies at advanced levels of inquiry are just beginning to test the effectiveness of different treatment interventions with rape victims. For example, Frank and Turner[4] are investigating the relative efficacy of three treatment modes: (1) individual counseling, (2) systematic desensitization, or (3) individual counseling combined with systematic desensitization. Kilpatrick and Veronen[8] are conducting an empirical investigation to ascertain the effectiveness of brief behavioral interventions. Findings from such empirical research will help improve the counseling of women.[6]

A review of the literature on rape indicates that the majority of research on rape suffers from a variety of problems resulting from design and methodology. For example, it is known that lower socioeconomic groups tend to seek rape care in traditional health care delivery systems, while middle and upper socioeconomic classes often obtain care from physicians in private practice and do not report the assault. Factors such as these result in confusion in an understanding of rape and its impact; and they limit the extent to which the results of studies can be quoted as reliable, valid "facts." Methodological problems in rape research create discrepancies in the data and limit interpretations about the nature of rape. Existing studies suffer from limitations in the following areas: (1) diverse definitions of what constitutes rape; (2) wide range of age groups of victims studied; (3) differences in the types of sexual assault included in studies; (4) differences in where study samples were obtained—for example, police files or hospitals; (5) inadequate selection or description of victims in the study sample; (6) failure to include a comparison group—for example, women who have not been raped; (7) absence of experimental designs to test hypotheses; (8) failure to use

*Information about research funding can be obtained by writing to: Research Support Section, Nursing Research Branch, Division of Nursing (Center Building, Room 3-50, 3700 East West Highway, Hyattsville, MD 20782); American Nurses' Foundation (2420 Pershing Road, Kansas City, MO 64108); Sigma Theta Tau (School of Nursing Building, 1100 West Michigan Street, Indianapolis, IN 46223).

standardized, reliable, and objective means of measuring responses to rape or subsequent interventions; (9) data made to fit existing theoretical frameworks—for example, crisis theory or "rape trauma syndrome"; and (10) inadequate descriptions of crucially important steps of the research methodology.[8]

The preceding list of limitations levels a strong critique of current research on rape and may seem discouraging to the beginning nurse researcher. In reality, nurses are challenged to implement refined research studies that modify such limitations and to ultimately produce and publish scientifically reliable data about the effectiveness of nursing care of victims of rape. Nurses who scientifically understand the nature and essence of rape and its impact on victims can take strategic action to implement and investigate the effectiveness of prevention and treatment programs. Keen states: "There is a way to end the game that can't be won/If we see where and why it began."[7]

### CLINICAL EXAMPLE

Marsha is an 18-year-old female brought into the local health clinic by her sister. She is dressed in jeans and a denim blouse. The sister shares with the staff nurse her concern that Marsha might be pregnant. The nurse proceeds to interview Marsha in private. Marsha relates the following:

She had been attending college away from home and decided to visit her sister who lives across the state. Being a student, she did not have enough money for transportation, so she decided to try hitchhiking since she does it to get to school every day. She never had any problems with hitching a ride to school every day.

A young man offered her a ride in his van. After going a short distance, he drove onto a side road and pulled a knife on her. He then raped her, beat her, and left her by the roadside. Marsha blames herself for the rape. She does not feel she can tell her parents because they have warned her about the risks of hitchhiking. "If I had only followed their advice!" she says and begins to cry. Marsha then asks the nurse what she can do.

The nurse in this clinic is 20 years old. Her feelings about the rape event are as follows:

1. I identify with Marsha. She is very close to my age (assessment of similarities).
2. I know about the dangers of hitchhiking. I would not hitchhike myself because it's a potentially dangerous situation (personal value).
3. Marsha definitely put herself in a risky situation by accepting a ride from a stranger (value based on fact about rape).
4. Marsha should have known better! In a way she asked for it . . . How could she be so naive? (anger: blaming the victim).
5. I would feel terrible if this happened to me. I know I'd blame myself and feel guilty (becoming more sensitive to victim).
6. I need to help Marsha realize that self-blame is a normal victim response (education).
7. I can't believe I was so incriminating! (acknowledges earlier state of ignorance).

The clinical example above illustrates the first two phases of the value clarification process of the professional nurse: self-exploration of thoughts and feelings concerning rape (choosing values) and education of the patient (action). The staff nurse examined and worked through her own values regarding the rape and the victim's behaviors.

Providing care to the victim was particularly difficult since the nurse was of similar age to the victim. The nurse chose values freely and worked through her values to the phase of action. In the action phase she educated the victim and realized her own ignorance. If the nurse had moved onto the prizing phase, she might have selected public education as a behavior.

## SUMMARY

Working with rape victims can be a positive growth experience. Nurses who work with these victims are encouraged to examine their own values to assess which values are influencing their responses. The value clarification process provides a conceptual framework from which nurses can analyze their responses. The three phases of nurse responses include (1) choosing values, (2) action, and (3) prizing.

The first phase, choosing values, is characterized by four responses: (1) denial of rape facts, (2) cognitive dissonance, (3) anxiety, and (4) anger. In this phase nurses choose values freely from several alternatives. The second phase is action, which is characterized by making values part of behavior. Nurses invest their energies in productive activities that accomplish valued goals. Activities in the action phase include data inquiry, emergency nursing care, counseling, education, and consultation.

The final phase of nurse responses is prizing, in which self-awareness deepens, values are cherished, and values are revealed publically. Not all professional nurses who work with rape victims proceed to this phase. However, many do demonstrate prizing behaviors such as volunteering at rape crisis centers, public speaking, and social action.

Expanded roles in nursing—such as advocacy, education, consultation, and research—offer nurses the opportunity to synthesize knowledge and skills into actions that are most useful to victims and to the field of rape. Expanded roles are self-actualizing, permit the nurse to act autonomously and interdependently, and offer some of the most challenging and satisfying experiences in being of service to fellow human beings.

We emphasize that there is no "right" or "wrong" way to experience the value clarification process. Being unique individuals, nurses will have varying responses as they care for rape victims; and sometimes it will not be easy for nurses to look at themselves. Because of their unique position in carrying for rape victims, nurses can help or impede victim adaptation.

Values give direction to life. When nurses discover what values they prize, life has definite meaning and direction. Uustal has stated:

> How you perform as a nurse depends on your philosophy. *Values form your philosophy and are the basis for your actions* [emphasis added]. If you do not take time to examine and articulate them, you will not be as clear or conscious of your beliefs and values and the significant impact they have upon your behavior. The price you pay for value conflicts is often confusion, indecision, and inconsistency. . . . Values provide a frame or reference, a basic comprehension of reality through which we integrate, explain, and appraise new ideas, events, and personal relationships.[15]

## Learning activities

The following brief exercises are intended to heighten the nurse's self-awareness and bring out many values concerning rape. As with many issues there are no "right" or "wrong" values. You are encouraged to evaluate your responses. If possible, share your values with peers, co-workers, or supervisors so that a range of values can be discussed openly.

### EXERCISE 1: Value clarification case study

Jane is a 36-year-old married woman with three young children. Her husband is a salesman. Jane is going to night school to complete a degree. One evening after class she goes out for a drink with several classmates. On the way home Jane stops at a red light. A man forces his way into her car and forces her, at gunpoint, to drive to a secluded park area. He rapes her and runs off.

Once free of her assailant, Jane drives to the nearest emergency room. At the hospital Jane approaches the nurse and tells her she was just raped. The emergency room has no private rooms available, so Jane is asked to wait in a quiet part of the waiting room. Jane waits approximately 1 hour to be seen.

*Directions:* Respond to the following statements according to *your* value system—how *you* think, feel or act about rape. Again, there are no "right" or "wrong" answers. Read each statement and put a checkmark in the column that best describes your position.

|  | Strongly agree | Agree | Disagree | Strongly disagree |
|---|---|---|---|---|
| 1. Jane should not be in school in the first place. Her first priorities should be her husband and children. | _____ | _____ | _____ | _____ |
| 2. Jane should never have gone out with classmates for a drink. | _____ | _____ | _____ | _____ |
| 3. If her door had been locked, a man could not have forced his way into Jane's car. | _____ | _____ | _____ | _____ |
| 4. If a man were pointing a gun at me, I would do whatever he wanted. | _____ | _____ | _____ | _____ |
| 5. Jane would not have been raped if she had shown *some* resistance. | _____ | _____ | _____ | _____ |
| 6. Rape will be hard to prove because Jane complied. | _____ | _____ | _____ | _____ |
| 7. After being raped, Jane was right in seeking medical care. | _____ | _____ | _____ | _____ |
| 8. If I were Jane, I would call my husband. | _____ | _____ | _____ | _____ |
| 9. I would be angry about waiting 1 hour to be seen. | _____ | _____ | _____ | _____ |

| | Strongly agree | Agree | Disagree | Strongly disagree |
|---|---|---|---|---|
| 10. A rape victim should have immediate medical attention. | _____ | _____ | _____ | _____ |
| 11. Surely Jane's husband and children are wondering where she is. | _____ | _____ | _____ | _____ |
| 12. The nurse is inconsiderate of Jane's feelings by letting her stay in the waiting room. | _____ | _____ | _____ | _____ |

The nurse checks back with Jane to see if she is managing okay. She encourages Jane to let her call the police, but Jane is hesitant to do so. She is not sure what to do. She is just glad to be alive.

Jane is uncertain about what to say to her husband and children. She has noticeable bruises. She thinks her husband will be upset, and she is not sure if the children will understand. She wonders what to say to neighbors. What will be said about her in the community? Jane starts to cry softly.

| | Strongly agree | Agree | Disagree | Strongly disagree |
|---|---|---|---|---|
| 13. Someone from the nursing staff should be with Jane because she needs emotional support. | _____ | _____ | _____ | _____ |
| 14. Jane should definitely inform the police so the rapist can be apprehended. | _____ | _____ | _____ | _____ |
| 15. If Jane does not, the emergency room staff should inform the police of the assault. | _____ | _____ | _____ | _____ |
| 16. The police are generally poorly trained in helping the victim. They can be informed later. | _____ | _____ | _____ | _____ |
| 17. Jane should definitely tell her husband. | _____ | _____ | _____ | _____ |
| 18. Husbands are generally very understanding in these matters. | _____ | _____ | _____ | _____ |
| 19. Jane's children should not be told of the incident. | _____ | _____ | _____ | _____ |
| 20. In general, children cannot understand the concept of rape. | _____ | _____ | _____ | _____ |
| 21. It is really none of Jane's neighbors' business to know of this incident. | _____ | _____ | _____ | _____ |
| 22. Jane's community is likely to blame Jane for the assault. | _____ | _____ | _____ | _____ |
| 23. In a way, Jane is to blame for the assault. | _____ | _____ | _____ | _____ |
| 24. The emergency room staff should notify Jane's husband of the assault. | _____ | _____ | _____ | _____ |
| 25. I feel sorry for Jane. | _____ | _____ | _____ | _____ |

## EXERCISE 2: Expanded nursing role options

The following exercise helps nurses to consider and set priorities for action in response to rape. The choices listed below reflect expanded nursing roles in the field of rape work.

*Directions:* Complete the following steps: (1) Place a checkmark next to all the choices that you have a personal interest in. (2) Next, rank these choices by placing a number 1 by the item you would act on first, a number 2 by the one you would act on second, and so forth until all items that were checked are numbered according to your priorities.

_____ a. Complete a *training* program in a rape crisis center to learn how to work as a volunteer in that setting.

_____ b. Volunteer to do *public speaking* about rape through programs offered by the local rape crisis center (e.g., to high school students or civic groups).

_____ c. Work as a *crisis counselor* on the hotline of the local rape crisis center.

_____ d. Develop a *research* proposal to implement in collaboration with the rape crisis center and/or local hospitals and rape task forces.

_____ e. *Teach* nurses about nursing care of rape victims through continuing education programs.

_____ f. Assist a local director of nursing in *developing protocol* for nurse practitioners to follow in administering rape or sexual assault exams to victims.

_____ g. Be available on an on-call basis to provide *consultation* to staff in rape crisis centers or hospitals regarding the care of rape victims with a history of psychiatric illness.

_____ h. Write and *publish articles* about nursing care of rape victims and identify areas for further work in the field.

_____ i. Provide *long-term conseling* to victims and/or families as needed or requested through the local rape crisis center or a community agency (e.g., victims or families prosecuting an assailant).

_____ j. Other (specify) _____

_____ k. None of the above.

## EXERCISE 3: Rape knowledge values

*Directions:* You are asked to set priorities for your values on rape. What information would you consider important before choosing these priorities? Rank your choices by placing a number 1 beside the most important item to know, a number 2 beside the second most important item to know, and continue until all items on the list have been prioritized from most to least important.

_____  a.  Psychology of the rapist
_____  b.  Impact of rape on the victim
_____  c.  Statistics on rape, such as incidence and prevalence
_____  d.  Rape law and legal process
_____  e.  Ways to counsel the rape victim
_____  f.  Research findings on rape
_____  g.  Social factors influencing rape
_____  h.  Psychologic care given to rape victims
_____  i.  Medical aspects of rape
_____  j.  Ways police respond to a rape
_____  k.  Other value _____
_____  l.  Other value _____

## EXERCISE 4: Rape victim care values

*Directions:* You are asked to help a rape victim in the emergency room. What values do you consider important to delivering quality care to the victim? Rank your choices by placing a number 1 beside the most important item, a number 2 beside the second most important item, and continue until all items on the list have been prioritized from most to least important.

_____  a.  Confidentiality
_____  b.  Immediate medical attention
_____  c.  Emotional support to patient
_____  d.  Help in notifying someone who can comfort the patient
_____  e.  Privacy
_____  f.  Collection of evidence for future use if necessary
_____  g.  Information regarding nature of the assault
_____  h.  Informing patient about her rights
_____  i.  Patient protection from further intrusions
_____  j.  Clear explanation of procedures to the patient
_____  k.  Other _____
_____  l.  Other _____

## REFERENCES

1. Caplan, G.: The theory and practice of mental health consultation, New York, 1970, Basic Books, Inc.
2. Diers, D.: Research in nursing practice, New York, 1979, J.B. Lippincott Co.
3. Fletcher, P., and Spoto, D.: Rape: awareness and prevention for educators, Syracuse, N.Y., 1980, Rape Crisis Center of Syracuse, Inc.
4. Frank, E., and Turner, S.: The rape victim: her response and treatment, Pittsburgh, Pa., Western Psychiatric Institute and Clinic, doctoral dissertation, 1979.

5. Graves, H., and Thompson, E.: Anxiety: a mental health vital sign. In Longo, C., and Wiliams, R., editors: Clinical practice in psychosocial nursing: assessment and intervention, New York, 1978, Appleton-Century-Crofts.
6. Hill, C.E.: A research perspective on counseling women, Counsel. Psychol. **6:**53, 1976.
7. Keen, S.: Beginnings without end, New York, 1975, Harper & Row, Publishers.
8. Kilpatrick, D., and Veronen, L.: Treatment of fear and anxiety in victims of rape, NIMH Study No. R01 MH29602, 1981, Medical University of South Carolina, Charleston, S.C.
9. May, R.: The meaning of anxiety, New York, 1950, Ronald Press.
10. PAAR-Spectives, newsletter, Pittsburgh, Pa., 1979, Pittsburgh Action Against Rape.
11. Robb, S.: Possible or impossible, Vital Signs (official publication of district No. 6, Pennsylvania Nurses Association), **6:**8, Sept. 1980.
12. Simon, S., Howe, L., and Kirschenbaum, H.: Values clarification: a handbook of practical strategies for teachers and students, New York, 1972, Hart Publishing Co., Inc.
13. Smith, M.: A practical guide to value clarification, La Jolla, Calif., 1977, University Associates, Inc.
14. Warner, C.: Rape and sexual assault: management and intervention, Rockville, Md., 1980, Aspen Systems Corporation.
15. Uustal, D.: Values and ethics: considerations in nursing practice—a workbook for nurses, Phoenix, Ariz., 1978 (privately published by the author).

## ADDITIONAL REFERENCES

Burgess, A.W., and Lazare, A: Psychiatric nursing in the hospital and the community, New Jersey, 1976, Prentice-Hall, Inc.
Frank E.: Psychological response to rape: an analysis of response patterns, doctoral dissertation, University of Pittsburgh, 1979.
Holmstrom, L.L., and Burgess, A.W.: The victim of rape: institutional reactions, New york, 1978, John Wiley & Sons.
Katz, S., and Mazur, M.A.: Understanding the rape victim: a synthesis of research findings, New York, 1979, John Wiley & Sons.
Kerlinger, F.: Foundations of behavioral research, New York, 1973, Holt, Rinehart & Winston, Inc.
O'Conners K.: Why don't women publish more journal articles? The Chronical of Higher Educ., Nov. 3, 1980, p. 25.
Polit, D., and Hungler, B.: Nursing research: principles and methods, New York, 1978, J.B. Lippincott Co.
Sheehy, G.: Passages; predictable crises of adult life, New York, 1976, E.P. Dutton and Co., Inc.
Uustal, D.: Value clarification in nursing: application to practice, Am. J. Nurs. **12:**2058, 1978.
Woods, N.: Human sexuality in health and illness, St. Louis, 1979, The C.V. Mosby Co.

## ANNOTATED SUGGESTED READINGS

Abbey, D.S.: Valuing Chicago, 1973, Instructional Dynamics.

This instructional kit emphasizes the value process as an approach to problem solving. It includes cassettes, booklets, and discussion guides for the small group.

Barrett, J.E.: Value clarification as a teaching strategy in nursing, J. Nurs. Educ. **17:**12, 1978.

This article discusses the basic concepts of value clarification theory, the goals of nursing education that make it an appropriate strategy to use in this field, and a rationale for its use based on the writings of educators. A clinical case situation is presented to illustrate application of the strategies. A variety of strategies and specific applications to nursing situations are also presented.

Burgess, A., and Lazare, A.: Psychiatric nursing in the hospital and the community, Englewood Cliffs, N.J., 1976, Prentice-Hall, Inc.

This text presents basic psychiatric nursing approaches to the care of mentally-ill persons. An important section emphasized nurses' need to be aware of themselves; it explains how feelings (role appropriate and subjective) can influence the nursing care of psychiatric patients.

Coletta, S.: Values clarification in nursing: why? Am. J. Nurs. **12:**2057, 1978.

This article briefly introduces the reader to the relevance of value clarification strategies in nursing education and practice today. It suggests how nurses can use value clarification strategies with patients to help them clarify their feelings.

Gordon, T.: Teacher effectiveness training, New York, 1974, David McKay Co., Inc.

This book presents the principles and skills of effective human relations—the ways to make relationships more human through honest interpersonal communications and constructive conflict resolution. It applies the principles and skills taught in courses on Parent-Effectiveness Training to teacher-student relationships and identifies constructive and destructive interactional styles.

Hall, B.: Value clarification as learning process: a guidebook, New York, 1973, Paulist Press.

This volume describes 46 exercises that can be used as strategies for learning about value clarification.

Kirschenbaum, H.: Advanced value clarification, La Jolla, Cal., 1977, University Associates, Inc.

This handbook explores the theory and current research in value clarification. A basic guide for educators or counselors, it is a comprehensive, annotated bibliography of value clarification.

Kirschenbaum, H., and Glasser, B.: Developing support groups: a manual for facilitators and participants, La Jolla, Calif., 1978, University Associates, Inc.

This manual describes the professional support groups as a framework for ongoing support and learning. It offers guidelines for starting a support group with suggestions for structuring meetings, learning modes to offer members, evaluation sessions, and forms for self-evaluation, group evaluation, and self-contracts. It is an application of theory and techniques in human relations training to integrate personal and professional development.

Maslow, A.: The farther reaches of human nature, New York, 1971, The Viking Press.

Maslow develops his theory of self-actualization by researching the values of self-actualized persons. He also seeks to identify objective values from subjective values.

Notman, M., and Nadelson, C.: The rape victim: psychodynamic considerations, Am. J. Psych. **133:**408, 1976.

This article emphasizes the consideration of psychodynamic influences that affect responses of rape victims. It discusses the impact of rape on the victim in terms of developmental life-cycle and situational issues.

Polit, D., and Hungler, B.: Nursing research: principles and methods, Philadelphia, 1978, J.B. Lippincott Co.

This book is highly recommended for undergraduate and graduate nursing students as well as for the entire nursing research community. It is designed as a basic text on the methods and techniques of resolution in solving nursing problems. It attends to both the consumer and the producer of nursing research and addresses the problems students often encounter in reading, understanding, and evaluating research reports. Technical jargon in avoided; problems students commonly experience are introduced gradually and discussed at length; learning is facilitated through a number of strategies and relevant examples, and each chapter offers supplementary readings and study suggestions.

Raths, L., Harmen, M., and Simon, S.: Values and teaching, Columbus, Ohio, 1966, Charles E. Merrill Publishing Co.

This classic book presents the theory of values, the value-clarifying method, and the use of value theory. It initiated the current interest in the value clarification approach.

Rokeach, M.: The nature of human values, New York, 1973, The Free Press.

This book presents various research in the area of value clarification: what values a person has, inducing value changes through cognitive and behavioral change, and survey instruments for values.

Satir, V.: Peoplemaking, Palo Alto, Calif., 1976, Science & Behavior Books.

This book emphasizes relationships within one's family and how interactional processes influence harmony. The author also presents various exercises for assessing one's own family's interactional dynamics.

Tobac, S.: The effects of a rape crisis center's training program on volunteers' rape-myth-fact awareness and their attitudes toward women, master's thesis, 1979, University of Pittsburgh, School of Nursing.

One strength of this study is its review of the literature on socialization patterns of women and sex-role stereotyping. The results indicate that liberal women's attitudes are basically unchanged despite training; and this may influence their behaviors in electing to work with rape victims.

Uustal, D.: The use of values clarification in nursing practice, J. Cont. Educ. Nurs. **8:**3, 1977.

This article discusses the theory behind the value clarification process. The author tells how the process can help nurses discover more completely who they are and understand themselves. Freedom of choice is emphasized, and nurses are encouraged to share their values and ideas with others.

Uustal, D.: Value clarification in nursing: application to practice, Am. J. Nurs. **12:**2058, 1978.

The author emphasizes that feelings and values significantly affect nursing care. After reviewing value clarification theory, the article presents strategies that are designed to increase awareness and appreciation of the self and to explore selected value conflicts and ethical dilemmas in nursing.

Woods, N.: Human sexuality in health and illness, ed. 2, St. Louis, 1979, The C.V. Mosby Co.

This book examines the biopsychosocial nature of human sexuality, including the changing nature of sexuality throughout the life-cycle. The author discusses roles for professional nurses in the delivery of sexual health services.

# CHAPTER 4

# Victim response to rape

No matter how terrible people think rape is, it's worse than they know. It's like a bomb going off at the center of your soul. . . .

Carolyn Craven, rape victim of The Berkeley Rapist, "Stinky"

## CHAPTER OUTLINE

Stress adaptation
  theory
Stress response
  syndrome
  Alarm phase
  Resistance phase
    Fear
    Shock, disbelief,
      and denial
    Anxiety
    Self-blame and
      guilt

Compulsive
  repetitions
Mastery and
  control
Recuperative phase
  Resentment and
    anger
  Sadness
  Realistic appraisal
    of assault

Sexual dysfunction
Post-traumatic
  stress disorder
Developmental
  stressors
  Adolescence
  Young adulthood
  Middle age
  Older adulthood
Summary

## LEARNING OBJECTIVES

After reading this chapter the student will be able to:

1 Define the important concepts of stress adaptation theory, which are steady state, stress, stressor, adaptation, and stress reaction

2 Explain the experiences of rape victims during three phases of the stress response syndrome

3 List three psychologic coping responses and describe appropriate nursing interventions during the resistance phase of the stress response syndrome

4 List two psychologic coping responses and describe appropriate nursing interventions during the recuperative phase of the stress response syndrome

5 Identify four diagnostic criteria for post-traumatic stress disorders

6 Explain the developmental stressors relevant to four phases of life: adolescence, young adulthood, adulthood, middle age, and older adulthood

7 Describe nursing interventions appropriate for rape victims in each of four developmental phases of life

Women, depending on their particular personalities and life circumstances, have variable responses following a rape experience. Similar to responses of other persons who undergo a physically violent and emotional trauma, rape victim responses include physiologic, psychologic, and sociologic disturbances. Rape victims are trying to cope with an unexpected, threatening disruption in their daily lives. Most women, given adequate medical care, emotional support, and legal assistance, have the capacity to cope with a rape experience.

Since rapes generally occur without warning, victims are in vulnerable positions because of limited time to react to the sudden stress. Consequently, many rape victims cannot mobilize themselves to fight their assailants, to run away, or to protect themselves. After the rape, most victims seek help for medical attention, police intervention, and psychologic intervention.

The most frequently cited victim responses are reported from clinical observations of rape victims. Recent clinical research studies, based on reliable and valid measurement instruments, show a high variability of psychologic response to rape. The stress response syndrome provides a clinical model within which nurses assess identifiable phases of rape-victim stress reactions, starting with an alarm phase (characterized by shock and disbelief), moving on to an emotionally resistive phase, and finishing with a recuperative phase. Most rape victims work through thoughts, feelings, and behaviors related to their rape.

Nurses can develop the abilities to recognize and assess victim response patterns and to intervene in victim adaptive processes in response to a rape experience. An understanding of stress adaptation theory and the stress response syndrome provides a knowledge base from which nurses can assess rape victim responses. Three important stress principles that relate to rape victim responses are: (1) stress is a universal human phenomenon; (2) stress influences behavior; and (3) intense stress is an agonizing experience.

This chapter ends with a close look at women in four developmental phases: (1) adolescence, (2) young adulthood, (3) middle age, and (4) older adulthood. Special emphasis is given to the interaction of the stress from a rape event with the biologic, psychologic, and social stressors of development. Nursing interventions unique to each phase of development are presented in an effort to assess individual differences in rape victim response.

## STRESS ADAPTATION THEORY

Rape is an unexpected and frightening experience. Victims are highly stressed and fearful, both during and after a rape. The concepts of stress and adaptation provide nurses with a theoretical framework from which to assess rape victim responses. Stress adaptation theory presents the person as a living system that has the capacity to maintain a balance (within fairly constant limits) between itself and the environment. The living system's regulatory processes maintain life and promote growth and development. Regulatory processes that maintain life include circulation, metabolism, seeking food, and elimination. Regulatory processes that promote growth and development include cognitive development, maturity of sexual organs, and childbearing processes.

A person is usually in a *steady state*. According to Bryne and Thompson,[6] this term refers to processes whereby the living system regulates the internal environment as a result of reactions to disturbances induced from within or without the living system. For example, a woman functions in her steady state by using her energy and capacities to adapt to internal needs and drives, life experiences, and environmental demands. Woman, student, wife, parent, lover, and worker are all life roles within the bounds of a steady state.

An individual experiences *stress* when there is a change in or threat to the steady state. Stress is an abstract concept that means that energy is allocated to the living system's functions or processes for the purpose of coping with a change or threat to the living system. It is always present and is generally not noticeable. Only when its intensity increases to a point that signs or symptoms occur is stress observed. For example, a woman needing to complete a task is stressed, so she mobilizes her energy to finish the activity. Her stress is not observed directly, but her internal energy is allocated to the skills needed for task completion. If she cannot complete the task or gets upset because of the poor quality of her work, a woman shows observable signs of stress such as irritation, impatience, shouting, or making angry comments.

The factor or agent causing the intensification of stress is a *stressor*.[6] A person feels a level of discomfort from a stressor and tries to resolve the situation. If resolution occurs, the stress is considered *constructive*. Then the person feels relieved, returns to a steady state, and has greater capacity to handle future stressors. If resolution of stress is not successful, the intensity of stress increases and is *destructive*. Then the person feels more discomfort, cannot return to a steady state, and has greater difficulty handling stressors. Fig. 4-1 illustrates the process of stress resolution to a common developmental stressor: whether a girlfriend should comply with demands for sex from her boyfriend. As demonstrated in the diagram, constructive resolution of the stress leads to reduction of discomfort. Destructive resolution of the stress leads to greater levels of discomfort.

A common observation of stress research is that of severe disturbances of adaptive functioning in people, animals, or social systems. These disturbances are generally regarded as *stress reactions*. When biologic, psychologic, or social disturbance results from threatening stress, a stress reaction is occurring. The living system usually can adapt to a stress reaction and return to a steady state. If it cannot adapt (maladaption) to the stress reaction, the living system will experience physiologic illness or psychologic disorder. Table 4-1 provides definitions of important stress adaptation concepts. As noted in this table, stress is neither positive or negative; it is a force. A person (living system) may react positively (constructively) or negatively (destructively) to the stressor.

What kind of rape victim response can nurses expect to observe during clinical

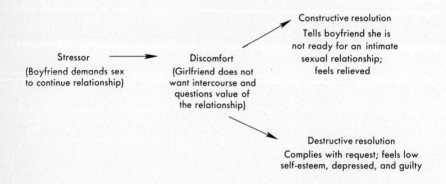

**Fig. 4-1. Stress resolution.**

## Table 4-1. Stress adaptation terms

| Terms | Definitions |
| --- | --- |
| Steady state | Processes involved in maintaining the living system within balanced limits. |
| Stress | A force that is always present in man. Stress is constant mediation between environmental demands and adaptive capacities. |
| Stressor | A factor or agent that causes a greater range and rate of activity or produces a state that is beyond a person's coping abilities. |
| Adaptation | The variety of actions or mental activities that a person uses to adjust to stressors. |
| Stress reactions | Those behaviors or responses that appear when the biologic, psychologic, or social well-being is threatened. The severity of stress reactions ranges from mild to intense disturbances in biologic, psychologic, and social functions. |

work with rape victims? Clinical observations of rape victims have lent evidence for organizing assessment data and observations into one model called the stress response syndrome.

## STRESS RESPONSE SYNDROME

Common physiologic and psychologic patterns emerge in victims after a rape experience. These patterns, documented in clinical studies of rape victims, make up the stress response syndrome. Beginning with the rape event, this syndrome follows three phases of progression: (1) alarm phase, (2) resistance phase, and (3) recuperative phase.

### Alarm phase

CLINICAL EXAMPLE

Diane, a married woman in her thirties, was at home with her infant daughter. Diane left the front door unlocked so her husband could let himself into the house. While whe was preparing dinner, a man suddenly grabbed Diane from behind. He had a knife and threatened to kill Diane and her infant if she did not cooperate with him. Diane was terrified and felt nauseated and faint. She begged the man not to hurt her or her baby. She complied with his demands for oral sex and intercourse. During the rape Diane could hear her baby crying.

As in this clinical example, most rapes occur *without* advance warning, and so the victim is in a vulnerable position. The *alarm phase* begins when the woman perceives a stressor and prepares for fight or flight. The woman is overcome with intense immobilizing fear. She cannot allocate her energy to fight-or-flight behaviors. She is concerned with personal safety and security. Physiologic responses during the alarm phase include hypotension and lowering of muscular tone.

### Resistance phase

The *resistance phase* of the stress response syndrome begins when the body's physiologic and psychologic responses are mobilized to cope with the stressor. In this phase rape victims use adaptive behaviors to alleviate intense levels of physiologic and psychologic stress. Common physiologic responses include elevation of blood pressure, tachycardia, increased sensitivity to sensory stimuli, and increased muscle tone. During a rape body tissues are often damaged, particularly in the genital area. The physiologic stress of injury has an immediate effect on body tissues, causing a reduction in body temperature and the lowering of blood pressure.[6]

The intense stress of a rape experience produces common psychologic coping responses, including the following:

1. Shock, disbelief, and denial
2. Anxiety
3. Fear and guarded behaviors
4. Humiliation and embarrassment
5. Self-blame and guilt
6. Anger
7. Emotional numbness
8. Compulsive repetition
9. Psychosomatic reactions
10. Need for mastery and control

It is during the resistive phase that nurses most often see rape victims. During this time rape victims seek, or are brought to, social service agencies for emergency medical care, police assistance, and psychologic intervention. The most common victim requests include the following:

1. *Medical attention.* Victims want emergency medical care to alleviate pain and physical discomfort. They have fears of disease, bodily harm, or pregnancy.
2. *Police intervention.* Victims want police assistance for support, protection, or legal action. Police are viewed as defenders of the community who should protect other women from the assailant.
3. *Psychologic intervention.* Victims express a need to discuss the incident with someone supportive. Some victims express relief in sharing their burden, while others (viewing the nurse as knowledgeable) ask for advice and guidance.[3]

While interacting with rape victims, nurses collect behavioral data to evaluate victim adaptive capacities. Behavioral data, in the form of overt statements and nonverbal responses, guide nursing interventions. The theoretical framework for the nursing care of rape victims is crisis intervention (see Chapter 7). This section presents and briefly discusses common victim responses and corresponding nursing interventions.

### Fear

Because the woman has experienced a violent rape event, which is also life threatening, the most common victim response is *fear*—fear of physical injury, mutilation, and death. Rape victims also fear that the assailant will return. The immediate need is for personal safety and protection.

CLINICAL EXAMPLE

Ethel is a 60-year-old homemaker who recently became active in her local community's political campaigns. After a political victory celebration, Ethel walked to her car outside the campaign headquarters. She had difficulty with the lock on her door. A man approached her from behind and offered his assistance. Ethel was startled at first (alarm phase), but she thanked him politely and replied that she had a jammed lock. She walked cautiously around the car to try the opposite door. Ethel then felt smothered by something over her head. She heard the man's voice again, "Scream and I'll kill you lady!" Terrified, Ethel was forced into a nearby van and raped. She could hardly breathe during the trauma. She was brought to the emergency room by two female campaign workers who found her in a state of shock in the parking lot. Ethel appeared cautious of anyone who approached her. She answered questions with brief statements. She did not want the police involved and insisted that the nurse remain with her. When the physician approached her for the medical examination, Ethel became frightened and screamed, "Don't touch me . . . please don't touch me."

The clinical example above illustrates that frightened rape victims may be guarded and wary of others. Effective nursing interventions with a frightened rape victim may include:

1. Remaining with the victim
2. Giving clear, succinct explanations of forthcoming procedures
3. Allowing extra time to complete procedures
4. Continually assessing the victim's readiness for procedures

5. Reassuring the victim that she is in a safe place
6. Encouraging expression of fears
7. Giving relevant information to dispel verbalized fears
8. Ensuring safe escort to home or shelter

### Shock, disbelief, and denial

Many rape victims are shocked, overwhelmed, and may hardly believe what has actually happened to them. Their coping behaviors indicate the traumatic impact of the rape experience.

> CLINICAL EXAMPLE
>
> Karen is a 34-year-old woman who called into the crisis center hotline and described being raped by her husband's best friend. She was shocked by the experience and stated, "This is unbelievable! I have known Jim for 8 years; I never suspected that he was capable of this. How could he do this . . . he's my husband's best friend?"

The clinical example above illustrates a common response post-rape: the victim has difficulty integrating the reality of the rape. Others may even question whether the experience was a rape. Effective nursing interventions with a rape victim in shock may include:

1. Acknowledging that rape is difficult to accept and that shock is a normal response
2. Empathic listening
3. Helping clarify thoughts and feelings
4. Presenting options for health decisions
5. Giving clear directions and explanations of procedures
6. Providing care in a quiet, nonstimulating environment

### Anxiety

Many rape victims feel anxiety ranging from a mild level to panic. Rape victim behaviors for varying degrees of anxiety are shown in Table 4-2.

**Table 4-2. Anxiety responses of rape victims**

| Degree of anxiety | Victim response |
| --- | --- |
| Mild | Alert, seeking information. Wishes to actively participate in solving problems related to the rape. Asks questions; seeks help. Able to focus on what is happening. Normal state. |
| Moderate | Energy is mobilized to solve problems of getting help. Able to attend to other problems as attention is called to them. Present is anger, mild hostility, irritability, repetitive questioning, constant need for reassurance. Limited ability to focus on what is happening. Unable to sit still for long periods of time. |
| Severe | Cannot focus on what is really happening. Does not hear directions or information clearly. Ability to cope with situations is temporarily suspended. Moves around a great deal. |
| Panic | Severe disorganization. Random activities show attempt to escape the situation. Unresponsive to voices or directions. Does not see clearly. May strike out at persons who offer assistance. Talks or shouts incoherently. |

CLINICAL EXAMPLE

Sharon is a 23-year-old, full-time graduate student. She generally studies late at the library because her dormitory is very noisy. One night on the way home from the library Sharon was jumped by two men who dragged her behind a building, beat her, and raped her several times. When found by the campus police in a disheveled and disoriented state, Sharon mumbled incoherently in response to their questions. The police escorted her to the emergency room, where she was examined for rape. Sharon was unresponsive to the nurse's voice or directions. The nurse touched Sharon to reassure her. Sharon jumped away and flung her arms in the air. She screamed, "Please, please, don't hurt me any more!"

The clinical example above demonstrates a victim experiencing a panic degree of anxiety. Effective interventions with anxious victims may include:

1. Assessing the degree of anxiety
2. Focusing on here-and-now events
3. Being clear, concrete, and explicit in directions
4. Speaking slowly and in short, simple sentences
5. Not hurrying the victim through procedures
6. Being kind and reassuring
7. Giving necessary information and assistance for decision making
8. Providing reality-oriented conversation
9. Using safety precautions as necessary

### Self-blame and guilt

Society generally holds rape victims responsible for their sexual assaults. Therefore it is not surprising that many victims demonstrate self-blaming behaviors.

CLINICAL EXAMPLE

Jean is a 42-year-old divorced woman. After a fight with her boyfriend, Jean decided to go out alone to a neighborhood bar. She was angry about the fight. She decided that several drinks with acquaintances in the tavern would mellow her. Jean wanted to leave the bar alone, but a man she had just met insisted on walking her home. Jean decided to accept the offer. At her home Jean thanked the man and proceeded to enter the house. The man kicked open the door, grabbed Jean, and forcefully dragged her into the living room. He forced her to have intercourse with him. In the emergency room Jean is tearful and blames herself for the rape: "It's all my fault; I should have never allowed him to pick me up."

Effective nursing intervention with victims who engage in self-blaming behaviors may include:

1. Helping the victim separate poor judgment from responsibility for rape
2. Clarifying distortions of reality
3. Redirecting anger for the assault toward the rapist
4. Presenting factual information to refute myths
5. Not joining in expressions of blame or worthlessness
6. Reassuring the victim of her worth

7. Providing care in a manner that demonstrates respect for the victim
8. Allowing crying and expression of feelings such as sadness, loss, and hurt
9. Believing that victim is not to blame for the rape
10. Avoiding moralizing and preaching

### Compulsive repetitions

Clinical studies indicate that major stress events are sometimes followed by compulsive repetitions. These repetitions involve stress-related content and occur in the form of thoughts, feelings, or behaviors. Repetitions in thought include nightmares, dreams, and obsessive ideas. Behavioral repetitions may involve compulsive verbalizations, gestures, or movements (such as being startled easily); fear of walking; and artistic productions of the rape event. Repetitive physiologic responses include sweating, tremors, or palpitations. Repetitive responses tend to occur in the resistance phase and alternate with periods when the rape victim successfully wards off the repetitions.

CLINICAL EXAMPLE

Barbara is an 18-year-old secretary in an industrial firm. Several days after being raped by her boss, Barbara had nightmares consisting of repeated scenes and images of her boss betraying her confidence in him and of the subsequent rape. She awoke frightened, with perspiration soaking her nightgown. After several weeks the nightmares decreased in frequency. Eventually Barbara slept the whole night without disturbance.

In the clinical example above, the rape victim (Barbara) had compulsive repetitions in the form of thoughts; her nightmares were highly specific to the rape event. Rape victims also describe symbolic dreams from which they awaken in a frightened state. Physiologic responses that accompany post-rape reactions often relate to the physiologic responses victims experience during their rape.

Effective nursing interventions with victims who experience compulsive repetitions include:

1. Helping the victim understand that repetitions are stress related
2. Reassuring the victim that repetitions usually dissipate in time
3. Demonstrating patience while dealing with the victim's fears
4. Encouraging verbalization of thoughts and feelings
5. Avoiding interpretations of dreams and nightmares (requires advanced training)
6. Considering referral for further treatment if repetitions last (more than 6 weeks)

### Mastery and control

Rape is a stressor over which victims have no control. Victims need to gain some *sense of control* over what has happened and a real control over what is happening to them in the present. Victims react differently to the loss of control. Some rape victims want to think things through and settle the crisis alone. Others want to sort out thoughts and feelings with someone in an attempt to put the incident in a realistic perspective. Often the victims hardest to assess are those who mask their feelings with a subdued or composed manner.

CLINICAL EXAMPLE

Marie is a 53-year-old woman who came to the hospital with a friend. She reported that she was raped in an indoor parking lot of a nearby shopping mall. Marie demanded to be examined immediately. Her friend's efforts to comfort her went unheeded. Marie shouted, "Why must I wait so long? I demand to see the supervisor!"

The clinical example above demonstrates a victim who attempts to control her environment through demanding behaviors. Effective nursing interventions with victims who attempt to master and control their environment include:

1. Avoiding anger and remaining calm in the face of abuse
2. Recognizing the behaviors as a stress reaction
3. Refraining from arguing with the victim
4. Allowing the victim some control over decisions ("Would you like to get dressed now or wait a few moments?")
5. Empathically relating to the victim understanding about the need for control
6. Helping the victim verbalize feelings and discuss concerns
7. Quietly explaining reasons for procedures

### Recuperative phase

The third phase of the stress response syndrome is the recuperative phase, in which rape victims recover from their physical and psychologic stresses. Physiologically, body processes mobilize to restore tissues to their previous integrity. Common physiologic reactions include a decrease in muscle tone, lowered locomotor activity, reduced blood pressure, bradycardia, and decreased sensitivity to sensory stimuli.

Psychologically, rape victims work through and resolve their thoughts, feelings, and responses to the rape event. Clinical studies reveal common themes that rape victims work through in the recuperative process, including (1) resentment and anger, (2) sadness, (3) realistic appraisal of the assault, and (4) sexual dysfunction. While working with rape victims who have progressed to the recuperative phase, nurses support adaptive responses and encourage victims to resume usual pursuits at home, work, or school.

#### Resentment and anger

Many rape victims experience anger and rage at their assailants for having used them for a violent, sexual assault. Some victims become frustrated that society encourages aggressive behaviors from men. In the recuperative phase victims also react with a need to blame and punish their assailants or others for the assault.

CLINICAL EXAMPLE

Lyn is a 16-year-old high school student who experienced a violent, abusive rape. Lyn felt angry and frustrated over the experience. She began to feel hatred toward all men, except her boyfriend and her father whom she knew were kind and gentle. Lyn was artistically talented, and when she was very angry, she drew grotesque pictures of men to symbolize her anger. When Lyn completed a drawing, she tore the picture into small pieces and verbalized her anger through profane language. She felt a need to "get back at him for what he did to me." Unable to get back at the assailant literally, Lyn worked through her feelings symbolically.

The above example illustrates the victim's adaptive process. Through her artwork the rape victim worked through her feelings of anger and the need to punish the assailant. Nursing interventions for victims in the recuperative phase who demonstrate resentment and anger include:

1. Reassuring the victim that angry reactions are appropriate responses at this time
2. Encouraging the victim to verbalize anger
3. Encouraging techniques to express anger (art, poetry, dance, sports, prose, or music)
4. Supporting resumption of usual pursuits (at work, home, or school)
5. Encouraging motor activity to release energy (exercise, sports)
6. Supporting turning to a family member, friend, or mate for support

### Sadness

Many rape victims experience sadness in the recuperative phase, sometimes to a degree of depressive symptoms. They feel a personal loss: of self, of respect, of virginity, or of self-esteem. Victims in a recuperative process of sadness need reassurance of worth and time to resolve conflicts. Some victims express fear that they will lose a significant person as a result of the rape event.

CLINICAL EXAMPLE

Joan is a 40-year-old administrative secretary who was raped on her way home from work on a dark winter night. She had stayed overtime to do extra work for her boss. Joan could not eat or sleep after the rape event. The sight of food made her nauseated. When she tried to eat, Joan soon became nauseated and vomited. At night she spent hours awake thinking about the rape. Joan confided to a friend, "I don't deserve to eat or sleep. I should suffer for what happened." Her friend tried to offer reassurance, saying that Joan was not responsible for the rape. Joan replied, "Only bad people get raped. If I had been more careful or was a better person, God would not have punished me like this. The rape would not have happened."

The clinical example above illustrates the victim's (Joan's) loss of self-esteem after her rape. Blaming herself, Joan perceives herself as bad and deserving of the rape. She experiences physiologic and depressive symptoms of poor appetite and insomnia. The victim's depressive disturbances will eventually remit after the victim works through her feelings in the recuperative phase.

Nursing interventions with rape victims who demonstrate sadness include:

1. Recognizing feelings and encouraging verbalization
2. Empathic listening to convey understanding of feelings
3. Reassuring the victim of her worth
4. Not joining in expressions of self-derogation
5. Conveying a respect for and concern about the victim
6. Tolerating silences
7. Allowing the victim to cry
8. Helping the victim recognize that sadness is a normal feeling in this phase

### Realistic appraisal of assault

Most victims come to accept the rape event as part of their history and develop a realistic appraisal of their complicity in the assault. Victims resolve their feelings about their relationship with the offender and their feelings about him as a person. By resolving doubt about their responsibility for the assault, rape victims can continue with their lives. Some victims engage in actions that they believe will prevent rape in the future (e.g., change in phone number or residence, joining rape prevention groups).

> CLINICAL EXAMPLE
>
> Pam is a 20-year-old staff nurse who works rotating shifts at a local hospital. She was in her apartment at 10:00 P.M. when she realized that she had no milk for her breakfast cereal the next morning. An all-night general store was nearby, so Pam put on her coat to dash quickly to the store. In the parking lot two men grabbed Pam and pushed her into a nearby car. The men drove to a neighborhood park. While each man raped Pam, the other man choked her. Warning her not to report the rape, the men left Pam in the park. Weeks later Pam could not go outside at night for fear of a repeated incident. She loved to take walks, but Pam could not pass the grocery store. Eventually Pam preferred to stay inside her apartment at all times because she felt safe from further attack. Pam thought about moving from the area because her feelings of insecurity only increased with time.
>
> Finally a friend convinced Pam to seek help from a local rape crisis center. At the center a nurse helped Pam work through her fears of repetition. Eventually Pam could walk by the grocery store without becoming anxious. She also came to accept the event as part of her history.

Effective nursing interventions with rape victims who have a realistic appraisal of the assault include:

1. Supporting resumption of usual pursuits (at work, home, or school)
2. Supporting adaptive strategies such as moving or changing phone numbers
3. Recognizing a victim's continued need for support from family, friends, or mate
4. Listening empathically as the victim integrates feelings and thoughts about the assault
5. Supporting realistic perceptions of the rape experience
6. Helping the victim realize that she may have reactivation of feelings of one kind or another, but that the emotionality and impact of the experience usually decreases over time

### Sexual dysfunction

Many adult victims experience concerns about sexual adequacy and sexual identity. The physical and psychologic problems include (1) aversion to all sexual activity; (2) reduction in vaginal lubrication; (3) loss of sensation in the genital area; (4) vaginismus; and (5) loss of orgasmic facility.

Not every victim develops any of the above responses to being raped, and if one of them does develop, it does not necessarily lead to the emergence of the others. Often a victim relives the rape when her partner makes an overt sexual approach. She may report now feeling less worthy of love from her partner. Sometimes sexual problems are elicited because of fear of rejection by her partner. If sexual practices outside the woman's normal experience were demanded during the rape experience, she is more likely to develop an aversion to sex and the sexual acts demanded during the rape in the post-rape resolution. Severely physically damaged women most commonly evidence signs and symptoms of vaginismus. Key factors in determining whether or not a victim will develop sexual dysfunction and the degree of severity include:

1. The partner's attitude toward the rape and subsequent developments in how he or she relates to the victim
2. The extent to which the crime can be desexualized for the victim
3. The amount of guilt and blame that other people attach to the victim

Nursing interventions with rape victims who experience sexual dysfunction include:

1. Encouraging open communication between partners
2. Avoiding overfocusing on sexual activity
3. Helping the victim gain a sense of control by assuming charge for when sexual activity occurs
4. Having the couple identify arousal and aversive sexual stimuli
5. Encouraging a relaxed, romantic atmosphere for foreplay activities
6. Encouraging integration of sexuality as part of a holistic partner relationship
7. Setting a realistic time-frame for working through sexual concerns
8. Evaluating for referral to counseling (if no progress is felt by the couple)

The usual outcome of the victim's stress response syndrome is a return to a steady state. Although most victims go through stress response syndromes, two points need to be considered. (1) *The types of responses demonstrated in each phase of stress response are highly individualized for each victim.* We have presented common reactions demonstrated by many victims in an effort to present guidelines for nursing interventions. However, a thorough physical and psychologic assessment of each victim is important prior to implementing quality nursing care. (Chapters 6 and 7 discuss this subject in more detail.) (2) *The length of each phase of stress response is unique for each victim.* A crisis state (see Chapter 7) normally lasts from 4 to 6 weeks, but victims usually take longer to thoroughly work through their rape experiences.

### Post-traumatic stress disorder

When a return to a steady state does not occur, the stressor produces more anxiety, which becomes an additional stressor. What happens if a rape victim cannot cope with the stressor? Phase two, resistance, is *not* successful at resolving the stress situation. The victim continues to feel intense stress; discomfort is so prolonged that she becomes exhausted. The self-system collapses under the strain of prolonged, intense stress. The victim shows a physiologic illness or psychologic dysfunction that interferes with her ability to carry out normal daily activities. An intense stress situation becomes a *threat* to the victim. The danger of physical and psychologic instability increases with time.

Presented below are diagnostic criteria for post-traumatic stress disorders, a well-described category of the *Diagnostic and Statistical Manual of Mental Disorders.*[1] Recent clinical observations of stress responses to rape indicate that many victim responses can be categorized as post-traumatic stress disorders.

DIAGNOSTIC CRITERIA—POST-TRAUMATIC STRESS
DISORDER*

A. Existence of a recognizable stressor that would evoke significant symptoms of distress in almost anyone
B. Reexperiencing of the trauma as evidenced by at least one of the following:
  1. Recurrent and intrusive recollections of the event
  2. Recurrent dreams of the event
  3. Sudden acting or feeling as if the traumatic event were reoccurring because of an association with an environmental or ideational stimulus
C. Numbing of responsiveness to, or reduced involvement with, the external world, beginning some time after the trauma, as shown by at least one of the following:
  1. Markedly diminished interest in one or more significant activities
  2. Feeling of detachment or estrangement from others
  3. Constricted affect
D. At least two of the following symptoms that were not present before the trauma:
  1. Hyperalertness or exaggerated startle response
  2. Sleep disturbance
  3. Guilt about surviving when others have not, or about behavior required for survival
  4. Memory impairment or trouble concentrating
  5. Avoidance of activities that arouse recollection of the traumatic event
  6. Intensification of symptoms by exposure to events that symbolize or resemble the traumatic event

Burgess and Holmstrom[2] have identified a *compounded reaction* with women who had a history of psychiatric, physical, or social difficulties. The compounded reaction was characterized by psychotic behavior, psychosomatic disorders, and acting-out behavior (alcoholism, drug abuse, and sexual promiscuity) combined with the previous history. The authors also discussed management of the *silent rape syndrome,* in which a woman has not told anyone about being raped, has not settled her reactions and feelings about the trauma, and carries alone a tremendous psychologic burden. The authors' historical data indicated that many of these women had been previously raped or molested, and that the current rape reactivated unresolved responses and reactions to the previous experience.

Nurses who care for rape victims recognize that the phases of victim response are not discrete entities and that victims may demonstrate behaviors from more than one phase simultaneously. Also, many victims may have a reactivation of the stress response syndrome triggered by life events such as the anniversary date of the rape, seeing a documentary or hearing a news report on a rape, being in a place or situation similar to the rape situation, or attending the court hearing.

*From American Psychiatric Association: Diagnostic and statistical manual of mental disorders, ed. 3, Washington, D.C., 1980, APA.

Each rape victim is also a unique individual. Nurses who work with rape victims are aware of individual differences and recognize that victims vary in physiologic, emotional, intellectual, and social factors. For example, nurses know that two rape victims of adolescent age may show great differences in physical and emotional maturity. The next section presents an overview of the changes and issues relevant to four phases of life: (1) adolescence (9-18), (2) young adulthood (18-35), (3) middle age (35-65), and (4) older adulthood (65+). Often it is the *interaction* of the rape event with other stressors from the victim's developmental phase of life that influences a rape victim's responses. (Childhood sexual abuse is discussed in Chapter 10.)

### Developmental stressors

Since the amount of literature on each phase of development is massive, this section is selective. Table 4-3 summarizes the interaction of rape and developmental variables and the areas of focus for nursing care in each of the developmental phases.

**Table 4-3. Interaction of developmental levels with rape event\***

| Phase of development | Developmental stressors |
| --- | --- |
| Adolescence (ages 9-18) | Search for identity<br>Conformity with peers<br>Choosing sex-role behaviors<br>Forming new relationships<br>Onset of puberty; increased body awareness<br>Dependence vs. independence<br>Parental power struggles |
| Young adulthood (ages 18-35) | Physical maturity<br>Leaving the family<br>Getting into the adult world<br>Settling down<br>Choosing life work and sexual partners<br>Parenting |
| Middle age (ages 35-65) | Adequate coping skills<br>Social interactions<br>Acceptance of adult responsibility<br>Power and control<br>Individuality<br>"Mid-life crisis"<br>Sexuality |
| Older adulthood (65+) | Attitudes toward aging<br>Health issues<br>Family and friends<br>Finances<br>Living arrangements<br>Safety and security |

\*Modified from Foley, T. S., The client who has been raped. In Lego, S., editor: Lippincott manual on psychiatric–mental health nursing, New York, J.B. Lippincott Co., 1983. (In press.)

### Adolescence

To become a fully mature adult in our culture, it is essential that everyone experience a phase of adolescence. It is during this period that tremendous changes take place. Adolescents search for identity and build their self-esteem upon the performance of social roles. As adolescents approach physical and social maturity, they face new demands: conformity with adolescent peers, choosing sex-role behaviors, and forming new relationships.

Adolescence is precipitated by hormonal changes that define the onset of puberty. Along with physical maturity of the primary and secondary sex characteristics, adolescents experience sexual and aggressive drives. Because the body is developing and changing its proportions at this phase, adolescents sometimes appear awkward and clumsy. Adolescents of the same chronological age may show great differences in physical maturity.

In girls, menarche appears to influence interest in sexuality and makes adolescents aware of their femaleness. As girls' bodies undergo changes in form, body awareness increases and girls experience being objects of sex attraction. Girls are usually adequately prepared for the physiologic changes of adolescence, if not by mothers then by siblings, girlfriends, or health education courses.

Adolescents demand to be treated as adults, yet they are afraid of the responsibilities of adulthood. Many times they still act like children. Wide swings in moods, impulsive and unpredictable behaviors, and sensitivity to inner turbulence are common experiences of adolescents. Although adolescents are dependent on adults for direction, shelter, and financial security, they mistrust adults. In their rebellious struggles for independence, adolescents often reject help even from those closest to them. Adult values are ridiculed or challenged; parents are treated coldly or hostilely.

Adolescents rebel against and separate from the affectional relationships of childhood. They find persons whom they can idealize, and they establish new peer social relationships outside the home. For girls, an admired figure may be a teacher, a public idol, or an older adolescent. The essential criterion is that the older person has qualities that the adolescent girl admires.

Emotional support and understanding comes from close relationships with peers who can understand one another, share feelings and experiences, and join in rebellious activities. Adolescent groups of the same sex eventually give way to heterosexual groups. Adolescents try out a variety of sex-role behaviors as they form heterosexual relationships.

The school-age rape victim will generally experience a disruptive school life, either changing schools or stopping school for a period of time following the rape. Some younger victims also experience school phobia reactions or may have academic difficulties.[4]

CLINICAL EXAMPLE

Jane is a 15-year-old who is a cheerleader at the local high school. After a rally Jane went with her group of friends to the football game. She became exhausted and decided not to go to a friend's party. Instead she walked home alone. On her way home Jane was approached by three boys from school who had obviously been drinking. Jane asserted herself as the boys tried to grab and caress her, "Leave me alone or I'll scream."

The boys mumbled abuses and went away. Very frightened and considering herself fortunate, Jane walked faster toward home. Several blocks later Jane noticed the same three boys behind her. This time they ran toward her and grabbed her. Jane decided to run for it. She could not outrun the boys, who caught her and dragged her between two buildings. They beat her and took turns raping her. After the rape Jane stumbled back into the street.

In the emergency room Jane cried bitterly and said to the nurse, "My parents told me never to walk home alone . . . I'm so ashamed . . . I'm a virgin . . . Please help me!"

As demonstrated in this clinical example, adolescent rape victims may demonstrate regressive behaviors such as crying or dependent clinging. Nurses may also notice that unresolved conflicts of adolescence emerge during the post-trauma phase. In this example Jane verbalizes several unresolved developmental conflicts: independence, parental power struggle with fears of disapproval and loss of autonomy, self-esteem, and sexuality. The adolescent usually views the nurse as someone to be trusted for physical care and emotional support.

Nursing interventions with adolescent rape victims include:

1. Recognizing that regression may occur and accepting its adaptive value
2. Allowing for dependency and recognizing difficulty in self-directed behaviors because adolescents have limited experience in handling complex situations
3. Fostering open communication by allowing for expression of confusion, outbursts of anger and other emotions, and fluctuations in the level of maturity
4. Recognizing that an adolescent may depend almost exclusively on family, peers, or a significant adult for emotional support
5. Recognizing the victim's struggle with issues of self-esteem or social role identity
6. Realizing that unresolved conflicts of adolescence may surface in the post-rape crisis situation
7. Giving factual information and answering questions related to risks of pregnancy and venereal disease
8. Avoiding power struggles: focusing on strengths and constructive adaptive behaviors
9. Acting as negotiator between the victim and family as necessary to facilitate the system's adaptation to the stressor of rape

### *Young adulthood*

Young adults make life choices that can influence their responses in the event of a rape. A closer look at the phase of young adulthood shows the disappearance of the turmoil and conflict of adolescence and the appearance of increased emotional control and general predictability. According to Burnside and others, transitions of young adulthood include physical maturity, leaving the family, entering into the adult world, and settling down.

Most young adults have healthy bodies that are physically mature. At this stage the body's capacity to mend itself is at an optimal level. Despite the high level of physical health, many young adults do suffer from physical illnesses, for example, colds, allergies, migraine headaches, and silent heart disease. Often unacknowledged are those young adults who suffer psychologic illnesses such as depressions, character disorders, or psychoses. Suicide is the third leading cause of death among young adults (many make suicide attempts as a way of asking for help). In general, the many stressors and changes of this period of life can influence the rate of illness.

Leaving the family is characterized by choices such as moving out of the family home and setting up an independent living arrangement. Young adults become more financially independent and move toward autonomy and adult responsibility. Many continue to have "home as base" but attend college, travel, or enlist in the military.[5] Other young adults assume adult roles of work and marriage. Sheehy[8] describes "rebounds" as not uncommon in young adults—persons who may return to home for a while before again setting out into the adult world.

In Western culture young adults are expected to take initiative in choosing life work and sexual partners. The social demand for a choice of a vocation can be a source of stress during this stage. Many choices are open and a choice determines the young adult's future way of life. Selection of friends and sexual partners depends in part upon the young adult's identity and conception of the kind of friend or mate a person should choose. Young adult women are determining role identities such as student, wife, homemaker, mother, or career woman.

Marcia[5] describes four "normal" positions in which young adults are likely to find themselves: (1) the moratorium position, (2) the identity-foreclosed position, (3) the identity-diffused position, and (4) the identity-achieved position. There is a possibility that young adults might adopt one position as a life-style or assume several positions concurrently.

Young adults who are in the *moratorium position* are actively struggling to find commitments or causes, while not making strong investments in relationships or vocation. Examples of behavior styles of young adults in this period include traveling, starting and dropping out of college, and experimenting with living arrangements.

Young persons in the *identity-foreclosed position* are very sure of life choices and make commitments to relationships, life-styles, and vocation. Those in this group passively accept predefined identity and roles and live their lives according to cultural standards.

Young adults in the *identity-diffused* group are not able to decide what they want or how they feel. They are not committed to anything or anyone. They perform well in social roles but feel like misfits.

Young persons who are in the position of *identity-achieved* have a sense of purpose and view their world as more stable and understandable. They are less anxious in their relationships and tend to survive the crisis of young adulthood because of a joyful outlook and healthy coping skills. The identity-achieved persons are in control of their lives and have a sense of identity and direction.

### CLINICAL EXAMPLE

Alison is in her early thirties and lives alone. She works in a large office building as a steno-pool secretary. She met John at work and dated him twice. John seemed to like her, and she was pleased when he asked her out for a third date. On the next date John invited Alison to his apartment for dinner. Shortly after her arrival John forced intercourse on her. Alison felt confused and ashamed. She did not know what to do about the rape. She *thought* John was a nice guy! Alison thought to herself, "How could I have been so stupid! I'm so gullible . . . so naive! I thought I was a loser before . . . but this takes the cake!"

As in the above clinical example, many women experience a loss of self-respect following a rape. Other psychologic responses include feelings of worthlessness, shame, guilt, or helplessness. Some women experience depression, and a portion of depressed women also report suicidal feelings.

Areas of difficulty with the young adult victim include schooling, employment, parenting, and homemaking. Within the first week after rape, many women regain their coping skills and resume usual parenting and homemaking patterns. However, within 6 months of the rape, many women either quit work or change jobs. Economic reality prevents some women from quitting jobs or changing work settings. Adult victims who are students are sometimes in conflict over acquiring a school credential and needing to make a living. In the absence of a social network or support system, it is not uncommon for adult victims to evidence flight or avoidance behaviors.[4]

As stated earlier, young adult rape victims are struggling with both the trauma of rape and the developmental tasks of self-definition. Nursing interventions with young adults include:

1. Avoiding giving advice or making judgments because these may turn young adults away or close off communication
2. Demonstrating an attitude of listening, having time, and caring
3. Assisting with problem solving by helping a young adult identify problems and explore alternatives
4. Allowing a young adult to decide which course of action seems workable
5. Supporting young adults who are working through decisions about who to tell about the rape event by exploring the dilemma with them
6. Helping identify supportive persons (friends, mates, parents) in times of crisis[5]

### Middle age

The "normal" middle-age phase covers several decades of life. Adult stressors change over time, but predictable patterns of change do emerge for most adults in this phase of development. The components of adult maturity include adequate coping skills, social interactions, acceptance of adult responsibilities, and individuality. Middle-aged adults are more able to control and channel their emotional drives, and they have adequate coping skills that protect them from excess anxiety. Adults in this phase also enter into social interactions with peers and mates, developing social roles within the framework of their choices. Middle-aged adults are generally more capable than younger persons of weathering personal storms, frustrations, and disappointments.

As individuality forms, adults make choices that are clearly their own. An inner sense of self-direction emerges as career, family, and social choices are stabilized. A "settling down" takes place as middle-aged adults invest time and energy in their selected life-styles.

During the middle years adults vary in their body awareness because there is a wide range of function, bodily development, and strength. When the body becomes dysfunctional, body awareness increases. Some adults in this phase exercise vigorously to maintain strength and physical attractiveness. Others have expanding bodies because they consume more than needed to nourish the body. Normal physiologic changes during this phase include decreased visual and auditory acuity and the emergence of chronic disorders such as arthritis, cancer, diabetes, and cardiovascular problems.

The physiologic changes of middle-aged women include hormonal changes with the beginning of menopause. Youthful appearance is supplanted by aging signs such as wrinkles and gray hair. Many women try to retain a youthful, energetic appearance and consider bodily preservation a primary goal.

Erickson stresses the importance of viewing the development of stressors in middle-aged adults through a historical perspective.[5] In other words, many stressors in this phase are precipitated by social changes that have been witnessed or experienced throughout the adult life. For example, those middle-aged adults who experienced the Great Depression and the World Wars, or struggled to achieve an affluent social position, have experienced a complex life situation that influences responses to stressors. In contrast, those who experienced peace, affluence, and educational opportunities may have different values, expectations, and responses.

While middle age is predominantly a stage of stability, it is not unusual for many middle-aged adults to experience a "mid-life crisis" between the ages of 40 and 50 years. Ebersole describes this decade as a period of transition and change in five areas: (1) role and goal orientation, (2) parental relations, (3) sexuality, (4) career suitability, and (5) self-definition.[5]

Many adults have an overwhelming goal in their lives that is often assessed, revised, or changed during middle age. There is still time left in life to be open to new roles and life-styles. Middle-aged adults ask, "Who am I?" "What am I doing?" and "Where am I going?" within the realistic framework that their years are limited.[1] Many review the past and reflect on their accomplishments and failures. Many middle-aged women disengage from mothering roles and try a new life-style, for example, entering the job market. Other women move into traditional female roles of grandmother, friend, community member, or volunteer.

Parental relations shift as middle-aged adults see their parents as individuals rather than in relation to one's needs as children. Adjusting to aging parents is a task, with the middle-aged adult often providing assistance in finances, residential placement, or physical care. As this group's children grow up, the intensity of identification with offspring increases and grandparenting is usually an enjoyed experience.

Identity gains strength during this phase when many middle-aged adults are happy with themselves, their roles, and their life-styles. Others have low self-esteem and may be anxious and depressed. Many middle-aged adults who are dissatisfied with traditional roles seek a change in their roles and life-style so that they can feel more significant.[5]

### CLINICAL EXAMPLE

Martha, who is 44 years old, has recently separated from her husband. She has been attempting to adjust to her new life situation and has begun fixing up her apartment. Martha reported that a "friend" of her husband helped her move some large furniture from a discount store to her apartment. She fixed dinner for him in return for the favor. While she had her back turned to him to do the dishes, he grabbed a kitchen knife and forced her to the bedroom where he raped her. Martha was furious that a "friend" would take advantage of her. How *could* he violate her? What kind of woman does he think she is? Martha wondered if her husband should be told of the incident. Her marriage was unstable and she wondered if the rape could destroy it.

Although divorce or separation can occur at any age, the above clinical example illustrates emerging conflicts for the *separated or divorced* woman. The rape experience often results in her credibility, morality, character, and life-style being questioned. Women in this group are prone to feel overwhelming guilt because of society's response to them, which also promotes failure to report the crime. Separated or divorced victims often await implications in the community for themselves and their children as a result of the rape being known, and they tend to worry about their adequacy as mothers.

The middle-aged rape victim is concerned with issues concerning her ability to maintain control in a situation and regard for her independence.[4] Husbands in comparable mid-life crises may not be as supportive and responsive to the sexual and emotional needs of their middle-aged wives who have been raped. The mid-life woman may be concerned with the demise of reproductive years and the redefinition of her sexuality. It is not easy for the middle-aged woman to quantify and explore feelings of shame, self-devaluation, and worthlessness often connected with the myth that her sexuality is minimally affronted by the rape (as compared with that of a younger woman) because of her age.

Nursing interventions with rape victims in the middle-age phase of development include:

1. Recognizing that generally the need to be helped is weak, while the need to help others is strong, which may lead some middle-aged adults to resist help
2. Allowing regression (middle-aged adults may become dependent and demanding)
3. Allowing middle-aged adults to talk about responsibilities and concerns (work, family, or community)
4. Understanding concerns about bodily functions, body image, and sexuality as developmental issues compounded by the rape
5. Recognizing "at risk" middle-aged women who are in mid-life crisis
6. Assessing problems being confronted and focusing on the victim's ability to cope
7. Assisting women to develop actions that constructively resolve the identified problem
8. Allowing women to seek supportive persons who can best help them through the crisis (spouse, friend, or mate)[7]

### Older adulthood

Presently there are some 22 million aged Americans. Recent efforts by clinicians and researchers indicate a new interest in what happens to persons through the normal aging process. To best understand the older adult, nurses recognize that past life experiences have a significant influence on the older adult's present circumstances. The past has shaped coping abilities and has set the groundwork for the older adult's survival skills needed in the present. This section will address the present circumstances of the older adult in terms of five areas of concern that may influence rape victim responses: (1) attitudes, (2) health, (3) family and friends, (4) finances, and (5) living arrangements.

A major element to consider in nursing care of older adults involves attitudes, values, and views of self. Some older adults view the latter years of life as a continuance of vital, useful living; others view them as a period of decrepitude and failure.

Another problem for older adults is society's role expectations and associated stereotypes for "the elderly." Many people devalue older adults and describe them as "old, decrepid, and useless." Prestige and status within the community are often lost; power is gradually relinquished to younger adults.

Good health is important at any age, but those in the older adult phase are especially aware of health concerns. Even those people who "never felt better" express concerns about their health in the future. Recently older adults have been in a very good position to preserve health and monitor their own well-being. However, as people age, chronic illness increases. Also, the sensory changes in normal aging can lead to difficulties in perceptual functioning (e.g., cataracts and glaucoma) and hearing loss.

Many older adults are fearful of losing physical health to a point where institutionalization is a forced choice. An alarming number who require extended care will die in a short time after admission to an institution. Recent increased news media exposure to mistreatment, misdiagnosis, and poor quality of care provided in settings for the elderly alarms and frightens older adults as well as younger adults facing old age.

Older adults gain strength and confidence from the support of family and friends. Many maintain an active social life and have families and relatives who provide satisfying relationships. However, not all older adults are fortunate enough to have supportive relatives and friends. The changing structure of many families in contemporary society has forced many older adults into isolation. Loss of a spouse or friend can also precipitate special problems for older persons.

Many adults in middle life plan and save for their financial security in old age. Unfortunately, costs and inflation have risen at such rates that what was considered adequate in middle-adult years becomes barely survival level in older adults years. Many aged adults live frugally from one Social Security check to another. Others have health problems because of poor nutrition, inability to pay heating bills, or poor housing conditions. Disillusionment and bitterness are common reactions as the task of daily survival becomes paramount.

Older adults who own a home have a decreasing need for a large family dwelling and sometimes feel burdened by increasing taxation and the need for upkeep of their property. A decision to sell and relocate is a significant one because of severing social ties or losing community recognition. Many older adults live alone and gravitate to urban inner-city, high-rise apartments for the elderly or geriatric ghettos.[7] There they often suffer from geographic isolation and loss of social interaction.

An important issue that emerges for older rape victims, particularly if the rape assault has occurred in the victim's home, is whether to remain in the present living situation. Many older adults love their homes or have a fear of change that keeps them where they are. Others are unable to look at their living situation objectively and instead base their decision on emotional reactions.[9].

Older adults are particularly concerned about, and vulnerable to, physical assault, vandalism, and criminality. One distressing aspect of seeking physical care and psychologic help after a sexual assault is that rape symbolizes a loss of power and control—an area in which many older adults already view themselves as personally inadequate. Cognitive distortions and depression are two reactions often evident among older adults who have experienced a rape event. Cognitive distortions occur because of disruption in the ability to control present circumstances and high anxiety levels, both of which interfere with cognitive skills. Depression results when internal feelings of hopelessness and helplessness are compounded by the rape event.[7] Depression can persist for months and can lead to isolation; elderly rape victims may shut themselves away and establish minimal contact with others. Such withdrawal is a maladaptive attempt to protect themselves.

In general, older women evidence a greater fear of people finding out about the rape than younger women do. Fears about disclosure may lead older women to exclude their own families from sharing and working out the experience with them. This drastically limits their supportive network, which may be already limited because of the demise of close friends, and taxes their resolution of the rape experience.

### CLINICAL EXAMPLE

Marie is a 65-year-old rape victim who lives in a single-room-occupancy hotel within an inner-city community. The hotel has a social community that places a high value on self-reliance and independence. Marie has several acquaintances within the hotel and identifies one other woman as a close acquaintance.

After the rape, Marie's nurse asked if a friend could be called or family summoned to provide Marie with support. Marie hesitated for several minutes and then asked the nurse to call her best friend, Lucy. When the nurse asked for Lucy's phone number, Marie gave a long-distance number from across the country.

Marie's nurse assessed Marie as needing someone nearby who could provide her with some support during the post-rape period. Exploring possible community supports, Marie decided to discuss the rape with her church priest. When the nurse offered to call the priest, Marie protested, "Please don't call him; I'll tell him in the confessional this Saturday. I go to confession every Saturday. My priest will help me, he's wonderful."

The clinical example above illustrates that Marie's social boundaries extended over many geographic miles. Her own social community, the hotel, provided Marie with a wide range of activities, such as visiting, advice giving, and provision of food and medical aid. However, her ties within the hotel did not extend beyond essential social activities. Reliable relationships with emotional attachment were limited by the social norms of independence and self-reliance. A friend many miles away was Marie's source of emotional support.

In this instance the nurse respected Marie's right to use whatever support she thought was most helpful. The victim identified her friend and the priest as understanding, supportive, and respectful of her right to privacy. For various reasons Marie did not summon her family or other hotel boarders. The nurse supported Marie's choice and offered the health agency as a continued service if additional help was needed.

Nursing interventions with an older adult rape victim include:

1. Recognizing that the past has shaped present coping capacities and survival skills
2. Adequately preparing the victim to adapt to present circumstances
3. Understanding as "normal" an older adult's responses of fear and apprehension about what can happen in any health care facility; giving clear, concise explanations of procedures
4. Recognizing symptoms of cognitive distortion and depression that can be assessed as a reaction to the rape event
5. Offering clear, direct communication, line-of-sight visual contact, and physical closeness
6. Touching the victim to reduce feelings of isolation
7. Offering or providing a close relationship as a professional who can provide security, restore trust, and reduce feelings of abandonment
8. Assisting an older adult to identify emotionally supportive persons who can help her through present crisis[7]

## SUMMARY

Prior to a rape, women generally live in balanced states; their personal energies are allocated to self-regulatory processes, activities of daily life, and coping abilities. Most women are successful at adapting to their internal and external environments. However, rape is a stressor that occurs suddenly and unexpectedly. It disrupts women's lives and influences their behaviors. Rape victims must cope with a frightening, traumatic experience.

Concepts from stress adaptation theory provide nurses with a knowledge base for assessing rape victim responses. Generally regarded as experiencing stress reactions, rape victims usually come to health care systems with observable signs and symptoms of biologic, psychologic, or sociologic disturbance. The stress response syndrome provides a model for nurses to use in organizing their clinical assessments, in making observations of the responses of rape victims, and in choosing appropriate interventions.

In general, rape victims experience three phases of a stress reaction: the alarm phase (fear and danger); the resistance phase (oscillating emotions), and the recuperative phase (working through thoughts, feelings, and behaviors). The outcome of stress reactions produces a return to a steady state. If maladaption occurs, victims experience increased stress, which becomes an additional stressor. If stress continues, discomfort becomes so prolonged that rape victims become physically ill or psychiatrically disturbed.

Nurses are in important positions to make skilled physical, psychiatric, and sociologic assessments of rape victim responses. An understanding developmental stressors and stress-reation phases indicates areas for specific clinical assessment and nursing interventions. Nurses can better support rape victims by reassuring them of the appropriateness of their responses, encouraging them to express their concerns, and helping them resolve their present situations. Referral to psychiatric–mental health nurses or appropriate care-giving agencies or persons for counseling is indicated if rape victim responses are maladaptive.

# Learning activities

## EXERCISE 1. Role-play situations

The following are illustrations of case situations handled by rape crisis centers in working with victims of rape. These cases are intended for two people to act out, with one person being the nurse and the other being the victim. A third person can act as an observer-recorder and offer feedback to the participants for discussion.

1. A victim is trying to decide whether or not to tell her family about being raped and how to actually go about telling them.
2. A victim is afraid to report the crime to the police. She knows the assailant, and he threatened to kill her if she reported him or to seek revenge when he got out of jail.
3. A victim is blaming herself for being raped. "If only I hadn't been out jogging by myself, this would not have happened."

## EXERCISE 2. Victim response patterns

*Directions.* Identify probable response patterns that would result from the following situations. List three nursing interventions appropriate for the situation. Next, how would you respond if you were the victim? Answers can be used for discussion.

## Example

Probable response pattern: *Shock and disbelief*
Nursing interventions:
1. Provide immediate help, clear directions.
2. Offer calm, supportive listening.
3. Stay with victim.
If I were this victim, *I'd go to an emergency room.*

## Situation 1

A victim was raped by her next-door neighbor. Now she doesn't feel safe at home alone. She calls you on a telephone hotline at a rape crisis center.

Probable response pattern: _____
Nursing interventions:
1.
2.
3.
If I were this victim, _____

## Situation 2

A rape victim is sleeping a lot and acting withdrawn. Her friends know that she is behaving differently, that something is wrong. But she hasn't told them what happened, and so they keep asking why she's acting so strange. She doesn't know what to tell them. The victim has been in counseling with you for several weeks.

Probable response pattern: _____
Nursing interventions:
    1.
    2.
    3.
If I were this victim, _____

## Situation 3

A victim's mother is blaming her daughter for the rape. Because the victim was raped on a date, the mother is accusing her of being naive and stupid about men. The victim feels ashamed to tell the nurse what happened.

Probable response pattern: _____
Nursing interventions:
    1.
    2.
    3.
If I were this victim, _____

## Situation 4

A 25-year-old high school teacher returns home from work and finds a strange man in her apartment. He has a gun, a camera, and a suitcase full of underwear. The man forces her to try on all the underwear while he takes pictures of her. Then he rapes her and leaves. The woman had been a virgin, and she doesn't want anyone to find out about the rape. You are her staff nurse in the emergency room.

Probable response pattern: _____
Nursing interventions:
    1.
    2.
    3.
If I were this victim, _____

### Situation 5

An 83-year-old widow is raped one night by the 24-year-old man who rents a room from her. While the woman is sleeping, he cuts the phone cord, rips her pajamas, and tries to smother her with a pillow. During the actual rape, the woman passes out. Now at the hospital she is suffering from extensive internal bleeding. She wants to prosecute. You are her staff nurse in the emergency room.

Probable response pattern: _____
Nursing interventions:
  1.
  2.
  3.
If I were this victim, _____

---

### EXERCISE 3. Intervention

The following situation is an account of one rape victim's experience. Her responses reflect the phases of trauma that follow a rape. Nurses are encouraged to complete the activities as indicated. Responses selected in completing the exercise can also be shared in open discussion.

---

### Situation

A 19-year-old, single, black female is brought into the emergency room by the police. She reports that she was just raped by her brother's boyfriend. She describes the following situation.

Rose has been working as a nurse's aide on a 3 to 11 shift. She got off work late one night and started home when her brother's friend (Sam) drove by and asked if she wanted a ride home. Sam said he called the house to see her and her parents said she was working, so he dropped by to give her a lift home. Rose had no reason to be suspicious because she knew Sam. Sam suggested that they stop at a bar to hear some live jazz and have a few drinks before going to her house. Rose agreed and said it would be a nice way to start her vacation, which began the next day. Instead of going directly to the bar, Sam stopped at his apartment, saying he needed to get some cash. Sam said he didn't bring any cash along because he didn't know if Rose would want to go out. Then he suggested that Rose come up and meet his roommate (Larry). Rose agreed. While there she called her parents to let them know she was going to be out late.

After Rose had talked to her folks, Larry said he was taking off for the night. Then Sam came into the room with a gun. He told Rose to get into the bedroom and take off her clothes. Rose protested, so he hit her across the face, knocking her to the floor and causing her mouth to bleed.

Rose started to scream and cry. Then Sam grabbed her by the hair and threatened to kill her if she didn't shut up. Sam shoved Rose into the bedroom, ripped her clothing off, and threw her on the bed, telling her to lie face down. He raped Rose anally and then flipped her over. Holding a gun on Rose, Sam tied her extremities to the bedposts. Sam then raped Rose vaginally and physically abused her by pulling at her breasts and hitting her. When Sam ended the rape, he urinated on her, humiliated and degraded her verbally, and threatened to kill her if she told anyone about the rape. Sam let Rose leave after she had sworn to secrecy.

1. When Rose enters the emergency department, the staff nurse assigned to her could expect which reactions? (Check the appropriate responses.)

    \_\_\_\_\_ shock                       \_\_\_\_\_ anxiety

    \_\_\_\_\_ disbelief                    \_\_\_\_\_ fear

    \_\_\_\_\_ depression                 \_\_\_\_\_ resentment

    \_\_\_\_\_ need to talk              \_\_\_\_\_ subdued appearance

    \_\_\_\_\_ anger at her assailant     \_\_\_\_\_ outward adjustment

    \_\_\_\_\_ dismay                    \_\_\_\_\_ guarded attitude

2. Rose is in what phase of response to the rape? _____

## Situation continued

Rose was rocking back and forth as she told the nurse this account. She asked the nurse to call her mother and cousin to come and be with her. The nurse notified Rose's family and returned to talk with her until they arrived. Rose said she was afraid that she might be pregnant because she was midcycle. She didn't know what she would do if she were pregnant. Rose had not yet made up her mind about prosecuting Sam. She said that if her brother knew about the rape he would be out on the street to get Sam, and she didn't want her brother in jail for trying to kill him.

3. The nurse identified the following needs for Rose. Put the needs in order according to their importance (make #1 the first priority).

    \_\_\_\_\_ medical care

    \_\_\_\_\_ police involvement

    \_\_\_\_\_ legal action

    \_\_\_\_\_ family and friends

    \_\_\_\_\_ comfort and reassurance

    \_\_\_\_\_ privacy and confidentiality

    \_\_\_\_\_ crisis counseling

4. The following statements are possible choices for the nurse's responses to Rose's needs and concerns. Indicate which responses the nurse could implement in intervening in Rose's case. Give reasons for the choices selected.

| Yes | No | Nursing intervention response statements |
|-----|-----|------------------------------------------|
| ____ | ____ | "I've been scared to death myself. Let me help you." |
| ____ | ____ | "You really should have had some karate or self-defense classes in high school to prevent this from happening." |
| ____ | ____ | Putting an arm around Rose, the nurse tells her, "Go ahead and cry. It must have been a living nightmare to experience all that." |
| ____ | ____ | "You'll have plenty of time to talk later about what to do if you get pregnant." |
| ____ | ____ | "I feel scared, too, when I walk home alone late at night. It could happen to anyone, including me." |
| ____ | ____ | "Oh, you poor thing. Come right in here where I have an empty room. Your poor mother is going to be so distraught." |
| ____ | ____ | Looking Rose in the eye and moving closer to her, the nurse suggests, "It's disheartening and hurts to have entrusted yourself to Sam only to be violated. What a miserable way to start a vacation!" |
| ____ | ____ | "Underneath the terror I can sense you must have felt deceived. You were trusting a friend and instead he abused that confidence; that would infuriate me!" |
| ____ | ____ | "I used to worry about that happening to me. Now I carry mace in my purse or a screech siren." |
| ____ | ____ | "We trust people we think are our friends. You just have to learn that there are times when you'll get hurt." |

## REFERENCES

1. American Psychiatric Association: Diagnostic and statistical manual of mental disorders, ed. 3, Washington, D.C., 1980, APA.
2. Burgess, A.W., and Holmstrom, L.L.: Rape trauma syndrome, Am. J. Psych. **131**:981, 1974.
3. Burgess, A.W., and Holmstrom, L.L.: Rape: victims of crisis, Bowie, Md., 1974, Robert J. Brady Co.

4. Burgess, A.W., and Holmstrom, L.L.: Rape: its effects on task performance at varying stages in the life cycle. In Walker, M.J., and Brodsky, S.L., editors: Sexual assault: the victim and the rapist, Lexington, Mass., 1976, Lexington Books.
5. Burnside, I.M., Ebersole, P., and Monea, H.E.: Psychosocial caring throughout the life span, New York, 1979, McGraw-Hill Book Co.
6. Byrne, M.L., and Thompson, L.F.: Key concepts for the study and practice of nursing, ed. 2, St. Louis, 1978, The C.V. Mosby Co.
7. Kalkman, M.E., and Davis, A.J.: New dimensions in mental health–psychiatric nursing, New York: McGraw-Hill Book Co., 1980.
8. Sheehy, G.: Passages: predictable crises of adult life, New York, 1976, E.P. Dutton & Co., Inc.
9. Uris, A.: Over 50: the definitive guide to retirement, Toronto, 1981, Bantum Books.

## ADDITIONAL REFERENCES

Ben-David, S.: Rapist-victim interaction during rape, paper presented at the Third International Symposium on Victimology, Munich, Germany, 1979; Department of Criminology, Bar Ilan University, Ramat Gan, Israel. Mimeographed.

Biddle, B.J., and Thomas, E.J., editors: Role theory: concepts and research, New York, 1966, John Wiley & Sons.

Brodsky, S.: Prevention of rape: deterrence by the potential victim. In Walker, M.J., and Brodsky, S.L., editors: Sexual assault: the victim and the rapist, Lexington, Mass., 1976, Lexington Books.

Burgess, A.W., and Holmstrom, L.L.: Rape: sexual disruption and recovery, Am. J. Orthopsychiatry **49:**648, 1979.

Feldman-Summers, S., Gordon, O., and Meagher, J.: The impact of rape on sexual satisfaction, J. Abnorm. Psychol. **33:**101, 1979.

Fosburgh, L.: The Berkeley rapist, New Times, p. 28, May 15, 1978.

Frank, E.: Psychological response to rape: an analysis of response patterns, doctoral dissertation, 1979, University of Pittsburgh.

Groth, A.N., with Birnbaum, H.J.: Men who rape: the psychology of the offender, New York, 1979, Plenum Press.

Horowitz, M.J.: Stress response syndromes, New York, 1976, Jason Aronson, Inc.

Katz, S., and Mazur, M.A.: Understanding the rape victim: a synthesis of research findings, New York, 1979, John Wiley & Sons.

Masters, H., and Johnson, E.: Human sexual inadequacy, Boston, 1970, Little, Brown & Co.

Selkin, J.: Rape, Psychol. Today **8:**71, 1975.

Skyes, G.M., and Matza, D.: Techniques in neutralization: a theory of delinquency, Am. Sociol. Rev. **6:**664, 1957.

## ANNOTATED SUGGESTED READINGS

Bart, P.: Unalienating abortion, demystifying depression, and restoring rape victims, paper presented at the 128th annual meeting of the American Psychiatric Association, Anaheim, Calif., May 1975.

The author studies the questionnaire responses of 1,070 women who reported they had been raped. Nearly 50% of the women reported a loss of trust in male-female relationships as a result of the rape. One third of the respondents were affected in their sexual responsiveness, had nightmares, and felt hostile toward men.

Brodsky, C.M.: Rape at work. In Walker, M.J., and Brodsy, S.L., editors: Sexual assault: the victim and the rapist, Lexington, Mass., 1976, Lexington Books.

The author discusses five case histories to illustrate the nature and consequences of a rape or attempted rape at a work setting. The author speculates that the effect of rape would be different in a nonwork setting. Brodsky found the sample studied had reactions resembling the post-rape symptoms identified by Burgess and Holmstrom.

Burgess, A.W., and Holmstrom, L.L.: Rape trauma syndrome, Am. J. Psych., **131**:981, 1974.

The authors analyze 92 interviews in a heterogeneous sample of victims diagnosed as experiencing a "rape trauma syndrome" and report a two-phase reaction: (1) disorganization displayed by emotional and somatic reactions, depending on styles of expressed or controlled responses, and (2) reorganization, affected by factors such as coping behaviors, the way people treated the victim, and social support network systems.

Burgess, A.W., and Holmstrom, L.L.: Rape: it effects on task performance at varying stages in the life cycle. In Walker, M.J., and Brodsky, S.L., editors: Sexual assault: the victim and the rapist, Lexington, Mass., 1976, Lexington Books.

The researchers report the effect of rape on a victim's expected task performance within varying stages of the life-cycle. Special areas of task disruption are cited for the grade school or adolescent victim and for adult victims.

Fletcher, P.: Criminal victimization of elderly women: a look at sexual assault, paper presented at Rape Crisis Center of Syracuse, Inc., April 28, 1977 (60 Allen St., Syracuse, NY 13210). Unpublished paper obtained by writing to the author at the Center.

The author identifies six postulates to consider when counseling elderly victims. Factors include (1) social differences in upbringing, (2) the effect of alteration in life-style, (3) feelings of helplessness, (4) confusion surrounding the assault, (5) sexuality, and (6) physical trauma.

Horowitz, M.: Stress response syndrome, Arch. Gen. Psychiatry **12**:768, 1974.

The author discusses common patterns in the progress of phases of a stress response syndrome. General strategems of treatment are presented with the general goal of preventing either extreme denial or extreme intrusion-repetitiousness.

Lazarus, R.S.: Psychological stress and the coping process, New York, 1966, McGraw-Hill Book Co.

The author presents the important viewpoint that psychologic stress production and reduction are different at various developmental levels. Physiologic stress and psychologic stress are paralleled to view formal similarities and interaction between the systems.

Queen's Bench Foundation: Rape victimization study, San Francisco, 1975, the Foundation.

  The study reports a detailed investigation of rape victimization describing the impact of rape on 55 female victims. A large percent (67%) of the sample felt that they suffered long-term psychologic effects as a result of the rape.

Schmidt, A.M.: Adolescent female rape victims: special considerations, J. Psychosoc. Nurs. Ment. Health Serv. **19**(8):17, 1981.

  This article describes the legal and social aspects of rape, with special emphasis on the adolescent rape victim. Main concerns of adolescents are described, such as concern about the family's perception of the event, defensive behaviors because of lack of credibility, and fear of indiscriminate conversation. Nursing interventions are presented with the primary focus as helping the adolescent integrate the experience into the family system.

Selye, H.: The stress of life, New York, 1976, McGraw-Hill Book Co.

  This book is a revised edition of an earlier classic on stress and reflects new research and theories on the subject. Stress is viewed as exerting its effect on all living things and influencing both mental and physical processes.

Sutherland, S., and Sherl, D.J.: Patterns of response among victims of rape, Am. J. Orthopsychiatry **40**:503, 1970.

  The authors report follow-up interviews with a small homogenous sample (13) of white female victims of rape in which three separate phases of response to rape are identified. The three phases include (1) acute reaction, (2) outward adjustment, and (3) integration and resolution. Supportive mental health interventions are discussed in relation to specific patterns of response.

# CHAPTER 5

# Family response to rape

I just didn't realize how pervasive an assault it was, how deeply it has affected us all . . . I cried and screamed, I was completely out of control . . . just plain crazy with the pain of it . . . I wanted to kill them all . . . my husband held me and let me cry, we *all* cried. I'm exhausted now. I didn't realize, until now, how pervasive a thing this was . . . the *whole* family was raped!

Mother of 15-year-old rape victim, 2 weeks post-rape

---

## CHAPTER OUTLINE

## LEARNING OBJECTIVES

After reading this chapter the student will be able to:

1 Describe different nursing roles in working with families of rape victims

2 Define a social network and differentiate between primary and secondary social networks

3 Describe the assessment process of families and significant others following the rape of a loved one

4 Differentiate between adaptive and maladaptive stress reactions of families to rape

5 Explain the two phases of family response patterns in resolving a rape

6 Relate principles of crisis intervention and basic counseling to the nursing care of families resolving a rape experience

7 Explain future directions needed in the care of families of rape victims based on current findings reported in the literature

Rape victims do not exist alone. The impact of their rape experience strongly affects those who are emotionally close to them. Nurses who work with rape victims discover that families, friends' and mates experience physiologic and psychologic reactions to the rape of a loved one. Do the responses of significant people influence rape victim responses?

Out of experiences in world wars and natural disasters, professional caregivers have learned much about victimization. "When a disaster or tragedy strikes, no one escapes."[12] When a person is raped, the family and significant others also live through resolving the tragedy with the victim. The term *indirect victim* is applied to anyone in a victim's social world who is emotionally close to the rape victim and who experiences a stress reaction after the rape experience, such as family members or peers. *Family* is defined in this text as those persons related to one another by blood relationship and/or having emotional commitment to one another. Family members could include, for example, a mother, father, and children; a woman and man or two women living together but not married; a single parent and children; or a parent, step-parent, and children. (Hereafter, to facilitate writing style, all indirect victims are referred to as family.) Often families do not recognize their own victimization because they are so involved in attempting to cope with or problem-solve the victim's crisis. Nursing interventions in the psychologic distress of families is particularly important when these individuals do not recognize that they are experiencing a post-traumatic stress reaction. Eventually the impact of the tragedy is felt, and the family is faced with working through the crisis in their lives. Effective nursing interventions are planned and implemented on the basis of understanding the meaning of behavior and the function the behavior serves in the family.

This chapter focuses on the responses of rape victims and the persons in their social world who react to the rape experience. First, the varying roles of nurses working with rape victim families are discussed, and social network theory is presented as a theoretical framework from which nurses can assess which persons are most emotionally close and significant to rape victims. The remainder of the chapter focuses on assessing rape victim families and the nursing care of family members who experience an acute reaction and long-term reorganization process in response to the rape of a significant other.

## ENTRY INTO HEALTH CARE SYSTEMS
### Nursing roles with rape victim families

Nurses work with many types of families in a variety of settings. The type of care provided to rape victim families will be determined in part by the setting and role in which the nurse is working. For example, nurses work as volunteer counselors in rape crisis centers and/or as team members employed in the emergency department where victims come for a rape examination.

Fig. 5-1 depicts a number of different settings and clinical practice roles in which nurses work with rape victims and their families. As depicted by the double arrows ($\longleftrightarrow$) in the illustration, nurses may function in more than one role in providing services to rape victims and their families. Some nurses see rape victim families in the emergency department during the immediate aftermath of a rape assault and may be primarily responsible at that time for providing medical nursing care to the victim during the rape examination. Other nurses may be assigned as members of a specialty rape team within the hospital, comparable to cardiac arrest teams, and be assigned responsibility for providing crisis intervention and counseling; the same nurses may provide follow-up care to victims and their families as part of their private practice. The level of preparation of nurses working in different roles varies. However, nurses who provide family therapy are clinical specialists prepared in psychiatric–mental health nursing at the graduate level and have graduated from programs that provide both theory and supervised clinical experience in this specialized area. Some families will be in need of family therapy on a longer-term basis. However, the majority of contacts with families of rape victims is for the purpose of crisis intervention or brief follow-up care, and professional nurses without master's level preparation are educated and trained to provide families with such care.

If nurses find that their work setting does not have an established mechanism for providing care to rape victim families in the emergency department and for follow-up care, they are encouraged to work with the administration to develop such a service in their setting. Too often rape victim families are left alone in the emergency department waiting room to cope with their own post-rape crisis while attention and care is given solely to the victim; such practice ignores the holistic and systems approach professional nurses are educated to apply in providing service to consumers. While one nurse might assume primary responsibility for the medical nursing care of a rape examination, the same nurse might notify a clinical specialist or specialty nurse on the rape team to come to the emergency department to provide nursing care to the family of the victim.

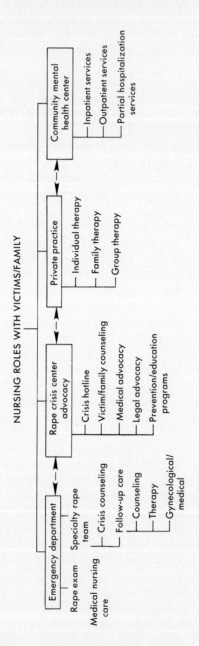

Fig. 5-1. Varying settings and nursing roles with rape victim families.

## SOCIAL NETWORK THEORY: WHO IS THE SIGNIFICANT OTHER?

In providing nursing care to rape victims and their families nurses need to assess which persons are important or significant to one another because these individuals are often deeply affected by the rape and can be supportive and/or destructive with one another in resolving a crisis precipitated by rape. Social network theory provides nurses with a knowledge base from which to assess social variables that influence a rape victim and her family's responses. A *social network* is defined as "that group of persons who maintain an ongoing significance in each other's lives by fulfilling specific human needs."[2] It is important for nurses to distinguish who is important to whom in the social network—for example, a peer or "gay" partner may be of more importance to a rape victim in the immediate aftermath of a rape than one's parents. Nurses are assisted in identifying who is a significant other to a person according to whether these individuals are within a person's primary or secondary social network. Fig. 5-2 depicts a model of primary and secondary social networks victims and their families may identify. Just as social relationships influence rape victims and their families, responses of rape victims and their families influence societal reactions. The mutually influential nature of social relationships is illustrated by the double arrows that depict a two-way influence within societal systems.

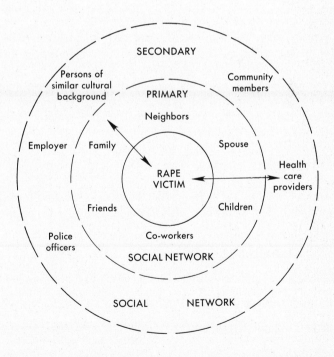

**Fig. 5-2. A model of primary and secondary social networks.**

## Primary social networks

A *primary social network* encompasses people with whom one has a strong emotional commitment and personal interaction. This network is unique for each person. Examples of people in primary social networks include family, friends, mates, spouses, children, co-workers, and neighbors. What is important is who a given person identifies as significant to them and not who the nurse thinks is significant or important to that person. For example, many victims live away from their families of origin in today's mobile society; thus a neighbor might be more important to a victim and her family than extended kin in the immediate aftermath of a rape. Relationships within a primary social network provide a variety of needs and support to living systems. For example, friendships are valuable in providing closeness, reassurance, social activity, and understanding. But friendships do not supply people with the *same* needs provided by a spouse or mate, such as intimacy, sexual satisfaction, love, and security. Likewise, a family provides for security, love, nurturance, and reassurance, thus overlapping the needs provided by friendships and mate relationships. For each person different types of primary social relationships provide different needs. These differing needs become apparent in counseling rape victims and their families, and they often assist nurses in identifying a person's primary social network. The needs provided for by primary social relationships are called *relational provisions*. Weiss [17] identifies six categories of relational provisions ordinarily associated with a particular type of primary network relationship:

1. *Attachment.* The individual gains a sense of security and place (provided by marriage, cross-sex relationship, or friendships).
2. *Social integration.* The individual shares with others common concerns, ideas, and interests. A network of these relationships offers a base for social activity (friends, co-workers, or peer groups).
3. *Opportunity for nurturance.* The individual assumes responsibility for a child, which provides a sense of being needed (care-givers, parents, or teachers).
4. *Reassurance of worth.* The individual's competency in a social role is recognized (associates, friends, co-workers, or family members).
5. *Sense of reliable alliance.* The individual expects continuing assistance regardless of affection or reciprocation (kin relationships, siblings, parents, friends).
6. *Obtaining of guidance.* The individual trusts a person who furnishes emotional support and help in problem-solving or advice (friend, teacher, adviser, or boss).

## Secondary social networks

*Secondary social networks* consist of persons with whom one has contact but not a strong emotional commitment. A secondary social network influences a person's responses but not as strongly as one's primary social network. Examples of people in secondary social networks include social community members, persons of similar cultural background, employers, health care providers, police officers, and teachers. Nurses providing care to rape victims and their families are identified as supportive persons within one's secondary social network. Frequently rape victims come to the emergency department escorted by the police or rape crisis center advocate and subsequently notify someone within their primary social network to come be with them. Deciding who to notify and how to talk to that person about the rape is particularly troublesome for many victims. Nurses have an important role in helping rape victims activate support systems within their primary social network and in helping these persons be supportive of the victim, as illustrated in the following clinical example.

> CLINICAL EXAMPLE
>
> Louise had some ambivalence about seeking her husband's support after her rape event. At the time of the incident, she had immediately summoned a neighbor friend for help. Louise had been raped by a man who gained access to her home by posing as a delivery man. Her husband, George, had lectured her on several occasions not to admit strange men into the home. However, Louise judged the man on his appearance and reported, "He was polite and looked well-groomed." The man threatened to kill Louise with a 10-inch knife that he pulled from under his jacket.
>
> Louise verbalized her ambivalence to the nurse: "I want to tell George, but he'll be so angry with me." Louise then continued with self-deprecating comments: "I'm so stupid and George will tell me so! Why didn't I listen to him?" The nurse provided Louise with reassurance of worth and then helped her explore alternative courses of action:
>
> 1. Louise could tell George and accept his lecturing which is highly predictable.
> 2. Louise could not tell George and try to keep the rape event a secret.
> 3. Louise could tell George about the event and verbalize her own needs for his support rather than his reprimands.
>
> In their problem-solving discussion Louise disclosed to the nurse that she had difficulty keeping secrets from George because their marriage was based on open communication. Deciding to tell George, Louise asked the nurse to call him to the health setting. Louise asked the nurse to stay with her while she told her husband. The nurse provided Louise with secondary support during her disclosure to George about the rape. Louise asked George for support and reassurance, telling him she realized her poor judgment. The nurse assessed the husband's ability to support his wife and provided him with answers to many questions. No additional referral was necessary.

As persons within a rape victim family's secondary social network, nurses can facilitate the family's resolution of a crisis precipitated by the rape by attending to many of their needs. These needs are similar to those often experienced by the victim. (Rape victim needs are discussed in Chapters 4 and 6.) Some of these needs are briefly listed here:

1. *Priority*. Explain to family members why the victim may not be seen immediately in the emergency department, such as a cardiac arrest patient taking priority in emergency care.
2. *Delays*. Explain to the family why an examination is being delayed (e.g., the physician is attending to another emergency) or why the rape exam takes so much time (e.g., to collect evidence).
3. *Privacy*. If possible, provide the family with a private room where they can explore their feelings and concerns with a counselor.

4. *Feelings.* Recognize that families experience intense feelings post-rape and the nurse may be the target of their anger. Respond with empathic listening and requested information that will help lower the family's high level of emotional reactivity.

5. *Primary care.* Assign a primary care nurse to meet the family's needs or contact a clinical specialist, hospital rape team member, or advocate from the rape crisis center.

6. *Tactless remarks.* Maintain professional behavior in the presence of family members; for example, avoid laughter that could be misinterpreted as ridicule or doubting the victim and do not reinforce family remarks that blame the victim.

7. *Social amenities.* Offer the family coffee of other refreshments while they wait for the victim to receive care, or inform them where they can obtain refreshments.

8. *Protocol.* Explain to the family what the rape exam consists of and "what will happen next" (e.g., a police interview when the exam is over).

One of the problems that arises in the family's resolution of the rape is that their reactions to the assault frequently differ from those of the victim or do not occur in the same sequence.[16] For example, the victim may report feeling recovered from her intense fear while her parents are just beginning to feel the impact of the life-threatening event; therefore conflict sometimes arises as the parents respond by overprotectiveness at a time when the victim is ready to return to an active life-style. Often family members can benefit from some short-term or longer-term counseling in trying to understand their own feelings about the assault as a preventative measure against long-term unresolved conflicts. Family members experience difficulty supporting the victim when their own thoughts and feelings are not identified or worked through. The next section discusses factors nurses consider in assessing families of rape victims and nursing interventions in the family's acute and long-term resolution of the rape.

## ASSESSING RAPE VICTIM FAMILIES
### Is this family healthy?

Rape results in family members experiencing intense emotional responses to the assault and these responses are seen in seemingly maladaptive behaviors of family members toward each other. Here, as with the victim's response, the nurse's guiding principle is to reserve value judgments about a family's response to the situational crisis of rape. Kliman[12] states that in an acute situational crisis people are "*entitled* to feel whatever they feel." The family's post-rape responses are an adjustment reaction to an acute stress state and are neither neurotic or psychotic. Rape heightens the family's vulnerability for experiencing dysfunction, but their adjustment reaction to the assault does not, in and of itself, imply pathology. The unit of observation and assessment becomes the *family system*. Victim responses are seen as adaptive functions within a family system of intimate relationships. By helping the family acknowledge their vulnerability, the nurse can help them explore the meaning and impact of the rape in their lives and seek out the most adaptive ways of mastering this crisis.[12]

The family's intense emotional and behavioral reaction can leave nurses questioning whether the behavior observed is "normal" in response to the rape of a member or loved one. Nurses intervene in the post-rape adaptation of both functional and dysfunctional families. Therefore it is useful for the nurse to assess the family's response in the context of what one would expect to observe about healthy family functioning in general, since family responses to rape are similar to their responses to other crises. Optimal healthy family functioning is characterized by the following:[14,15]

1. Warm, caring, and close association of family members with one another, fostering high levels of self-esteem in the members
2. Respect for the unique way in which individual family members perceive their experiences, that of others, and the world
3. Open, direct, clear, specific, and honest communication with one another
4. Cooperation and a strong emotional alliance between the parents
5. Understanding and appreciation of the fact that human beings act in response to multiple needs and motivations
6. Flexible, humane, and appropriate rules that are subject to change
7. Spontaneity and laughter
8. Viewing the world beyond the family as rewarding, exciting, and adventurous with an open and hopeful linking to society
9. Creative contributions to society with individual members having impressive characteristics

Families have adaptive and maladaptive coping responses to rape. Although some response patterns are more adaptive than others, adaptiveness needs to be defined within the family's unique context and more broadly than in terms of the behavior alone. For example, some parents do not want to disclose the rape to relatives because they anticipate stigma or rejection and their assessment of such reactions is accurate. Thus protecting the victim from further victimization by relatives is a healthy response by a caring family. On the other hand, some families keep the rape a secret because they view the act as sexually motivated and do not want others to know that the victim "engaged in illicit sex." Healthier family responses generally consist of caring, concern, and support for rape victims. Healthy families direct anger at the attacker, may even threaten to kill him, and show the ability to give emotional support to the rape victim. Unhealthy family responses include blame and anger directed at the victim or other family members. Unhealthy family responses focus on the family's welfare rather than the victim's welfare. For example, family members may say, "What will other people think of us?" These families are unable to give the victim support because the family's needs exceed or override the victim's needs. Table 5-1 presents family stress reactions to rape that the nurse needs to assess as adaptive or maladaptive within the context of a given family. To facilitate the nurse's assessment process, family stress reactions to rape are presented in categories most often identified by counselors as adaptive or maladaptive.

Nurses further assess families and significant others by a review of the following questions:

1. How much history taking is necessary at this time? Nurses are aware that the "here and now" may be the only factor that is necessary to assess in crisis resolution.

2. How does the family define the problem?
3. How intact is the family system? Who are the present family members? Who are the absent family members? Why are they absent?
4. What is the degree of anxiety in the family system?
5. What alternatives are being planned to help the rape victim?
6. Is the family capable of following through on recommendations?

Because family members experience their own post-rape responses, nurses who interact with families need to assess the type of family responses and the effect of family reactions on victim responses. Nurses observe family and victim interactions, gather information, and make the following assessments:

1. What is happening in the family members' lives right now?
2. How do family members respond to one another?
3. What are the effects of family members' statements on other family members?
4. How is the family responding to the nurse or their caregivers?
5. Can the family benefit from some help or counseling?

The mates and spouses of rape victims have been clinically studied regarding their ability to support the rape victim. Partners, like families, have difficulty focusing on victim concerns when they have their own needs and concerns. Communication breakdowns occur when partners cannot discuss the rape event and its impact on their lives. Nurses observe partner interaction and make the following assessments:

1. Can the man provide the rape victim with positive support?
2. What are the mate's reactions to the rape and toward the rapist?
3. What is the nature and quality of the dyadic relationship?
4. Could the couple benefit from some help or counseling?

Special problems sometimes arise in the family's response when the victim has been raped by a family member. The family may focus on the person who raped the victim and the meaning of that relationship in the family system, or the family may focus on the welfare of the victim. One mother called the nurse 1 week post-rape to discuss the following concern over her daughter's welfare.

CLINICAL EXAMPLE

I just want to know if she's all right . . . it's been a week now and she's sleeping all the time, won't eat much either. He bashed her head around and I'm afraid she's sleeping because he hurt her head. It was her brother-in-law that did this! She just can't get over it. He told her he's been watching her for some time and was determined to get her, no matter what. Now she's afraid to live alone. She just moved into this apartment and it was burglarized a week ago, now this. It's not a very good neighborhood, but she was trying to get out on her own. I'm worried about her and feel so helpless. Should I take her back to the emergency department?

Mother of 22-year-old rape victim
Crisis call to nurse on hotline

As the above clinical example illustrates, the welfare of the victim was the predominate concern of this mother. The mother was concerned about her daughter's health status and medical care needs and reached out to a nurse for crisis counseling. Responding to the mother's concern, the nurse talked with her about common victim

## Table 5-1. Adaptive and maladaptive family stress reactions to rape

| Adaptive stress reactions | Maladaptive stress reactions |
| --- | --- |
| Care and concern for the victim | Concern primarily about how others will think of the family |
| Support of the victim | Contested feelings over who was raped, hurt most, or victimized |
| Feelings of shock, disbelief, dismay | Minimizing the victim's feelings or response |
| Feelings of helplessness and disequilibrium | Feeling guilty or responsible for not having protected the victim |
| Physical revulsion which may parallel the victim's affective responses | Rape trauma syndrome |
| Distraction tactics to keep the victim and themselves occupied | Patronizing or overprotecting the victim |
| Reacting to rape as a violent act | Viewing rape as a sexually motivated act and the victim as "damaged goods" |
| Anger and rage directed at the rapist or society | Direct or indirect anger and resentment as seen in communication difficulties |
| Blame directed at the rapist | Blame directed at the victim or family members |
| Thoughts about violent retribution or active retaliation | Act out violent retribution toward assailant or victim |
| Reaching out to extended family/significant others for support | Emotional cut-offs with extended family/significant others |
| Empathic with each other | Absence of empathic responses with each other; emotional isolation or withdrawal |
| Use of crisis counseling as needed | Failure to seek professional counseling when needed |
| Supportive of victim's medical or gynecological care needs and follow-up care | Failure to seek medical or gynecological care and follow-up care |
| Cooperation with criminal justice system to prosecute rapist | Inability to cooperate with criminal justice system |
| Participation in rape prevention programs | Belief in rape myths |
| Supporting the victim's decisions and wishes | Action pressured against victim's wishes, such as forced or pressured sexual relations with victim, informing others, dropping charges, or insisting that prosecution be carried out |
| Reevaluating previous relationships with the victim | Divorce/separation |
| Unit stays intact | |

Based on Burgess, A.W., and Holmstrom, L.L.: Rape: victims of crisis, Bowie, Md., 1974, Robert J. Brady Co.; Halpern, S.: Rape: Helping the victim, Oradell, N.J., 1978, Medical Economics Company Book Division; Silverman, D: Sharing the crisis of rape: counseling the mates and families of victims, Am. J. Orthopsychiatry **48**:166, 1978.

responses post-rape, such as depression and hypersomnia, and supported her in keeping a scheduled appointment for follow-up medical evaluation. It is important for nurses to recognize that what is upsetting to the nurse—for example, rape by a relative—is not necessarily the presenting problem of the family. Nurses assess and intervene in the *family's* presenting crisis or counseling request.

A rape awakens each family member to different problems as the feelings of crisis mount to a peak. The stress may be defined differently by each member, but each one is experiencing change that results in a temporary state of disequilibrium. For example, one member of the family may experience the rape as a loss, while another may view the rape as a threat to safety. Regardless of individual reactions, the family's methods of problem solving begin to work as the family looks for ways to resolve the crisis of rape. During this phase nurses are often in a position to provide crisis intervention and counseling to such families. Family responses to rape and interventions are discussed in more depth in the section that follows.

## NURSING INTERVENTION IN FAMILY RESPONSE TO RAPE

In intervening in a family's post-rape crisis state, the nurse may observe two phases of response commonly experienced: (1) an acute reaction, and (2) a long-term reorganization process.[4] No one phase of response is discrete—that is, concerns experienced in one phase may overlap with another phase, depending on the particular conflict or issue the family is working through. The following section presents family response patterns frequently seen in each of the two phases and suggests effective nursing interventions for use in working with rape victim families.

### Acute reaction

The period of acute reaction includes (1) physiologic distress in response to the traumatic event, and (2) psychologic distress involving a variety of emotional, cognitive, and behavioral responses that arise in an effort to reestablish family equilibrium.[4]

#### Physiologic distress

Frequently the experience of stress in response to news of the rape is so intense that those closest to the victim report symptoms of physiologic distress. Common physiologic symptoms of stress include insomnia; gastrointestinal disturbances such as anorexia, nausea, and diarrhea; genitourinary disturbances such as urinary frequency, which accompanies intense anxiety; headaches; and extreme fatigue.[4] Some family members request medication such as tranquilizers or sleeping pills to assist them through the immediate impact phase of the rape crisis.

#### Psychologic distress

The most obvious symptoms of the family's stress response to news of the rape can be seen in their immediate emotional, cognitive, and behavioral reactions. At this stage nurses can apply principles of crisis intervention (see Chapter 7). One strategy used in preventive and crisis intervention with families of rape victims is *anticipatory guidance*. This is the process of preparing a person for a stressful event so that when a potentially hazardous event is experienced one has developed what Caplan[5] describes as a certain degree of "emotional innoculation" to the anticipated event and is less likely to experience the situation as a crisis.

Recognizing that those closest to the rape victim can facilitate or impede resolution of the rape (and that they have their own crisis response to the rape to resolve as well) volunteers and staff at the Washington, D.C. Rape Crisis Center have developed a "note" that provides anticipatory guidance to the victim's significant others to assist them in resolving the rape crisis. The letter is given to the victim's significant others, or to the victim to give to them, when seen in the emergency department during the impact phase of the crisis or during follow-up care. "A Note to Those Closest to Rape Victims" as developed by the Washington, D.C. Rape Crisis Center is shown on pp. 134 and 135.

When intervening in a family's post-rape crisis state, the nurse's actions are directed toward (1) clarifying the family's perception of the event, (2) activating the family's support network, and (3) facilitating the use of adaptive coping mechanisms. For example, the nurse helps a family open up communication by discussing the meaning and impact of the rape on their lives and encourages contact with their extended family during this stressful period (support system activated). Nurses educate family members about the nature of rape and the motives of rapists in an effort to prevent them from blaming the victim for the crime. They also encourage members to critically reevaluate their sense of responsibility for not preventing the rape in realistic terms so as to decrease the family's tendency toward blaming themselves for the assault (perception of event clarified). Furthermore, nurses encourage family members to maintain or resume usual activities of daily functioning or work. They use empathic listening to convey to the family an understanding of their sense of stress at a time when they have reached out for help (coping mechanisms activated).

Goals of crisis intervention frequently implemented by nurses in their work with families post-rape are presented in the box shown on pp. 136 and 137. These goals, as applied to counseling rape-victim families in an acute reaction phase, are elaborated on in the discussion that follows. Note that the discussion is intentionally limited to frequent post-rape responses experienced by families because a comprehensive presentation merits fuller attention in a separate volume.

*Shock, disbelief, dismay, and helplessness.* These feelings are commonly experienced by family members in the immediate aftermath of the rape. The family's response to rape is similar to other crises in this respect. One mother stated:

> I don't recall much about that night (of the rape), I was in a fog. It seemed unreal, like we would wake up and be back to normal. My boss said I was acting strange so I had to tell him what the matter was and he's been real understanding.

Another mother stated;

> You never expect this to happen to you . . . you just can't believe it's real. It's something you think only happens to *other* people . . . even now sometimes it doesn't seem like it could possibly have happened.

Referring to the disruption of the initial impact of the rape, one mother said:

> It's been a bad week, kind of a roller coaster effect. I told Pat we would just have to take it one day at a time. I told her it would be up and down hill for awhile and she reminded me of that when I got to feeling so awful. I told her to give me time to react and adjust. I'll just have to make decisions later about all the stuff she's pressing me about.

In the above case the nurse asked, "What happens when your upset feelings get triggered?" The mother replied, "I flash back to how awful she looked the night she came home and the terror I felt."

Effective nursing interventions with families experiencing shock, disbelief, dismay,

*Text continued on p. 138.*

# A NOTE TO THOSE CLOSEST TO RAPE VICTIMS: FAMILIES, LOVERS, AND FRIENDS*

How does rape affect a woman? How does rape affect those closest to a victim? How can those closest to a rape victim do "the right thing"? We have some ideas which we wish to share with you, and we hope they will offer a beginning for giving effective support to rape victims. More than anyone else, it is those closest to a victim who influence how she will deal with the attack.

Most women who have been raped do not react to the sexual aspects of the crime, but instead they react to the terror and fear that is involved. Often an immediate reaction of the woman is "I could have been killed." Many of those around her, particularly men, may find themselves concerned with the sexual aspects of the crime. The more this pre-occupation is communicated to the woman, the more likely she is to have difficulties in dealing with her own feelings. Probably the best way to understand her feelings is to try to remember or imagine a situation where you felt powerless and afraid. You may remember feeling very alone, fearful and needing comfort.

Often the raped woman needs much love and support the first few days. Affection seems to be important. Stroking or caressing can be comforting. They help break down the loneliness and alienation. This, of course, leads to the question of sex. It is impossible to generalize about how the woman will feel about sex, nor should you guess. If you have been involved sexually with the woman, try to discuss, at an appropriate time, how she feels in general about the attack, about you, and about sex. (An appropriate time is not right after the rape. Let her comments to the first two questions guide you in deciding whether you have chosen a good time to discuss it or whether you would be pushing the point too soon.) Some women will be anxious to resume normal sexual relations as a way of forgetting the rape; others will be more hesitant.

In the case of virgin rapes, female support seems most important. It is a good time to discuss the pleasure involved in sex—as well as to reassert the woman's right to decide when and with whom she wishes to have sex. Hopefully, a woman's mother will feel comfortable about this; if not, a friend or sister—especially if she has been raped, might help.

It seems advisable for the woman to talk about the rape; however, it is not possible to generalize about how much she should be encouraged to talk about it. Women do not seem to appreciate specific questions; they tend to be too probing and callous. To probe in these

*Reprinted with permission and courtesy of the Washington, D.C. Rape Crisis Center, P.O. Box 21005, Kalorama St. Station, Washington, DC 20009.

areas may only worsen any problems the woman may have in dealing with the rape.

Instead, questions about how she feels now and what bothers her the most are more useful. They are not threatening and should allow her to talk about her most immediate concerns. Remember, too, the woman wants to talk about other things. Often the rape may leave a woman concentrating on other problems and it is important that she talk about these. Probably the most practical suggestion is that you communicate your own willingness to let her talk. Because of your closeness to her, the woman may be more sensitive to your feelings. If the rape distresses her, it may be impossible for her to talk to you. She may also try to protect you. In these and other cases, where she really will not be able to talk with you, encourage her to speak with someone she trusts. Remember that the rape has brought up feelings of powerlessness, and encouraging her to talk to whom she wants, when she wants, is more helpful than feeling that it is necessary to talk to you.

If the rape is treated as a serious crime and not a heinous experience, women would probably have less difficulty in dealing with it. The woman survived the attack and one would suppose that she would want to resume living a "normal" life as quickly as possible. In a healthy, supportive environment, most women will find the rape meshes with other unhappy experiences in their lives. Because of others' reactions, or their own life situations at the time of the rape, other women will find the rape was indeed a traumatic milestone. If after a reasonable amount of time, a woman seems unable to cope with the day-to-day problems of life, professional help may be sought.

Whether or not professional counseling is sought, it is not a replacement for warm, concerned, loving communications. A professional counselor may help, but he or she cannot replace your role in the relationship. Rape not only affects the woman, but also you, as it plays upon your own fears and fantasies. Try to recognize the fears for what they are; otherwise you may end up projecting them on the woman and cause some serious problems for her and your relationship.

Finally, it should be noted that, if the woman has pressed charges, the whole process involves numerous hassles and stresses. Your awareness of the legal processes and problems involved and your support will be helpful.

## GOALS OF CRISIS INTERVENTION FOR FAMILIES
## OF RAPE VICTIMS

- Helping the family to openly express their immediate feelings in response to a rape—as a shared life crisis
- Helping the family to be supportive of and reassuring to the victim
- Helping the family work through immediate practical matters and initiate problem-solving techniques
- Helping the family develop cognitive understanding of what the rape experience actually means to the victim and to the family
- Explaining the possibility of future psychologic and somatic symptoms that characterize a rape trauma syndrome and what the family can do to minimize these symptoms
- Activating qualities characteristic of healthy family functioning during the impact and resolution phases of the shared crisis
- Educating the family about rape as a *violent crime,* not a sexually motivated act, and eliminating focus on the victim's guilt or responsibility
- Eliminating the family's sense of guilt for not protecting the victim by assuring them that they could not have anticipated or prevented the rape
- Discouraging violent, destructive, or irrational retribution toward the rapist (under the guise of being on the victim's behalf) by encouraging a sharing of feelings of helplessness, sadness, hurt, and anger
- Encouraging discussion of the sexual relationship between partners; suggesting that the man let the victim know (a) that his feelings have not changed (when this is true) and that he still sexually desires her, (b) that he will wait for her to approach him, and (c) that sex therapy is available if they have difficulties that persist and want assistance in reestablishing normal sexual relations
- Explaining the possibility of venereal disease and pregnancy that may result from a rape, the preventive care necessary for the victim and spouse or boyfriend, and the follow-up care indicated

Sources: Burgess, A.W., and Holmstrom, L.L.: Rape: sexual disruption and recovery, Am. J. Orthopsychiatry, **49:**648,1979; Burgess, A.W., and Holmstrom, L.L: Rape: victims of crisis, Bowie, Md., 1974, Robert J. Brady Co., pp. 59-63; Halpern, S., editor: Rape: helping the victim, Oradell, N.J., 1978, Medical Economics Company Book Division, pp. 51-54; Kliman, A.: Crisis: psychological first aid for recovery and growth, New York, 1978, Holt, Rinehart & Winston; Lewis, J.M., Beavers, W.R., Gossett, J.T., and Phillips, V.A.: No single thread: psychological health in family systems, New York, 1976, Brunner/Mazel Publishers.

- Explaining that early crisis intervention often prevents long-term problems in resolving the crisis and that to seek counseling at this time does not imply mental illness (the nurse specifies that crisis intervention usually lasts for 3 to 6 hours during the first few weeks post-rape)
- Giving families, lovers, and friends a copy of "A Note to Those Closest to Rape Victims"
- Referring the family for direct counseling when members' shared responses to the crisis interfere with their ability to cope adaptively
- Providing factual data, resource lists for counseling, and follow-up care *in writing* (because highly stressed persons do not hear or recall information verbally communicated)
- Letting families know that some decisions, such as whether to prosecute the rapist or move to a safer residence, can be postponed while more immediate needs, such as medical care, are taken care of (This action helps the family (1) set priorities and organize decisions about what has to be done now, and (2) gain emotional distance from the urgency and confusion felt during a crisis state to permit sound decision making later.)
- Identifying how the family has handled crises in the past and encouraging members to use adaptive coping mechanisms for this crisis
- Encouraging contact with persons identified as supportive to the family and offering to contact such persons
- Assigning a primary nurse to spend time talking with the family in the emergency department waiting room while the victim receives medical care
- Allowing time for thoughts and feelings in a decision-making process
- Using empathic listening to convey understanding of the family's feelings and concerns
- Asking if the nurse can check back with the family the next day to see how they are getting along and answer any questions they may have

and helplessness include (1) assistance with practical matters and information, such as medical care and persons that need to be notified; (2) referral of families for follow-up crisis counseling—to the rape crisis center, the hospital rape crisis specialty team, the community mental health center, or the professional with whom they have an ongoing relationship.

Nurses will find that families also experience a sense of shock and disbelief as they cope with rape-related issues—such as pregnancy, abortion, and prosecuting the rapist—that arise weeks after the initial impact of the rape. At these times the family may need help in solving what is for them a problem great enough to create a sense of disequilibrium and crisis.

For example, one couple sought follow-up counseling with the nurse who had seen them in the emergency department to determine how to handle the news of their daughter's rape and consequent pregnancy with the other family members. When asked how they handled similar crises in their family in the past, the mother replied, "I don't know what to do. We've *never* had a crisis like this before! I'll bet you find that hard to believe. I just need some rest from this situation." The nurse assessed that this family member lacked coping mechanisms to handle the crisis situation or was unable to recall coping mechanisms used during past stressful events. In the counseling session the mother identified her main stressor as not being able to mother her 16-year-old daughter (who was away from home for the first time at a residential high school academy out of state) rather than the pregnancy itself. When planning the home visit, the nurse had thought that the question of pregnancy and abortion would be the parents' main concern. Instead, the mother's first experience in being deprived of a known role and coping behavior (mothering) and the husband's confusion about how to be helpful to his wife were identified as the stressors precipitating the couple's crisis state. After the counseling session, the mother agreed to tell the daughter the results of the pregnancy test (she had contemplated withholding the information until the school vacation) but not to inform other family members about the pregnancy at this time. Expressing her sense of resolution, the mother then stated, "I feel alright now. I'm exhausted! But I think we'll be okay. Thank you for helping us."

The above clinical example illustrates the importance of the nurse assessing the family's crisis or counseling requests and following the family's lead in problem-solving the identified concerns. Nurses need to encourage the family to ventilate their sense of frustration and helplessness, to become aware of their response as one triggered by a desire to help "undo" the victim's plight or their own sense of guilt or responsibility for not having protected her from the rape, and to arrive at some realistic options about what they can or cannot do that are acceptable to them or meet their needs in a situation. Families usually resolve their sense of helplessness when they are able to (1) acknowledge their feeling state, (2) identify the psychodynamic forces triggering their stress state, and (3) determine ways to handle the presenting stressor. The above example also shows the importance of the nurse in providing follow-up care to rape-victim families. Many times people in crisis will seek out persons who have been helpful to them in other crises (such as this nurse had been in the emergency department). They will also seek out the professional who is familiar with their case and thus can provide continuity in their care. Knowing that continuity of care has been a problem for many rape victims and their families, nurses can strive within their work settings to establish policies that will ensure that such care is received.

 *Blaming or finding a scapegoat.* When misfortune befalls us, we cope by using psychologic mechanisms of defense that are "the mind's protective device, nature's way of allowing us to continue functioning."[12] One defense frequently activated by the crisis of rape is *projection* expressed in the form of *scapegoating*—that is, finding someone to hold accountable (blame) for the calamity. In Webster's dictionary projection is defined as the "attribution of one's own ideas, feelings, or attitudes to other people or to objects . . . *the externalization of blame, guilt, or responsibility as a defense against anxiety."* This defense is apparent when the family attempts to make the victim or another family member feel responsible for the rape.

 Blaming the victim or themselves for the rape is a frequent family response to rape. Frank[7] found that family members demonstrated less blaming behavior and more empathy if the victim was more brutalized during the assault or if a weapon was used. Strong support by the family appeared related to their ability to view the victim as not culpable for the assault. The result of blaming the victim is that a vicious negative interaction cycle is established when the victim counterreacts to a lack of understanding from her immediate significant others (see Fig. 5-3).

 As shown in Fig. 5-3, the victim, in response to being blamed by the family, psychologically and/or physically distances from others, concluding that those she once trusted did not meet her expectations. The victim is not always able to recognize that the persons blaming her for the rape are also indirectly feeling raped by the experience and reacting to their own sense of crisis. Disappointed, the victim frequently withdraws from her social network, which creates even more stress for her: isolating herself only deprives her of the support she so desperately needs at this time and elevates her level of anxiety, fear, and depression. The victim's stress reaction then creates further tension in the social network and impairs her own adjustment and that of the family to the crisis. The family or support system compounds resolution of the rape by continuing to blame the victim for the assault, being angry at her, or focusing on their own self-doubts and concerns. Blaming the victim for the rape sets off a series

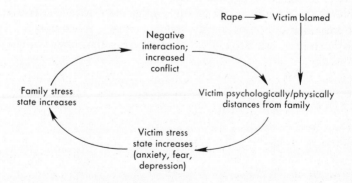

**Fig. 5-3. Negative family interaction cycle when victim blamed for rape.**

of increasingly negative interactions among family members who are feeling hurt, angry, irritable, frightened, and rejected.[7]

*Triangulation.* Sometimes the tension between two people in the family will be so great or uncomfortable that a third person is "triangled in" to reduce the family's tension to a more comfortable level. The process of involving others to reduce tension is called *triangulation.*[8] For example, a victim who anticipates that her parents will blame her for the rape may "triangle in" a peer to help reduce her sense of anxiety. A nurse may be "triangled in" as a counselor to help the family reduce their anxiety about protecting the victim in subsequent social engagements. The family may "triangle in" a number of persons to blame (scapegoat) for the rape in an attempt to reduce their sense of guilt for their misperceived responsibility for the rape. One illustration of multiple triangulation by families in reaction to rape is shown in Fig. 5-4.

In the figure the victim and family (parents) triangle in three different persons (boyfriend, girlfriend, and nurse counselor) to reduce the family's level of tension. This family also triangles in the school system to blame for the rape. Nurses can intervene in the processes of blaming the victim and triangulation by:

1. Exploring with the family the feelings they project onto others
2. Assisting the family in realistically appraising projected feelings, particularly guilt and a sense of responsibility for the rape
3. Providing a climate in which the family members feel safe enough to ventilate feelings hidden by a projection process (e.g., feelings of sadness, hurt, vulnerability, helplessness, anxiety, and fear)
4. Helping families acknowledge a sense of being raped by the experience although they were not directly victims of the assault
5. Encouraging family members to express feelings they vigilantly try to contain, such as rage, helplessness, hurt, and a sense of crisis or disequilibrium[16]

Once the family is able to get their feelings out in the open, they are better able to resolve their crisis. By denying their own sense of crisis, the family only postpones solving the problem. When the family has been given permission to express intense feeling responses such as rage and hurt, other issues that have escalated—for example, overfocusing on the victim's lack of sound judgment—tend to subside and the family's level of tension and dysfunction generally decreases. When nurses acknowledge and give the *family* permission to express their felt crisis, the family is often then able to go

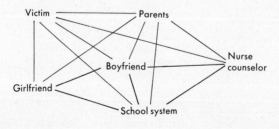

**Fig. 5-4. Triangulation process in response to rape.**

home and *share* what is basically a common experience. Sharing a crisis experience with significant others often activates readily available support systems and results in reestablishing a sense of well-being.

*Overprotecting or infantilizing*. In response to feeling helpless some families rally around the victim, overprotect and infantilize her, and even enlist the support of others in their social network to do so. Overprotective behavior expresses the family's attempt to protect themselves, the victim, and others from the pain, discomfort, and confusion they feel. However, such pseudo-protection only revictimizes the person being "protected." It is a disservice to the rape victim to assume that she cannot cope with the events and decisions in her life. Kliman states:

> We rationalize it as for their own good, but by denying them their rightful functioning within the family network we are revictimizing them. . . . We . . . play out a charade . . . and . . . pretending steals energy . . . for . . . problem-solving. . . . The more we treat people as unable to cope, the less able they are to cope.[12]

Overprotective behaviors commonly seen post-rape include (1) parental efforts to restrict and intensely survey the victim's activities or friends; (2) moving an elderly victim from her apartment back into the family home, thereby making her dependent on the family under the pretense of what is "best" for her welfare; (3) not disclosing the rape to others in the social network because "they'd be too upset"; and (4) taking the victim places or forcefully trying to get her to talk with others when she may not be ready to do so or feel the need to do so.[16] The following example demonstrates how one mother, through infantilizing behaviors, usurps the right of her daughter to direct, control, and participate in those events that affect her life at a time when self-care decisions and sharing would expedite her recovery.

### CLINICAL EXAMPLE

Gwen is a 16-year-old black female who was raped one evening following attendance at a jazz concert at a university student union. Her mother had felt comfortable permitting her to attend the concert, but her step-father disapproved as he felt the campus was in an unsafe area of the city. Following the concert Gwen lost her friends in the crowd and two college students offered to help her locate her friends. They directed her down a deserted corridor, shoved her into an empty classroom, and raped her. About 6 weeks post-rape Gwen wanted to try attending another concert at the student union and was feeling a bit anxious about being in the building where she had been raped but wanted to try getting out again. When she asked her mother for permission to attend the concert, her mother flatly refused, asked her how she "could even consider such a thing," and brought her into the rape crisis center for counseling even though Gwen felt she was not in need of counseling.

Effective nursing interventions for the family members who demonstrate overprotective or infantilizing behaviors such as in the above example include:

1. Helping family members identify what feelings they are having in response to the rape that are prompting their behaviors.

2. Helping families identify what they expect or hope their behavior to accomplish because often they have erroneous assumptions about their actions. (For example, they may insist that the victim talk with the nurse in order to recover from the assault when involuntary counseling can impede such an outcome. It is not unusual for a rape victim to experience the exact opposite result of what family members have done "in their best interest.")

3. Talking to family members alone in the absence of the victim to provide them with an opportunity to share their feelings without additionally stressing the victim by requiring her to listen to their distress. Separate sessions permit family members to freely ventilate feelings, explore concerns and hidden agendas—for example, how to cope with feelings about a sexually active adolescent—at a time when they feel unable to contain these feelings or concerns. Separate sessions can help prevent an escalation of intense or conflictual feeling states in the family and avert the reactive use of each other as a depository for emotionally charged issues that can overload an already stressed system.

4. Conveying to the family that in their efforts to be helpful their overprotective behaviors are, in reality, intrusive and create further distress for the victim which only adds to the whole family's distress.

5. Stressing the importance of respecting the victim's need for privacy, confidentiality, and freedom to personally determine what she will disclose about the rape, to whom and at what time or under what conditions.

6. Combining the use of individual counseling sessions with the victim or family members and counseling sessions together with the entire family/significant others.

The intervention approach implemented by the nurse is often based on subjective clinical judgment, varying theoretical frameworks, and experience in working with rape victim families.

*Disclosing or keeping the rape a secret.* It soon becomes clear that no single family response to rape is an isolated phenomenon. For example, keeping the rape a secret can sometimes also be an overprotective behavior. However, secrecy about rape is a frequent family response that merits exploration in itself. Families report as a rationale for secrecy the belief that others will "not be hurt" if they do not know about the rape. Often the "need" for secrecy is linked to a view of rape as a sexually motivated act (discussed below). Nurses will hear directives from families such as "Don't tell dad because he'll kill the guy," or "You better not let your boyfriend know, I don't think he could handle it," or "I don't think sissy (younger sister) should know about it," or "Grandma would just die if she heard about it." Keeping the rape a secret saps people of energy they could otherwise use for adaptive coping; secrets add an additional burden, draining valuable energy family members could use for sharing and problem-solving.[12]

Families will give a great variety of reasons to substantiate the "need" for a secret conspiracy about the rape—the parents' discomfort with their child's sexuality, fear of being blamed for negligence, or long-standing problems in family functioning. Secrecy is usually based on the firm opinion that if the family discussed the pain of the rape trauma openly it would only keep disorganizing memories alive in a nonconstructive way.[11] In reality, the net effect is to deprive both the victim and her family or significant other of the opportunity to share their sense of pain, to mourn the loss inherent to the assault, and to deny each other needed support and communication by implying that "what has happened is too traumatic to talk about," thereby confirming the victim's most devastating fears, fantasies, and doubts.[16] For example, because many victims believe rape myths, they feel guilty about the assault and expect that others will blame them for the crime. The victim often feels that others will think she has "done something terrible or despicable" and, if she cannot talk about her traumatic experience publically, "It must be true that others are ashamed of me and think I am to blame." The victim feels helpless in trying to establish the truth about her actual integrity and credibility. The problem becomes, "How can I establish my credibility if I can't even talk about what happened to me. People do not believe I was indeed raped, not even my family if that is the position they take."

Some rape victims anticipate that the family system will respond by overprotective behaviors if they know about the rape and therefore prefer not to disclose the assault. The victim's assessment of how others will respond to the rape sometimes extends to persons who are not related by blood but significant to her. In the following example, one victim describes her rationale for not initially disclosing the rape to her girlfriend's mother; finally the mother has to be informed that the daughter is testifying at the trial.

### CLINICAL EXAMPLE

*Victim:* Nancy (the girlfriend) was fearful that her social life would be restricted if she told her mom. So, we didn't tell her and that didn't happen. Now her mom realizes she can't rule Nancy's social life because the rape happened so long ago and she's seen that we've been safe ever since. When my mom found out there was no need for rules, I didn't go out. She didn't have to set down barriers. I used to be social and friendly but I stopped that. She let me get back to myself gradually.

*Nurse:* You're really lucky. Some moms get pretty upset.

*Victim:* If she would've said, "You can't do this, or you can't go there, or be home at this time," I would've been scared that I'd get raped again and again. I was always with Nancy, or two or three girlfriends. She knew I wouldn't take a chance. If she'd hovered over me I would've been more scared.

Frequently a situation will arise that requires the victim to disclose the rape even though she would prefer to keep it a secret. Events prompting disclosure of the rape include (1) need of parental signature for medical care, (2) indiscreet appearance of the victim's name in the newspaper, (3) sexual relations that deteriorate with one's partner or are so traumatic (aversion, vaginisimus, flashbacks, physical discomfort with sex, inorgasmic response)[4] that the partner seeks an explanation, (4) a decision to prosecute the assailant and desire for support from one's social network, and (5) stress reactions that are so severe that the rape cannot be concealed from others. A previously concealed rape presents a new set of problems to cope with. Persons not confided in often feel hurt, reevaluate their relationship with the victim, and wonder where they have failed because the victim did not confide in them.

In the following clinical example, the nurse provided counseling to a family while they were in the process of supporting their daughter in prosecuting a rapist. The family prepared for the trial by talking about all the events that had transpired at the time of the rape, including questions the rapist's defense attorney would ask about why the victim had not immediately told her family about the event. The mother talked about her feelings of having been "protected" from the upsetting news. In this situation the victim had wanted the family's support in resolving the crisis she felt, but she did not know how to tell her parents about the rape. So she came to the crisis center where the nurse working as a volunteer counselor talked with her. The victim was raped on the weekend and waited until Monday morning to call the crisis center from school at which time an appointment was scheduled for her that day. The victim's concerns were explored during the counseling session. Then she was assisted in filing a complaint with the police charging the assailant with rape, and she was accompanied to an emergency room for a rape examination. Her parents were notified from the detective's office to meet their daughter at the emergency department. When they arrived, the nurse volunteer counselor from the crisis center talked with them in the waiting room. The parents did not know about the rape until 3 days later.

CLINICAL EXAMPLE

*Nurse:*   What do you recall about how the family found out about the rape?

*Mother:*   I was upset.

*Victim:*   I told the detective to tell my dad. I kept crying everytime I tried to tell him so I told the detective to do it.

*Nurse:*   (to mother) What were you upset about?

*Mother:*   Jenny (the victim) hadn't told me that this even happened, it was three days before I knew about it. I always thought this happened to someone else. She told her brother about it and he hadn't told me either!

*Nurse:*   What do you recall about our conversation at the hospital?

*Mother:*   Not much, I was upset.

*Victim:*   You were angry with me! You called me Jennifer and you only do that when you're mad at me! (Laughed warmly acknowledging mother's feelings.)

*Mother:*   Well, I wouldn't have known what to do anyway.

*Nurse:*   Why do you think you would not have known what to do?

*Mother:*   I'm not prepared for anything like this.

*Victim:*   I didn't even know what to do (empathizes with mother). My brother said to tell the cops but we didn't know which ones to tell, and I didn't want them putting my name in the newspaper.

*Mother:*   I'm no good in emergency rooms; I fall apart. We haven't had any big emergencies except this one.

*Nurse:*   When Jenny talked with us at the crisis center she was trying to figure out what to do. She said she didn't want to tell you because she'd upset you.

*Mother:*   Wouldn't any mother be upset?

*Victim:*   Yeh, but I couldn't handle your being upset.

*Nurse:*   When Jenny talked with me she said she didn't want to upset you. She had some sense that if she told you, you'd fall apart. So, she came to the crisis center to get some help on what to do.

*Mother:* Sometimes I get more upset not being told.

*Victim:* (defensively replied) The detectives said Dan (the brother) knew and that Dan had told you.

*Nurse:* (to mother) What about not being told was upsetting?

*Mother:* I thought Jenny should have told me instead of her brother. Later on I thought I wouldn't know what to tell her or what to do anyway. I never knew about the rape crisis center and he did.

*Victim:* Dan (the brother) said to call the cops. I knew that if I told you I'd have to help you, and two bawling people (mother and victim) are useless.

*Nurse:* (to mother) Were you feeling inadequate that night?

*Mother:* Yes.

*Nurse:* Were you feeling left out by Jenny in being able to be a mother?

*Mother:* Very much so.

*Victim:* If more women knew about the rape crisis center it would be easier for them to tell their parents. In health class in 10th grade we had a talk about rape, but not about what to do if you were raped.

In the above clinical example, the nurse helped the mother openly express feelings about not being immediately informed of the rape by the victim. The nurse activated qualities characteristic of healthy family functioning: (1) open and direct communication with one another, (2) respect for the unique way each person perceived his or her experience, (3) warm and caring association with one another, and (4) spontaneity and laughter. In the counseling session with the nurse, the family members arrived at a cognitive understanding of what the victim's decision to delay disclosure meant to one another and an appreciation for the other's feelings about that action.

Effective nursing interventions with families concerned about disclosing the rape include the following:

1. Reserving personal judgment about whether the family "should" disclose the rape to others. Evidence suggests that the family's assessment of anticipated responses and the consequences of informing their family or friends about a traumatic event is accurate; the family is generally the best judge of how significant others will react, whether that is positive or negative.[13]

2. Helping the family identify *who to tell* among friends and relatives. This involves deciding who will be supportive and understanding so that the family can share the rape event and their feelings.

3. Exploring *how to tell* others about the rape. This might include answering such questions as: Should I be matter-of-fact? What will they think of me if they see me this upset and crying? Can I seek their help? I'm just numb from all this—what will they think if I'm not looking upset? Can I depend on them to keep this confidential?

4. Discussing *what to tell* others about the rape. This might include answering these questions: Should I tell them all the details of what happened? Should I tell them only essential information? What terms or words can I use? Can they tolerate hearing about it and how I feel?

5. Exploring the *type of help requested*. This might include questions such as: Will I be forced to report or make the victim report? Can I depend on them? Will they feel sorry for me? I don't want to be a burden to them—should I ask for help? Should I expect them to be supportive?

6. Helping the family identify the persons they do not want to know about the rape, their fears and fantasies about expected repercussions, and their rationale for these decisions.
7. Discussing the ways in which a felt sense of crisis is reduced by sharing traumatic events with significant others (activate support systems) or, alternately, how stress is increased when people attempt to handle traumatic events alone.
8. Exploring concerns about a partner or parents misperceiving the rape as a sexually motivated act (see discussion below).
9. Exploring concerns about relationships in the family being negatively affected if others (such as mates, siblings, or grandparents) know about the rape.

*Reacting to rape as a sexually motivated act.* Husbands and boyfriends frequently view rape as a sexually motivated act rather than an act of violence. This attitude often stimulates conflict in their relationship with the victim.[11] However, parents, extended kin, or significant others in the victim's social network may also express similar beliefs about rape. Families are subject to the same mythology about rape that the general populace believes. They may firmly believe that "only promiscuous women get raped," "no woman can be raped against her will (consent)," "all women really want to be raped (have sex)," or "real rapes only occur between total strangers."

Whether or not the victim remembers the details of the rape, if the family needs to see her as having consented to illicit sexual relations, that is the reaction the nurse will observe. Often when families believe that the victim consented to sex, their response is emotional, firmly held, and not amenable to interventions that counter their position by logic. It is important for the nurse to intervene by focusing on the family's misperception of rape as a sexually motivated act and on their feelings about the victim having been subjected to a sexual crime or offense. Often the family's angry reaction serves to mask a partner's feelings of insecurity about sexual adequacy or prowess, or feelings about the emergence of a child's sexuality with others, which they have not previously confronted. The following clinical example illustrates this point.

CLINICAL EXAMPLE

*Victim:* Marian is a 14-year-old who was raped one evening at a party following a volleyball game. She was an attractive young girl who was captain of her team. Marian states she resented her mother's need to know where she was all the time because she felt her mother did not trust her. She said that her mother's behavior made her feel that the rape was all her fault, not the assailant's. To cope with her parents Marian said she kept quiet and busy. She reported that she had no memory of most of the rape.

*Mother:* Mrs. N. reported having a lot of feelings about the rape she had not been able to get out very well. She said she had been feeling fearful, depressed, having crying spells, increased agitation, and sleep disturbances.

*Father:* Mr. N. told his wife that she spent too much time thinking about the rape and that she needed to "find something to distract" herself from thinking about it all the time. He said the rape was "taking up

> too much of his valuable time" and he did not understand why his wife just didn't get over it.
>
> *Mother:* Mrs. N. said that Marian should not have been in the role of team captain, that "if only" she had not been in that role this would not have happened because she would have been with a different crowd. Mrs. N. felt guilty for not having chauffeured her daughter to the party.
>
> *Victim:* Marian said she resented being grilled at the dinner table about what she did or didn't do all day and the unreasonable rules her parents had put upon her.
>
> *Father:* Mr. N. said that as long as Marian wasn't upset and went about her business he wasn't sure she was *really* raped. He wasn't sure if he *really* believed her.
>
> *Victim:* Marian was stunned by her father's statement. She did not reply and withdrew from the conversation.
>
> *Parents:* Mr. and Mrs. N. continued to focus on not trusting or believing Marian because she had not been where she was supposed to be on the night of the rape. To the parents Marian's change of plans meant she had had "illegitimate" sex, and they were unable to view her changing plans as typical or normal adolescent behavior.

In the above clinical example, Marian was not upset over the rape because she was coping with the event by blocking it from her memory. Mrs. N. was experiencing post-rape stress responses that victims report, particularly since her husband was coping by disengaging himself and by minimizing her feelings. His attitude left her feeling a lack of understanding and support. Mrs. N. blamed Marian for the rape and thus avoided her own sense of guilt stemming from a misperception that she had not "properly" carried out her role as family manager of activities (chauffeuring). She coped by an "If only . . . this would not have happened" reaction (discussed below). Marian felt upset about causing her mother to feel upset (responsibility issue: Who is the *real* victim?). Mrs. N. wanted Marian to "feel upset," otherwise she could not believe her because "legitimate" victims are upset or hysterical and certainly remember the rape (rape mythology operating). Because Marian was not upset, the family system adapted by Mrs. N. paradoxically expressing post-rape symptoms. The faulty assumption operating here was that the impact on Marian had to be the same as the impact on Mrs. N. Otherwise Mr. and Mrs. N. could not believe that Marian had been raped— that is, she had "illegitimate" sex in their viewpoint.

Concern over sexual adequacy is seen in the reaction of men who insist on having sex with the victim on the night of the assault in order to: (1) test their sexual prowess and feelings toward the victim, (2) focus exclusively on their own sexual needs, (3) test whether their sexual relationship with the victim has changed as a result of the rape, and (4) confirm that if the woman is available to the rapist she is similarly available to the partner.[11] It is not uncommon for family members who perceive rape as a sexually motivated act to doubt the victim's account of what happened to her, criticize (scapegoat) her for using poor judgment (assuming she could have avoided the rape), and even accuse the victim of enjoying the encounter (which they may attempt to verify by questioning whether she reached orgasm).[16] Victims find doubtfulness on the part of significant others an expression of anger that is insulting and distressing; they can hardly believe they are hearing such retorts. When family members are highly overreactive, some victims counter the feeling state by withdrawing and underreacting. Unfortunately, the family tends to see the victim's seeming nonreactivity as an implication of her guilt. Finally, when rape is viewed as a sexually motivated act, the family or significant others frequently view the victim as *their* "damaged" property (see discussion below).

Effective nursing interventions with families that misperceive rape as a sexually motivated act include the following:

1. Assessing value systems related to sexuality that are potentially harmful in relationships, particularly because these values escalate post-rape:
   a. The double standard (it is okay for men to have more than one sexual partner but not women), which establishes asymmetrical sexual exclusiveness in the relationship and fosters victim guilt
   b. Expectations of a mutually exclusive sexual relationship
   c. The premise that a sexual relationship is "sinful" unless the woman is married to the man and/or the woman is an "adult" according to the family's rules[11]
2. Helping the family members become aware that they are responding to the rape as though it were a sexually motivated act as seen in their expressed value system.
3. Avoiding open criticism of families that express beliefs that differ from those of the nurse. Attacking family members for their beliefs only heightens their sense of victimization: first by the rape of a loved one, and second by a critical attack from the nurse. The net effect of such an attack is to close off the nurse as a potential support system and to reduce the nurse's potential effectiveness as a crisis intervention agent.
4. Establishing and maintaining a climate of understanding, acceptance, and noncritical judgment in which the family feels free to ventilate or express their concerns.
5. Recognizing statements that express a "damaged property" perspective: "No one will want to date her now," "I don't think I want to stay in this relationship," or "What if my friends find out my wife was raped!"
6. Reassuring the family that although the victim will not forget what happened, her memory of the event will not be so intense or painful in time, particularly if she is given the emotional space needed to heal psychologic wounds and if she has their support.
7. Exploring the family's basic sense of hurt, injury, disappointment, and helplessness.
8. Helping the family focus on their pain and loss.
9. Helping the family recognize that they too are suffering from the tragedy their loved one endured.
10. Indicating that when we view people as able to cope or recover they generally do, and that to expect them to be handicapped for life only sets up a potentially damaging self-fulfilling prophecy.
11. Identifying and fostering direct expression of rape myths in a nonjudgmental manner.
12. Identifying and fostering direct expression of misapprehensions about the

victim's sexuality or the partner's concerns over sexual prowess in a nonjudgmental environment.

13. Assisting parents of an adolescent or young adult with their struggle to resolve overprotective behaviors or surveillance of their child's (sexual) activities by talking over their fears about repeated rape, sexual promiscuity, discrimination in judgment or decision-making, or emotional separation.

14. Talking with the family about normal family-life tasks that they must work through (such as feelings about a child's emerging sexuality with others) and showing them this is something they would have to do at some point; that is, the rape crisis is giving them the "opportunity" to work through this life task sooner than otherwise. Here the nurse's goal is to shift the focus from rape as a sexually motivated act to normal developmental issues within the family.

15. Referring the family for therapy if reactivity, restrictiveness, and unreasonable rules persist, creating high levels of family conflict or victim maladaptation.

*Viewing the victim as "damaged" property.* Traditional views of rape assert that the woman is the man's property and thus he (not she) is the injured party in the rape experience. Men who hold such beliefs experience a personal sense of devaluation and shame about the rape. Conflict arises in the family over who is the "real" victim or the "more injured" party and this impedes mutually supportive behavior in resolving the crisis. It is important for the nurse to be aware that these feelings are multiply determined because of the way people have been socialized. Silverman suggests that these feelings reflect

> male attitudes about feminine sexuality, the veneration of virginity, and a sense of entitlement to "exclusive rights" to that sexuality . . . unconscious concerns about homosexuality stirred by having been "had" by the rapist when "he took my woman," or discomfort associated with the excitement of "sharing a woman with another man."[16]

The family's anger masks their belief that the victim permitted herself to become "tainted" or "damaged goods" unsuitable for "trade" in marriage or that the victim needs purification to reestablish acceptability to her partner. Clearly these reactions increase the victim's sense of humiliation and worthlessness.

Effective nursing interventions with families that view the victim as "damaged property" include:

1. Self-awareness in relation to family attitudes the nurse believes to be chauvinistic, traditional, unenlightened, provocative, or "dumb."

2. Encouraging the family to be hopeful and to believe in the victim's healing capacity.

3. Pointing out (when possible) that this crisis is like other crises they have already survived and recovered from (which suggests that they will recover from this one as well).[16]

*Thoughts about violent retribution.* "Well, what do you expect? Isn't it normal to go after someone who has badly hurt someone you love?" This frequently expressed attitude represents the family's identification with the victim as well as their effort to cope with a shared sense of crisis. For example, one father threatened to "send out a hit man to get every guy on the list," but later he disavowed that he would carry out such a plan. Some men get weapons and drive around the neighborhood or the rape site, not just on the night of the assault but many nights, "looking for the bastard" so they can "blow his brains out." Meanwhile the victim is often left alone with no one to comfort her in her crisis state. Such actions by "protecting avengers" only serve to heighten the victim's already-intense fear and anxiety; the victim becomes further burdened in calming down the rage of those about her, placating them, and trying to convince them that their efforts "in her behalf" are in fact harmful.[16]

Effective nursing interventions with families that respond to rape of a loved one with thoughts about violent retribution include:

1. Helping the family recognize this response as masking a sense of utter helplessness, rage, and vulnerability that they share with the victim
2. Helping the family express feelings of guilt for not having protected the victim
3. Encouraging, through empathic "active" listening, the expression of feelings of hurt and sadness
4. Gently pointing out that acts of retribution might make them feel better but fail to be supportive of the victim
5. Encouraging cooperation with the criminal justice system to ensure that the rapist is convicted and receives treatment

In general, the nurse attempts to redirect the energy from intense feelings toward active participation in programs for rape prevention, public education, assistance to other victims and their families, and revision of the legal system toward more equitable and sensitive treatment of victims.[14]

*"If only" reactions.* "If only" reactions are a form of magical thinking characteristic of childhood years. Magical thinking consists of *believing* that if we simply wish, think, fear, dream, or say something it *will* come true or be *made* to happen. With adults this type of thinking is an adjustment reaction resorted to when they are severely stressed, and it is frequently expressed as self-imposed guilt.[12] Often family members will express a sense of responsibility for the rape because "if only" they had been available to the victim "this wouldn't have happened." Some families express their "if only" reaction through overprotection, as shown in the example below.

CLINICAL EXAMPLE

*Nurse:*   Are you going to the prom?
*Victim:*   If she (mother) lets me go! I'll have a date but she's worried and it spoils my fun knowing she's at home stewing about me.
*Mother:*   I don't know the kid.
*Nurse:*   Have you talked about how you'll get rides to the prom?
*Victim:*   She'll drive. She (mother) won't let me go with others.
*Mother:*   Your fun is more important than mine at the club (punishing herself). And you know I hate chauffering!
*Nurse:*   What's your reaction to your mom giving her night up for you?
*Victim:*   I think it's very considerate of her. I don't think you *need* to stay home.
*Mother:*   (humorously) You don't sound very convinced.
*Father:*   (to mother) I think you've got to get over this. You don't *need* to stay at home. You've got to get over being so overprotective.

> *Mother:* Oh, I know that. What bothers me is that on the night of the rape I wasn't home, I was out with my friends.
> *Nurse:* And if you had been there it wouldn't have happened?
> *Mother:* I know it's baloney! It would have happened anyway. We're even going out to a show tonight and leaving Terry alone (reporting active attempt to counter her fears and guilt).
> *Victim:* (humorously) Wow! You mean you're gonna leave me alone!
> *Nurse:* (to mother) You're punishing yourself.
> *Mother:* Yeah, I know. I'm doing better though. I know it's not my fault. I just feel so awful about it.

Family members may feel responsible for the rape if it occurred after an argument that spurred the victim to act in a way she otherwise would not have acted. For example, one woman reported going jogging late at night by herself after a heated argument to "run off some steam" and "get off by myself for awhile so I could think things through." When people are stressed, they are more at risk; since they are less aware of their environment, they may find themselves in situations that they would ordinarily avoid. For example, one victim's husband said, "If only I hadn't let her go by herself, this wouldn't have happened. It was such a dumb argument. I wish I hadn't been so bull-headed."

Effective nursing interventions with families that respond to rape with "if only" reactions include:

1. Helping the family understand their feelings as an attempt to relieve their sense of guilt and responsibility for the rape
2. Helping family members explore feelings of failure in protecting the victim from the assault
3. Exploring family members' feelings of helplessness, hurt, and pain
4. Helping the family members to realistically evaluate events related to the rape in order to reduce self-blame
5. Exploring what the family might have done differently to correctly evaluate neglect, destructive behaviors, or high-risk situations
6. Pointing out that "if only" responses imply to the victim that without her protector, she is a "defenseless" person
7. Indicating that "if only" reactions infantilize the victim, thereby interfering with her adaptive coping behaviors that would support her autonomy and self-esteem[16]

Every family responds differently to the rape of a loved one. Although post-rape responses are not pathological, they imply a state of vulnerability and risk as the family works to reestablish a state of equilibrium. Some of the responses experienced in the acute reaction phase may continue into or be reactivated by varying stimuli in the long-term reorganization process that follows.

## LONG-TERM REORGANIZATION

The long-term effects of rape on the victim's social network are only beginning to be researched and reported in the literature. After recovering from feelings and reactions of the acute crisis, families face issues related to (1) the victim's sexuality, (2) disrupted relationships, (3) coping with the victim's phobic behaviors or rape trauma syndrome, and (4) the court process.

## Sexuality

It is not surprising that the victim's sexuality becomes a troublesome issue for those closest to her. Recall that some people view the victim as having solicited her own victimization, as having gone "looking for sex," and subsequently perceive her as "damaged merchandise." In addition, many people view sexual intimacy with another person as a confirmation of emotional attachment to that person. The "waters are muddied," therefore, when family members misperceive rape as a sexually motivated act in which emotional attachment exists between offender and victim. In such cases the victim has a hard time convincing her partner that her love for him is real, that it has not been "tainted."

It is understandable that victims may have an initial *aversion to resuming sexual activity* with their partner. Sexual behaviors that were previously satisfying and pleasurable to the woman were forced on her during the rape. Therefore many victims report an aversion to sexual behaviors that occurred during the rape episode because these acts are specific to the pain and fear they experienced when they were forced on them. In general, women report no disturbance in their level of satisfaction with behaviors that did *not* occur during the rape. Acts not part of the rape usually consist of primary affectionate behaviors (such as hand-holding) or autoerotic behaviors (such as clitoral stimulation).[6] Resuming sexual activity may precipitate the experiencing of flashbacks of the rape for some women. One victim reported, "Every time I close my eyes I feel like it's happening all over again." Other distressing factors victims report having to cope with include (1) difficulty reaching orgasm or experiencing sexual feelings, (2) vaginisimus, (3) decreased or increased sexual activity, (4) physical discomfort during sex, and (5) coping with their partner's reaction.[3,16]

If the rape involved an assault on an adolescent or young adult, the parents are confronted with the issue of the child's sexuality. Because many in this age group are not sexually active, it may be necessary for the nurse to explain to the parents that rape does not imply a sexually active life-style. In instances in which young rape victims have been sexually active, they are often sensitive to their sexual behavior as an issue that would arouse parental disapproval. In addition, many mothers who have young adult or adolescent daughters who are raped will use the rape episode to talk about how they learned about sex, their views on premarital sex, their own experience with rape or sexual abuse, and fears that their daughter will think that all sexual relations are like the rape. For example, one mother stated:

> I kept trying to tell her that making love was different than the rape, that she would find sexual relations enjoyable. Even if she couldn't believe that now, I wanted her to know that at some time it would be different for her.

Effective nursing interventions with families that are working through conflicts related to the victim's sexuality or disrupted sexual satisfaction include:

1. Role-playing with family members about how to talk about the rape and acts that transpired during the assault
2. Encouraging increased empathic responses among family members or between partners

3. Exploring the potential relationship between worrying over a partner's reaction to the rape and difficulty in recovering sexual satisfaction in the relationship, rather than focusing on post-rape sexual difficulties as necessarily or only related to the rape
4. Conveying that the family will develop greater control over damaging overt and covert communications by coming to terms with their feelings and by being open to information about the nature of rape as a violent rather than sexual act
5. Helping family members desexualize the rape episode
6. Discouraging overfocusing on sexual activity
7. Suggesting that the victim assume charge of when sexual activity occurs
8. Encouraging a relaxed, romantic atmosphere for foreplay activities
9. Having the couple identify sexually arousing stimuli and avoiding sexually aversive stimuli
10. Encouraging integration of sexuality as part of a holistic partner relationship
11. Developing positive experiences by successive approximations of satisfying sexual experiences that reshape the relationship for the couple
12. Establishing a realistic time-frame for working through sexual concerns and refering to experts in sexuality counseling if no progress is felt

At this time very little empirical data is available regarding the impact of rape on the victim's sexual behavior or sexual satisfaction. However, it is clear that comprehensive treatment of rape victims needs to include sexual counseling to ameliorate the negative impact of rape on sexual satisfaction with one's partner; or, at the very least, information needs to be provided about where to obtain sexual counseling or therapy from a reputable professional.[6]

## Disrupted relationships

Regardless of the nature of the family unit or social network, rape is disruptive to the relationships of those whose lives it impacts. The literature indicates that between 50 and 80% of women who are raped suffer the loss of their boyfriend or husband as a result of the assault.[10] If relationship difficulties existed prior to the rape, the crisis precipitated by rape usually exacerbates these problems. The rape then becomes triangled as the issue over which the couple or family then focuses on and is symptomatic of long-standing difficulties that preceded the rape. If more families availed themselves of preventive counseling services, the severing of many relationships could be prevented and the losses sustained as a result of rape could be resolved.

Effective nursing interventions with families that experience disrupted relationships as a result of rape include:
1. Identification of families that are a high risk for familial disruption
2. Preventive counseling for families as standard protocol in post-rape counseling
3. Implementing counseling interventions according to the presenting problem of the family (e.g., sexuality or blaming)
4. Referral to family therapists experienced in working with families and victims of violence

5. Divorce or separation counseling that includes supportive measures for families working through grief and mourning processes

## Coping with phobic behaviors

Following rape many victims experience a variety of fears: (1) of being alone, (2) of being in crowds, (3) of going outside the home, or (4) of people walking behind them.[4] This phobic behavior is an expression of the victim's intense fear and an attempt to regain control over her life by avoiding situations that she defines as threatening. Likewise, family response can include phobic behaviors. For example, if a young adult was raped in her home, the parents or other family members may have difficulty leaving her alone.

Some families also report counterphobic behaviors. Family members may repeat certain actions in an attempt to convince themselves or others that they are in control of the conflictual situation. For example, one father repeatedly walked by the location where his daughter was raped "just to prove" to himself or others that he was in control of the situation. Phobic and counterphobic behaviors often indicate that the family has not resolved conflicts precipitated by the rape. Generally, phobic behaviors seen in an acute reaction phase are understandable as an expression of intense fear and anxiety in response to the rape. If phobic behaviors persist after a crisis period or for several months, they are symptomatic of a more serious difficulty that often requires professional intervention.

Phobic behaviors often discourage family members because they seem to represent a setback in the family's recovery process. The family may report feeling discouraged, depressed, annoyed, or intolerant of the phobic behavior. Frequently family members have given a great deal of support to the victim during the immediate crisis. Therefore they may feel emotionally drained and unable to continue being supportive to anyone working through phobic responses. The strain on the family is even greater when family units are without the immediate support of extended kin.

Effective nursing interventions with families coping with phobic behavior include:

1. Enlisting the help of the family with a treatment program specific to phobias
2. Explaining the nature of the phobic behaviors and the function they serve for family members
3. Participating in a behavior modfication program designed to desensitize the family to the phobic behavior
4. Teaching families cognitive restructuring strategies to refute thoughts that reinforce phobic behaviors (see Chapter 9 for discussion of such strategies), to invalidate unrealistic fears, and to facilitate coping with anxiety
5. Offering counseling to provide an opportunity for the family to express concerns to an understanding professional

### The court process

The court process is as upsetting for the family as it is for the victim. The victim finds the court process, particularly the cross-examination, a symbolic repeat rape. When the family members closely identify with the victim's rape, they often report experiencing a repeat rape.[11] Likewise, the family's responses to court proceedings are often similar to those of the victim (see Chapter 9). Delays and insensitive treatment take their toll on the family members as well as on the victim. In the following account, one victim reports her parents' response to the delay of her trial.

CLINICAL EXAMPLE

*Nurse:*  How did the delay affect your family?

*Victim:*  My mom went back to work and my dad went to the bar to drown his sorrows. He went to a Little League game and back to the bar again. My dad said, "Why all the delay? Just cancel the trial and forget it!" I said, "No, I've done the toughest part. I won't drop it now." He was really mad. He said, "So now we *all* have to go through it two months more!" I asked my mom if she wanted me to drop it too. She said, "No, I'm behind you all the way." If dad hadn't been drinking, he could have been more serious and we could have gotten somewhere in the discussion. He's really upset. I told him, "If you don't want me to talk about it, I won't mention it in front of you." Dad said, "This puts us *all* through it. We *all* go through this, not just you." Later I asked if I could use his bus pass. He wanted to know where I was going. I said, "Nowhere." But I knew I was coming down here to see you . . . just wouldn't talk about it anymore in front of him. Then I got a phone call and I said, "Wait a minute. I have to leave the room." I was being sarcastic and humorous. My mom knew what was going on, she started to chuckle.

*Nurse:*  So the *whole family* is affected by it and needs some way to wait out the two months.

*Victim:*  Yeah. Like Tuesday I couldn't stand waiting at home for the call to come down to the courthouse. I said. "Let's go down there!" My mom said, "Ask your dad." Dad said, "Sure, if you want to go let's go. Whatever you want to do." Both my parents took the whole day off work.

Nurses will find that families cope with the stress of the court process as they have handled other highly stressful situations. The stressor (court process) activates the use of coping mechanisms that have been helpful in the past, and those variables that characterize the family's degree of health or dysfunction become prominent. For example, in the above clinical example, the victim was able to understand her father's reaction to the court delay in terms of the stress it created for him. The family used humor and sarcasm to cope. They openly shared feelings and disagreements, were sensitive to each other's feelings, and were supportive of one another's needs.

The court process differs from other stressors because the family must cope with the guilty or not-guilty verdict and its meaning in their lives. Most often the family is upset by a not-guilty verdict. The account that follows shows one family's reaction to a not-guilty verdict. In this case the victim had waited 18 months for the trial to be held. During that time the courts heard petitions regarding whether or not a victim's record of counseling at the crisis center could be subpoenaed without her consent for the defense attorney's use. By the time the trial was scheduled to start, the family had begun to resolve the rape crisis and were "thrown back into" intense feelings about the rape. Yet at the same time they were anxious to see the trial take place because they had waited a long time.

CLINICAL EXAMPLE

*Mother:* I can't believe they came up with a not-guilty verdict. It just doesn't seem real.

*Victim:* How can they arrive at such an absurd conclusion! The defense attorney made me look like an idiot. He had this map that made it look like I was a couple blocks from home, when it was several miles in the dead of winter! He made it look like I could get out of the car with great ease, when in fact every time I unlocked the door he (the rapist) slapped the lock back down and restrained me even tighter.

*Father:* I called my brother out West and told him it looked like it was time to take the law into our hands again, like in the old times. There's no justice in the courts. It just isn't worth it.

*Victim:* There he is, out on the street again scot-free. I'll bet he's just snickering his head off. He did it again: first, the rape he got away with, and now he got over at the trial! I have some friends with a revolver who said they'd shoot him for me, but I told them "no," if anybody did it, it would be me. The rape happened to me, not them.

*Mother:* You can't do that. You can't shoot him. He'll get his justice in time.

*Nurse:* Who else have you been able to talk to about what happened at the trial?

*Mother:* I talked with my brother and my mother.

*Nurse:* Was that of any help to you?

*Mother:* Some, but not much. What can anyone do to make you feel good about injustice?

*Nurse:* How have you handled your feelings other times when you've been real upset?

*Mother:* Well, I usually talk with my brother and mother, and my husband some. Sometimes I let my boss at work know what is going on.

*Father:* We just talk about it here in the family. Sometimes I talk with the men I bowl with, and sometimes I just get drunk.

*Mother:* I'm worried about Celina (the victim).

*Nurse:* What have you done to settle your worries.

*Mother:* Well, I told her I would commit her before I would let her shoot him. Enough harm has been done, she doesn't need to spend her life in jail.

Nurses intervene in a family's distress surrounding a not-guilty verdict by applying principles of crisis intervention and basic counseling (see Chapter 7). They foster the family's expression and ventilation of feelings and reinforce adaptive coping behaviors—for example, sharing feelings with each other, the nurse, and significant others in the family. At times it is necessary to ease the family's grief and mourning, redirect anger into constructive activities such as work or sports, and help the family arrive at a perspective of the rape and the trial as one of many events in their life.

Families resolve the impact of rape on their lives through varying periods of growth and recovery. There is no way to predict how long it will take the family to recover from the rape; resolution depends on the family's ability to work through the issues that confront them. According to systems theory, what affects our fellow man ultimately affects each one of us. It is important, therefore, that nurses help families of rape victims to regain an optimal degree of healthy functioning and happiness in life. Ackerman has aptly stated:

> None of us lives his life alone. Those who try are foredoomed; they disintegrate as human beings. Some aspects of life experience are, to be sure, more individual than social, others more social than individual; but life is nonetheless a shared and a sharing experience. . . . The family is the basic unit of growth and experience, fulfillment or failure. It is also the basic unit of illness and health.[1]

## SUMMARY

In response to growing awareness of sexual assault as a problem and to the needs of victims, services have been primarily victim-oriented. Therefore the crisis and adaptation of indirect victims in the rape experience often have been ignored. Current research has marginally investigated family response to rape, and the majority of reported studies are retrospective in design. Current studies, which often report conflictual family response to rape, are biased because the clients seen for treatment are in distress when they seek help; in most cases their response patterns, as well as the therapeutic interventions implemented, are not compared to those of families with similar characteristics and experiencing an equivalent traumatic event.

An increasing amount of clinical evidence supports the importance of the victim's social network in post-rape counseling. Indirect victims clearly experience a response to rape that is comparable to the victim's own response. The social network has a tremendous potential for both negative and positive influence: for either revictimizing the victim and increasing her burden in resolving the rape, or providing the victim with support and finding support themselves in resolving a shared crisis. Interventions for families of rape victims generally are of two types: one encourages the expression of feelings in response to a shared life crisis; the other refutes misconceptions and offers strategies for coping with the crisis. Pivotal in restoring the victim's equilibrium is the response of those closest to her. However, often she and they are in self-imposed isolation or shamed into silence.

Clinicians and researchers are interested in what happens to the families that do *not* seek counseling post-rape. Are they more disturbed than those that do? Are they healthier and more able to resolve the crisis than families that seek help? If so, what makes it possible for them to get along so well in the aftermath of rape? The answers to these questions are not available yet because caregivers and researchers have not even reached all the direct and indirect victims that come into their system for care—let alone the many persons at large who have never sought help.

Current literature disagrees on the type and interpretation of response to rape by indirect victims. Subjective impressions offer only a weak base for planning effective intervention approaches. Researchers in the field generally concede that indirect victims of rape would benefit from some help in understanding their own feelings and those of the victim in relation to the assault.

As yet nurses do not know if the needs of indirect victims are best met through individual counseling or through intervention approaches designed for couples or families. Nurses need to know more about the value of family intervention approaches for victims living with parents, in single-parent families, or in blended or alternative family forms. Nurses *do* know that development of cognitive understanding, ventilation of feelings, and crisis intervention principles are essential in providing care to families regardless of their structure.

It is disappointing and hurtful for victims to discover that they cannot count on those persons that mean the most to them, and that trusted persons may also victimize them. However, nurses and other professionals who try to help families with their pain are generally optimistic that the difficulties experienced by direct victims and those closest to them can be resolved. Kliman has poignantly expressed the importance of providing nursing care to families in crisis in this way:

> In this age of plastic products, pocket computers, and supersonic transportation, human values and interactions need ever more tender nurturing and conservation. We can commit ourselves to saving an endangered species of wildlife, or preserving a tract of wilderness, but how unecological of us to waste our nearest and most precious natural resource—our own families.[12]

## Learning activities

Below is a case situation followed by exercises related to primary social networks. Follow the instructions as indicated.

### Situation 1

Anne is a 19-year-old, white, single college student of middle-class background. She has been attending a university away from her rural hometown. Anne never lived in a metropolitan area before, and her parents were quite anxious about her safety. She was raised to believe that bad things only happen to "bad" people who deserve what they get. Since arriving on campus, Anne has made only a few acquaintances. She lives in a boarding home with several other girls. The landlady is motherlike and Anne likes her very much. Anne's teachers seem competent and Anne relates well to them. Anne misses her boyfriend and writes to him every day.

*Exercise 1:* Identify Anne's primary social network based on the relational provisions provided by these persons:

1.                          4.
2.                          5.
3.                          6.

### Situation 1 (continued)

Anne reported to the nurse at the student health clinic that after a late class she had smoked some marijuana with a girlfriend and relaxed. As she was returning home that evening, two men asked her for directions and then dragged her behind a campus building where they raped her. The men threatened to kill Anne if she did not comply and to take revenge later if she reported the rape to the police.

Anne says she does not want her parents to know about the rape. She is afraid they will withdraw financial support for her education unless she returns to live at home and study at the local community college. The nurse tells Anne to notify her parents so they can be a support to her, and she insists that Anne obtain medical care.

*Exercise 2:* Answer the following questions.

1. What new positions and roles has Anne assumed?
2. What primary network relationships are influencing Anne's responses?
3. In attempting to help Anne cope with variables affecting her stress state, the nurse intervenes in which of the following ways:
   a. Suggests that Anne talk with at least one close peer about her experience; says she might find the advocate at the rape crisis center helpful in this respect.
   b. Recommends that Anne take a hot bath, listen to music, or read a book when she gets home to help her relax and forget the incident.
   c. Tells Anne all she needs to do right now is talk with the police, sign the consent forms, and complete the remainder of the interview.
   d. Suggests that Anne pull herself together so she can decide about whether or not to take the morning-after pill (DES).
4. When Anne regrets not fighting and blames herself for the rape, the nurse intervenes in which of the following ways:
   a. Agrees that it wasn't very smart of Anne to smoke a "joint" and go walking alone late at night, that she set herself up for the assault.
   b. States that Anne reported being threatened with her life if she resisted and that she did all anyone could do under terrifying circumstances.
   c. Suggests that Anne get into therapy to sort out her role in the incident and resolve her guilt feelings.
   d. Says: "I don't think you should've smoked a joint, but don't worry because everything always works out for the best."
5. Explain the rationale for the answers selected in questions 4 and 5 above.

### Situation 1 (continued)

At the hospital the ED staff encourages Anne to report the assault to the police to help protect other young women on campus. However, Anne isn't really sure she wants to report the rape and defers the decision. During the rape examination Anne appears to be quite calm, conveying an attitude of "No problem, I can handle anything, including this." The doctor tells Anne that if she misses her period she has several options, which he lists for her. After the doctor leaves the room, Anne is in a state of shock and mumbles in a barely audible voice, "Oh my God! What'll I do if I'm pregnant? I don't believe in abortions. What do you think I should do?" Exhausted, Anne then begins to cry uncontrollably. She rebuffs the nurse's attempts to be supportive by saying, "I'm fine. Really . . . I'm fine and I'll be okay . . . This is stupid of me to be so upset . . . Why didn't I fight back more? . . . It wouldn't have happened if I hadn't smoked a joint . . . Maybe I should go home . . . No, I'm really just fine. I guess I'll go back to the boardinghouse. Nobody here really understands me."

*Exercise 3:* Answer the following questions.

a. Based on Anne's behaviors, what nursing assessments can be made?

b. How can the nurse help Anne with her primary social network?

c. What types of primary social relationships does Anne need at this time?

d. Who can provide Anne with needed emotional support?

## Situation 1 (continued)

Anne copes by rebuffing the nurse's attempts to be supportive. The nurse tries to be supportive, understanding Anne's responses to the rape experience.

*Exercise 4:* Select the most appropriate nursing responses and give the rationale for your choices.

The nurse shows the best understanding of what Anne is experiencing by:

a. Telling Anne she should share her plight with others because research shows victims resolve the crisis better if they do.

b. Inquiring about why Anne thought she would be safe out alone at night in that part of the campus.

c. Commenting: "Obviously Anne's not 'just fine' after what she's been through, so she needn't try to hide it."

d. Stating: "It must be pretty scary to be alone in a strange city and wondering who to rely on at a time like this."

## Situation 2

Jessica is a 36-year-old, black, married woman with three children. Her husband works for a computer firm and is just beginning to get ahead in his career. Jessica has been going to night school to complete a B.S. degree, and her husband is able to stay with the children. Occasionally she takes advantage of the opportunity to be "out from under the kids" and stops to have a beer with a few classmates before returning home.

One such night on her way home, Jessica is stopped at a red light. Suddenly a man forces his way into her car, holds her at gunpoint, and makes her drive to a secluded park area. There he rapes her and then flees.

Once free of her assailant, Jessica drives to the ED for care. She is concerned about the "attitudes" she might encounter, especially since she had been drinking. Jessica tends to not trust whites because she has lived with so much discrimination. She expects not to be taken seriously at the ED and to be accused of inviting her own victimization (by drinking, being alone, leaving car doors unlocked).

At the ED Jessica tells the nurse that she was just raped. The nurse finds a comfortable place for her in the crowded waiting room (no private rooms are available). It is a busy evening in the ED (cardiac arrest case, a man with a stab wound), and Jessica waits 1 hour to be seen. She feels terrified from the assault but is glad to be alive. While waiting to be seen, Jessica struggles with how to tell her husband about the rape. She knows she is precious to him and that he will be upset. She has managed many upsets alone before and does not want to add her own difficulty to his efforts to manage the home, the children, and a career right now. Jessica also wonders what she will say to the children and how she should explain her brutalized appearance. She wonders what to say to the neighbors and what others would think about her. As Jessica waits, she becomes increasingly angry about what happened to her and about waiting so long for medical care. Jessica asks the nurse to call her husband to be with her. The nurse escorts her to the first available exam room, where she begins to cry and talk about the assault. As the rape exam is about to begin, Jessica's husband arrives along with her mother, sister, aunt, and mother-in-law.

*Directions:* Answer the following questions in relation to the above case situation. In each question identify the best responses the nurse could make. Explain your rationale for the choices made.

1.  After preparing Jessica for the physical exam, the nurse would:
    a.  Tell Jessica her family just arrived and ask if she would like one or more of them to be with her in the examining room.
    b.  Tell Jessica: "I asked your family to sit with you in the examining room because just think what it would do to them to worry about you in the waiting room!"
    c.  Suggest to Jessica that she stop crying so the nurse can talk with her and have her answer questions needed to complete the medical report.
    d.  Offer to bring Jessica and her family coffee or soft drinks while they are waiting for the physical exam to begin.
2.  When Jessica tells her family how she felt helpless and terrified, the nurse would:

    a. Reinforce that rape is a terrifying experience in order to encourage family members' support and reassurance of Jessica.

    b. Suggest that, just like in other crisis situations, Jessica is probably exaggerating her feelings a bit now and will feel less upset later.

    c. Not discourage family members' anger directed at the attacker or their need to blame someone, including themselves.

    d. Suggest that the family would be more helpful to Jessica if they were less expressive about their own sense of alarm because it only intensifies Jessica's feelings.

3. While the family members are sitting in the waiting room during the rape exam, the nurse would:

    a. Give them popular magazines to read to distract their attention from the crisis; ask them to help answer parts of the medical questionnaire.

    b. Call another nurse or advocate from the rape crisis center to be with them, explain what is happening, and answer their questions.

    c. Suggest that it is necessary for only one family member to remain and that the others can return home to get some rest.

    d. Allow the "strongest" family member to be with the victim during the exam.

4. During the physical exam, when Jessica's mother expresses regret that Jessica was not more careful—that she stopped for a drink and did not resist more—the nurse would:

    a. Comment that it would be difficult to prosecute and get a conviction because Jessica's character would be defamed as a result of her drinking.

    b. Tell the mother that many people believe the myth that they are responsible for the rape or could have prevented it "if only" the victim or family had done something different.

    c. Suggest that the family keep Jessica at home this week until she feels safe going out alone again, not let Jessica push herself.

    d. Ask the mother if she thinks Jessica needs to feel regret or shame when she was so terrified and hoped only to save her life.

5. When Jessica wonders if she is "going crazy," how she will manage her mothering functions in the next few days, and what the neighbors will say, the nurse would:

    a. Tell Jessica, in front of her family, that it would be best to schedule an appointment for counseling with the nurse or rape crisis center.

   b. Tell Jessica that her reaction is quite normal and reassure her family that many victims feel this way after the assault.

   c. Suggest to the family that they encourage Jessica to resume her normal activities in order to distract her from thinking about the rape and to minimize her depression.

   d. Tell the family that Jessica should pull herself together before going into the community because others *would* wonder if she was "going crazy" by acting uncontrolled.

## Situation 3

Judy is a 21-year-old single woman who comes from a very conservative home. She has been a stable person with a normal developmental history. When Judy graduated from college with honors, her parents gave her a trip to Mexico as a gift.

While in Mexico, Judy decides to do some backpacking for fun and to cut expenses by staying at youth hostels. She is looking forward to a rendezvous with her parents the next day and to attending a bullfight. However, that night, on her way to use the common bathroom in the hostel, a man grabs Judy, puts a knife to her throat, and pulls her into his room. The man threatens to put the knife "up her ass" and "cut her tits" if she does not comply with his demands. Judy struggles against being raped, but the man hits her on the head until she is nearly unconscious. Limp and scared to death, Judy complies with his demands, figuring it is better to be alive than dead. The man tells Judy to turn on her stomach and forces anal intercourse on her despite her cries from the pain of it. In terminating the rape the man urinates on Judy, takes her ID and travelers checks, and tells her not to report the assault or he will track her down and get revenge.

Judy waits until the man is gone. She thinks that she is to blame for the rape because it was stupid of her to travel alone. Judy grabs some clothing and makes her way to the front desk, where she tells the clerk that a stranger has just assaulted her. The desk clerk takes Judy to the local hospital for care. Judy is so scared—being in a strange country, her money and ID stolen, and her body invaded. She doesn't know how she can tell her parents about the rape, stating "they are really Victorian about sex." The nurse encourages Judy to contact her parents at least for financial support and to accept overnight hospitalization.

When the parents arrive, the ED nurse escorts them to Judy's room. The parents had thought Judy was only robbed, so they are stunned to find out about the rape. The parents feel responsible for Judy's rape because they let her travel alone. The mother expresses a sense of alarm and revulsion that Judy is "no longer a virgin" and insists that Judy keep the rape a secret to protect others from being upset.

Judy decides to cut her travel plans short and returns home. There she becomes a recluse around the house. She is afraid to go anywhere alone, even with her college friends, and refuses to go for counseling. Judy's parents try to keep her busy with activities and escort her wherever she wants to go.

*Directions:* Answer the following questions in relation to the above case situation. Explain your rationale for the answers selected.

1. In helping Judy cope with the rape crisis, the nurse would intervene in which of the following ways?
   a. Acknowledge that the rape was a terrifying experience and that Judy is not to blame simply because she traveled alone.
   b. Encourage Judy to get into counseling with her family and discuss with her the ways she can help her parents cope with the rape.
   c. Allow Judy to be dependent on the hospital overnight (regress), to ensure her safety and comfort.
   d. Notify the authorities so they can trace Judy's identification and travelers checks.

2. While assisting with the rape examination, the nurse would talk about which of the following matters?
   a. That it is not uncommon for family members to respond with a sense of shock and disbelief and to blame someone for the assault.
   b. That both Judy and her parents may feel that "if only" they had done something different the rape never would have happened.
   c. That Judy may find it tempting to permit others to infantilize her while she is recovering from the rape, but to do so will only prolong her recovery.
   d. That parents and lovers commonly feel the victim is "damaged" property and that she had better be prepared to refute traditional attitudes that view a woman as a man's property.

3. Recognizing the family's immediate reaction to Judy's rape, the nurse would intervene in which of the following ways?
   a. Arrange to see the parents alone, before they talk with Judy, to explain that rape is a violent act, not a sexually motivated act.
   b. Provide an opportunity for the parents to talk about their basic sense of sadness, hurt, and anxiety in response to the rape.
   c. Discuss the fact that many parents feel guilty and responsible; that in reality they are normal parents respecting Judy's independence.
   d. Tell the parents where to obtain a hotel and assure them

that after resting they will view the situation from a better perspective.

4. When Judy's parents seek out the nurse for counseling at the community mental health center, the nurse would intervene in which of the following ways?
    a. Convey to the parents that their overprotectiveness is intrusive and disregards Judy's need for privacy.
    b. Confirm that it is entirely Judy's decision to seek counseling, that their role is to remain available and supportive.
    c. Talk about the rape as an event that prompted the parents to work through their feelings about Judy's sexuality as a young adult.
    d. Tell the parents that Judy's response is quite normal, that there is no cause for concern because her behavior will return to "normal" in time.

## Situation 4

Ellen is a 35-year-old married woman of Irish heritage. One night her car breaks down in a deserted, run-down part of the city. Ellen starts to walk across a bridge toward a gas station when a man pulls up and offers her a ride. She hesitates a minute, wondering about her safety. But it is a cold night and Ellen is feeling distressed by the car trouble, so she accepts the offer. The man quickly pulls a gun on Ellen, telling her not to make a move or scream because he will "blow her brains out." The man frightens Ellen by telling her about the many people he has assaulted and that he has no qualms about hurting her. Then the man drives Ellen to an abandoned apartment building in a strange part of the city. There he rapes her and made her perform embarrassing sexual acts. Just before dawn the man tells Ellen to get dressed and drives her back to her car. Ellen walks to the nearest gas station in a state of shock and tells the attendants what happened. The police are notified, and Ellen is taken to the ED where medical care is provided.

Weeks later Ellen finds out that she is pregnant. When Ellen tells her parents what happened, they reject her for having "illicit sex" and tell her to get an abortion. Because an abortion would violate Ellen's value system, she decides to carry the child to full term and give it up for adoption (without ever seeing the child).

Fifteen years later Ellen contacts a rape crisis center for counseling and is seen by a nurse. Ellen states that her request for counseling was precipitated by a routine visit to the gynecologist, which coincided with the anniversary of the child's birth. She reports that she was tearful and that the physician inquired about what was upsetting her. Ellen told the doctor about the pregnancy and the adoption, and the doctor, dismissing her feelings, callously replied, "You ought to be over that by now." Ellen says that she recently read *The Bereaved*

*Parent* and has found herself grieving (for the first time) over the loss of her child and the loss of her "self" from the rape. She says, "No one wants to listen! No one wants to hear my feelings! Even my best friends tell me the adoption was the luckiest thing that could have happened to me because I won't be reminded of the sexual incident every time I look at the kid. Can you believe that?"

In the next few counseling sessions, Ellen talks about deciding to marry a man (Jim) 15 years post-rape. At the time one of her "friends" (Rita) said, "Oh, you're *not* going to wear white are you?" A second "friend" (Mary Ann) told her husband (Joe) about Ellen's rape and that Ellen had shared the event with her husband (Jim). Joe replied, "What did she tell Jim for? I would feel she was second-rate. I don't think I'd want to marry a raped woman." Ellen explains her feelings about Joe's reply: "I felt so alienated and unwanted when I heard that. I thought it was responsible of me to tell the man I was about to marry about all that . . . it still impacts my life." Now Ellen's husband says, "I have no control over what happened 15 years ago," and asks Ellen to stop crying, claiming that she is upsetting the two children. Ellen says she is even more upset because her husband is moving out of state (a promotion) and the relocation is in the city where she was raped. Ellen doesn't feel able to move there because it is still too painful to return to the vicinity of the assault.

In another counseling session Ellen reported having seen a male graduate student in a counseling program for therapy prior to contacting the rape crisis center. Because the therapist had limited knowledge about rape, Ellen had been afraid to talk about her residual feelings in response to her rape. Ellen told the therapist that she needed more than an hour to talk and she didn't feel able to wait a week for another appointment: "I have a lot of needs right now that have *got* to be met. I want to get rid of this experience, put it behind and get on with my life." The therapist told Ellen that everyone was limited to an hour and that was all she could get. Ellen recalled: "He assured me no one would notice me crying in the lobby as it is such a busy building." To the nurse Ellen wails, "All of a sudden it's all coming out and I can't stop it. I can't eat or sleep, I throw up. I'm beginning to realize the enormity of all the losses I've had: the pregnancy, the adoption, the insults at my wedding time, no family support, my distant husband, the gynecologist's insensitivity, and not being able to talk about any of it because no one will hear my feelings." Ellen reports that the male therapist reassured her that she was not "unique, tragedy happens everywhere—for example, six million Jews were killed. God lets things happen we can't ever understand." When the nurse asks how Ellen felt about that therapy, she replies: "I'm afraid of being cut off in the middle of opening up my guts and spilling out all my feelings. I can't stand rejection right now. I am afraid to cry for fear I won't be comforted or understood. Just like my husband . . . he cuts me off when I cry and says to stop crying . . . I need someone to listen to me, to give me *enough* time." Ellen asks the nurse if she should stop seeing the male therapist.

*Directions:* Answer the following questions in relation to the above case situation. Explain the rationale for answers selected.

1. Indicate the type of relationship between Ellen and the persons in her primary social network.

| Persons | Relationships (check all that apply) | | |
|---|---|---|---|
| Person | Affectional | Instrumental | Relational provisions |
| Ellen | | | |
| Ellen's parents | | | |
| Doctor (GYN) | | | |
| Jim | | | |
| Rita | | | |
| Mary Ann | | | |
| Joe | | | |
| Male Therapist | | | |

2. Indicate the type of response to rape expressed by persons in Ellen's life. Place a check in the appropriate boxes.

| Response | Persons | Ellen | Parents | Doctor | Jim (husband) | Rita | Mary Ann | Joe | Male therapist |
|---|---|---|---|---|---|---|---|---|---|
| 1. Shock, disbelief, dismay, helplessness | | | | | | | | | |
| 2. Blaming, finding a scapegoat | | | | | | | | | |
| 3. Triangulation | | | | | | | | | |
| 4. Overprotecting, infantilizing | | | | | | | | | |
| 5. Keeping the rape a secret | | | | | | | | | |
| 6. Reacting to rape as sexually motivated | | | | | | | | | |
| 7. Viewing the victim as "damaged" property | | | | | | | | | |
| 8. "If only" reactions | | | | | | | | | |

3. Identify Ellen's feelings in response to remarks made by persons in her primary and secondary social networks.
4. Discuss what the nurse would do to intervene in Ellen's long-term resolution of the rape experience, as well as Ellen's response to significant others in her primary and secondary social networks.

## REFERENCES

1. Ackerman, N.: The psychodynamics of family life, New York, 1958, Basic Books, Inc.
2. Adams, B.: Interaction theory and the social network, Sociometry **30:**64, 1967.
3. Burgess, A.W., and Holmstrom, L.L.: Rape: sexual disruption and recovery, Am. J. Orthopsychiatry **49:**648, 1979.
4. Burgess, A.W., and Holmstrom, L.L.: Rape: victims of crisis, Bowie, Md., 1974, Robert J. Brady Co.
5. Caplan, G.: Principles of preventative psychiatry, New York, 1964, Basic Books, Inc.
6. Feldman-Summers, S., Gordon, O., and Meagher, J.: The impact of rape on sexual satisfaction, J. Abnorm. Psychol. **33:**101, 1979.
7. Frank, E.: Psychological response to rape: an analysis of response patterns, doctoral dissertation, 1979, University of Pittsburgh.
8. Gersen, M., and Barsky, M.: For the new family therapist: a glossary of terms, Am. J. Family Therapy **7:**15, 199.
9. Grace, H., Layton, J., and Camilleri, D.: Mental health nursing: a socio-psychological approach, Dubuque, Iowa, 1977, Wm. C. Brown Publishing Co.
10. Halpern, S., editor: Rape: helping the victim—a treatment manual, Oradell, N.J., 1978, Medical Economics Company Book Division.
11. Holmstrom, L.L., Burgess, A.W.: Rape: the husband's and boyfriend's initial reactions, Family Coordinator **7:**321, 1979.
12. Kliman, A.: Crisis: psychological first aid for recovery and growth, New York, 1978, Holt, Rinehart & Winston.
13. Lazarus, R.: Psychological stress and the coping process, New York, 1966, McGraw Hill Book Co.
14. Lewis, J.M., Beavers, W.R., Gosset, J.T., and Phillips, V.S.: No single thread, Psychological health in family systems, New York, 1976, Brunner/Mazel Publishers.
15. Satir, V.: People making, Palo Alto, Calif., 1972, Science & Behavior Books, Inc.
16. Silverman, D.C.: Sharing the crisis of rape: counseling the mates and families of victims, Am. J. Orthopsychiatry **48:**166, 1978.
17. Weiss, R.S.: The provisions of social relationships. In Rubin, A., editor: Doing unto others, Englewood Cliffs, N.J., 1974, Prentice-Hall, Inc.

## ADDITIONAL REFERENCES

Burgess, A.W., and Holmstrom, L.L.: Rape: crisis and recovery, Bowie, Md., 1979, Robert J. Brady Co.

Henderson, S.: A development in social psychiatry: the systematic study of social bonds, J. Nerv. Ment. Dis. **188**:63, 1980.

Metzger, D.: It is always the woman who is raped, Am. J. Psychiatry **133**:405, April 1976.

Shore, B.: An examination of critical process and outcome factors in rape, report to the public, December 1979, and final summary report submitted to NIMH, January 1980, National Center for Rape Prevention and Control, Washington, D.C.

Speck, R.: Network therapy: a developing concept, Family Process **8**:182, 1969.

Washington D.C. Rape Crisis Center: A note to those closest to rape victims: families, lovers and friends, Washington, D.C., Jan. 1976, The Center.

## ANNOTATED SUGGESTED READINGS

Beavers, R.W.: Psychotherapy and growth: a family systems perspective, New York, 1977, Brunner/Mazel Publishers.

    The author, a noted researcher and clinician, presents a conceptual framework for therapeutic interactions that promotes healthy growth in families. Combining systems concepts and analysis-of-behavior patterns observed in competent and incompetent families, the author describes a growth-oriented approach in family therapy that calls forth various psychotherpeutic techniques. This book is recommended reading for nurses who provide counseling to rape victim families.

Burgess, A.W., and Holmstrom, L.L.: Rape: sexual disruption and recovery, Am. J. Orthopsychiatry, **49**:648, 1979.

    The authors report a longitudinal study of 81 adult victims of rape interviewed 4 to 6 years post-rape. The effects of rape on the victim's subsequent sexual functioning are descriptively analyzed. Most victims who were sexually active pre-rape reported changes in frequency of sexual activity and in sexual responsiveness. Victim responses to interview questions are reported, and suggestions are presented for counseling rape victims and their sexual partners.

Burgess, A.W., and Holmstrom, L.L.: Recovery from rape and prior life stress, Res. Nurs. Health, **1**:165, 1978.

    The authors report a longitudinal study in which four life stresses are examined for their association with recovery from rape: (1) prior victimization; (2) chronic life stressors; (3) family grief stressors; and (4) recent life-change stressors. The study results indicate that the recovery process can be hastened or inhibited by prior life stress.

Davis, L.: Rape and older women. In Warner, G., editor: Rape and sexual assault: management and intervention, Germantown, Md., 1980, Aspen Systems Corp.

    The author sensitizes the reader to the prevalence and problems of victimization of older women. Factors contributing to the vulnerability of older women to victimization in all violent crimes are described. The aftermath of rape on the social network is discussed. Psychodynamic issues—anxiety, resistance, independence, isolation, mental functioning, self-per-

ception regarding groups one belongs to, and acculturation into aging—
are discussed for consideration in planning prevention programs.

Dohrenwend, B., and Dohrenwend, B., editors: stressful life events: their
nature and effects, New York, 1974, John Wiley & Sons.
    The authors present general research findings on stressful life events.
Some observations are made on the role of stressful life events in the
course of physical illness and psychiatric disorders.

Feldman-Summers, S., Gordon, P.E., and Meagher, J.R.: The impact of
rape on sexual satisfaction, J. Abnorm. Psychol. **83**:101, 1979.
    The authors report the results of responses of 15 rape victims to retro-
spectively rating satisfaction with 23 sex-related activities both pre-rape
and post-rape. The results indicate that post-rape sexual satisfaction sub-
stantially decreased for a wide variety of sex-related behaviors but that
autoerotic and primarily affectional experiences appeared unaffected by
the rape. Rape victims reported significantly less satisfaction with their
current sexual relations than a sample of nonraped women did.

Fleck, S.: Family functioning and family pathology, Psychiatric Annals,
**10**:17, 1980.
    The author defines the family as a social grouping with dynamic inter-
action. In the family, an individual grows, develops, and relates to others.
Beyond the family, the person relates to society.

Frank, E.: Psychological response to rape: an analysis of response patterns,
doctoral dissertation, 1979, University of Pittsburgh.
    The author specifically designed a study to determine which factors in a
rape situation affect victim response and found essentially no relationship
between rape situation variables and psychologic response. The researcher
discusses the need to study other variables, including social supports, noting that their response pattern impacts the victim's response to rape.

Goldenberg, I., and Goldenberg, H.: Family therapy: an overview, Monte-
rey, Calif., 1980, Brooks/Cole Publishing Co.
    The authors present the theory and process of family therapy through a
balanced presentation of major theoretical frameworks and clinical practices, the text provides a good introduction to the field for beginning
practitioners. The book offers an overview of evolving viewpoints in family therapy as well as perspectives, values, intervention techniques, and
goals of family therapy.

Gunderson, S.: Advocacy in family therapy, J. Psychiatr. Nurs. **9**:24,
1980.
    The author discusses the nature of advocacy and the use of this concept
as a framework for the nurse in a professional role with families. The
compatibility and complementarity of family systems theory and the concept of advocacy are briefly discussed. The author presents a case example
in which a systems approach to conflict was applied. The principles outlined by the author are adaptable to work with rape victim families who
are in conflict and unable to meet their needs within their social network.

Holmstrom, L.L., and Burgess, A.W.: Rape: the husband's and boyfriend's
initial reactions, Family Coordinator, **7**:321, 1979.

The authors present the results of interviews with 16 couples in which the reactions of husbands and boyfriends to the rape of their wives or girlfriends were reported. The authors noted two main components in the man's response to the rape: (1) his own response to the rape—perceptions of who was victimized, a desire to seek retribution, and "if only" reactions; and (2) his interaction with the raped woman—ability to freely discuss the rape with his partner, coping with the woman's phobic behavior, and resuming sexual relations.

Katz, S., and Mazur, M.A.: Understanding the rape victim: a synthesis of research findings, New York, 1979, John Wiley & Sons.

The authors review recent rape research (1966-1976) and the explanations for rape outcome. Almost all rape research is noted in this study, which shows the rape event as a major variable affecting rape victim responses. Methodolgic limitations of the research are well presented. Definitions of rape are not uniform, and research conclusions about rape need to be carefully deduced from sexual assault studies.

Lewis, J.M., Beavers, W.R., Gossett, J.T., and Phillips, V.A.: No single thread: psychological health in family systems, New York, 1976, Brunner/ Mazel Publishers.

The authors present a long-term study of how healthy families function. They describe the characteristics of optimally functioning (or healthy) families, focusing on variables that are interactional: power structure of the family; tolerance for individuation and autonomous function of family members; affect or feeling tone of the family; the family's perception of reality; and the family's capacity for acceptance of loss. The authors show how it may be possible to make a significant contribution to primary prevention as well as treatment intervention. Therefore the work is valuable to nurses counseling rape victim families.

Pilkonis, P.A.: Current social support and chronic difficulties in attachment, research plan from grant application, Pittsburgh, Pa., 1980, Western Psychiatric Institute and Clinic.

The author discusses the need to study social relationships and their influence on physical illness and psychologic disorders. Particular emphasis is on the attachment process and the needs provided by this type of relationship.

Satir, V.: Conjoint family therapy: a guide to theory and technique, Palo Alto, Calif., 1964, Science & Behavior Books, Inc.

The author presents content intended to prepare students for effective family therapy work. The individual is seen in the context of the family as a system having regular and predictable rules that govern behavior of the family group. The author presents, in a training manual format, a step-by-step approach to conjoint family therapy that addresses (1) family theory, (2) communication theory, and (3) theory and practice of therapy. The text is useful to nurses counseling rape victim families.

Smoyak, S., editor: The psychiatric nurse as a family therapist, New York, 1975, John Wiley & Sons.

The author presents a collected edition of papers, developed over 5 years, from workshops with nurses committed to clinical practice as family therapists. The contributing authors first present an overview of theoretic perspectives and then operationalize concepts related to recurrent family dynamics that result in disruption, states of crisis, or malfunctioning of individual family members. The selections address (1) changing the therapist, (2) expanding frames of reference, (3) covert communication modes, (4) scapegoating and labeling processes, (5) focus on children, and (6) problematic family patterns. Nurses counseling rape victim families will find the practical content useful in their work.

Silverman, D.C.: Sharing the crisis of rape: counseling the mates and families of victims, Am. J. Orthopsychiatry, **48:**166, 1978.

The author discusses counseling techniques for mates and families of rape victims. An attempt is made to understand and describe from a psychodynamic framework the responses among husbands, boyfriends, and family members. The author encourages efforts to explore and articulate feelings and concerns about the rape crisis.

Weiss, R.S.: The provisions of social relationships. In Rubin, Z., editor: Doing unto others, Englewood Cliffs, N.J., 1974, Prentice-Hall, Inc.

The author makes a supposition that individuals require interpersonal relationships for adequate personal adjustment. Identified are six categories of relational provisions that individuals must maintain to establish conditions necessary for well-being.

Weitz, S.: Sex roles: biological, psychological and social foundations, New York, 1977, Oxford University Press.

The book takes a social psychologic view of sex roles. The author emphasizes the need to consider both individual factors and societal structure when explaining the origins of sex roles, the systems that keep them going, and problems in introducing sex-role change. The emphasis is on both female and male sex roles, since they operate as a system and one cannot be understood or changed without the other.

# PART III

# Nursing Care

## CHAPTER 6

# Hospital care of the rape victim

To live is to suffer, to survive is to find meaning in the suffering. If there is a purpose in life at all, there must be a purpose in suffering and dying. . . . Each must find out for himself, and must accept the responsibility that his answer prescribes. If he succeeds he will continue to grow in spite of all indignities.

Preface remarks by A. Adler. In Frankl, V.: *Man's search for meaning.*

## CHAPTER OUTLINE

| Intrauterine | Diethylstilbesterol | Paying the bill and |
| devices | (DES, | compensation |
| Menstrual | Stilphostrol) | The legal process |
| regulation or | Gonorrhea and | and victim |
| early abortion | syphilis | advocacy |
| | After-care referrals | **Summary** |

## LEARNING OBJECTIVES

After reading this chapter the student will be able to:

1 Describe three technical and five interpersonal guidelines in providing nursing care to rape victims

2 Describe eight measures a rape victim can take to preserve evidence of and cope with a sexual assault

3 Describe the importance of obtaining a rape victim's consent to treatment as it relates to the judicial process, role position of the patient, and psychologic healing post-rape

4 List and describe the nine phases of the physical examination in providing medical nursing care to a rape victim

5 Discuss the similarities and differences of a rape examination of a male patient, victim or accused, as compared with the examination of a female victim

6 Describe the role of the nurse with a rape victim during the examination phase of a rape exam

7 Explain why evidence of a sexual assault is collected according to the same procedure used in homicide cases, and describe what that procedure consists of

8 Describe the major elements in establishing a chain of evidence throughout a rape examination, beginning with the preexamination phase and ending with the postexamination phase

9 List and discuss ten treatment, follow-up, and after-care considerations in the care of rape victims

Hospital emergency departments are frightening places for rape victims. They are often impersonal and filled with sick and injured people. Therefore it is important that emergency department staff provide a supportive environment for rape victims, one in which staff are sensitive to the victim's crisis state and needs. Immediate care is directed toward reducing the rape victim's stress state and meeting physiologic and psychologic needs.[14]

All too often emergency department personnel are trained only in selective techniques of rape examination and evidence collection; many times they lack awareness of the procedures required by police officials, crime lab experts, and the judicial system. An accurate, comprehensive medical examination of the rape victim that reflects communication between professional groups is critical in providing competent care to the victim, prosecution of the assailant, and the victim's resolution of the rape experience. This chapter presents one procedure as a model for an accurate and comprehensive medical examination—one that is sensitive to the rape victim's needs and meets criteria of legal admission for court evidence.

Hospital care of the rape victim is presented within the framework of nursing that conceptualizes the victim's response as an adaptation to the stressor of rape. Treatment is based on the nurse's findings about the patient's adaptive or maladaptive responses. Three distinct treatment phases in the medical care of rape victims are discussed in this chapter: (1) the preexamination phase, (2) the examination phase, and (3) the postexamination phase.

The *preexamination phase* begins with the rape victim's entrance into the hospital system and extends to the rape examination. It includes activities that transpire prior to the victim's examination for injury and the collection of evidence of sexual assault. The *examination phase* includes these steps: meeting the medical examiner; the initial interview describing the assault; obtaining a medical and gynecologic history; an oral examination; a physical, pelvic, and rectal examination; collection of whole blood samples; and examination for motile sperm. Attention is also given to the medical care of the male patient, victim or accused. The *postexamination phase* addresses these needs: establishing a chain of evidence; health teaching with rape victims, including follow-up care and after-care referrals; and criteria for eligibility for compensation for expenses and injury. (Often nurses answer victims' questions about the legal process, which is discussed in Chapter 8.)

It is important for nurses to be aware of their own responses when providing care to rape victims and accused rapists. Nurses are encouraged to review Chapter 3 to refresh their memory of the types of emotions that arise in providing nursing care to rape victims; these emotions can, if communicated to the victim, facilitate or impede the victim's resolution of the rape experience. It is particularly important for nurses to be self-aware of belief in rape myths; blaming the victim for the assault; anxiety while providing nursing care to rape victims; and anger at the victim, the rapist, and others for the rape. Further, providing care to an accused rapist is difficult for some nurses. It is important for nurses to remember that the accused offender is only a *suspect,* not yet proven guilty of the charges, and deserves the same nonjudgmental care and respect as is given to any patient seeking treatment. Self-awareness and value clarification are important cornerstones to the provision of sensitive, competent, and comprehensive nursing care to patients and clients. Finally, nurses will also find that principles of crisis intervention and basic counseling are interwoven into the nursing care of victims seeking a rape examination. (See Chapter 7 for a discussion of crisis intervention and basic counseling of rape victims.)

## GUIDELINES FOR NURSING CARE

Nurses who provide medical care to rape victims and assist physicians with the rape examination implement crisis intervention approaches and the core qualities of helping relationships: empathy, respect, nonpossessive warmth, genuineness, and concreteness. The response and treatment a rape victim encounters can increase her distress or, preferably, facilitate physical and psychologic healing. It is important for emergency department personnel to offer support and technical assistance to rape victims. Nurses who feel disturbed by the rape victim's condition are unsure about how to be most helpful to the victim emotionally.

Increasingly, hospital emergency departments are developing guidelines for nursing care of rape victims and protocols for a rape examination. In Webster's dictionary a *guideline* is defined as "an indication or outline of policy or conduct." The following are recommended guidelines that are helpful in providing nursing care to victims of rape, the families of rape victims, and in working collaboratively with medicolegal health care providers.

## Technical guidelines
### Priority

Nurses need to assess the level of illness or injury of all persons seeking emergency care and indicate their priority for treatment. For example, a person experiencing a cardiac arrest would take priority over a rape victim seeking a medical examination. However, many persons seek care in an emergency department for problems that are not of an emergency nature (for example, a cold or the flu) and could be treated in a general practitioner's office. Nurses need to be alert to the need of rape victims for priority in receiving treatment because of their crisis state.

### Privacy

A rape victim should not be subjected to waiting in a crowded public waiting room where she can be embarrassed or ignored. The victim has just suffered a humiliating, degrading experience and at this time must *not* be treated in an impersonal manner. The privacy of an unused office or examination room provides an atmosphere in which the victim can describe the assault and express her distress.

### Registration

Registration is the process of completing a written form containing information about the patient. A registration clerk or nurse can complete this process. If registration clerks are assigned to complete records on patients, it is recommended that such clerks have in-service training on rape victim care to heighten their sensitivity to the needs of the rape victim. Registration of rape victims for medical care should be completed in the privacy of the examining room or a private waiting area.

### Case assignment

Increasingly, nurses are finding that primary nursing is the best model for providing care to rape victims. Within the context of the nurse-patient relationship the victim finds the understanding, acceptance, respect, and support that are critical to psychologic healing of a rape experience. A primary nurse provides the victim with a constant person to relate to at a confusing time—many medical procedures to undergo, decisions to be made, a busy emergency department, and relatives to face. The primary nurse identifies with the victim goals to be achieved and collaborates with the team members (usually a counselor, a medical examiner, and the police) in planning comprehensive care and in ensuring effective communication among concerned parties.

### Referrals

If the victim refuses treatment in the setting where the nurse is employed, the victim is to be advised of other facilities in the community where she can obtain care. A rape victim should not be turned away from medical care even when the setting in which the nurse is employed has not yet developed a protocol for a rape examination. A rape victim has a right to quality medical care and safe transportation to a more appropriate setting.

## Interpersonal guidelines
### Attitude

Research has shown that victims vividly recall remarks made by persons with whom they come into contact immediately after a rape assault.[12] It is essential, therefore, that emergency department personnel remain respectful, calm, and nonjudgmental. The victim of a rape is to be given as much credibility as a victim of any other violent crime. Nurses need to assume that the victim is telling the truth, regardless of any factor characterizing the rape situation that inclines the nurse to doubt the victim's assertion (for example, the victim's relationship to the assailant).

### Tactless remarks

When nurses blame the victim for the rape, any attempt to establish a therapeutic relationship is sabotaged. It is important that nurses avoid remarks that are disbelieving, judgmental, tactless, or hostile—for example, "You gotta be kidding!" or "You don't really expect anyone to believe that, do you?" or "You ought to know better than to hitchhike—what do you expect?" The nurse's role is to provide nursing care, not to function as a detective or to pass judgment on the moral values and behavior of the victim. Also, using the word *rape* as *infrequently as possible* in the emergency department can alleviate the victim's stress. Developing a code, such as Code R (for rape) or Code A (for assault), to refer to rape victims is more discreet than asking, "Where's the rape case?"

### Empathic listening

Sharing her distress helps the victim to bear painful feelings about a rape experience and gain control of her situation in a climate of understanding. (See Chapter 7 for a discussion of empathic listening.) Nurses therapeutically intervene in a victim's response to rape by carefully listening to the victim's feelings and thoughts. In an effort to interview and obtain information about the rape assault and the victim's response to having been raped, it is important to *listen to what the victim says*. For example, if the victim does not want to talk with anyone, or wishes not to disclose the rape to anyone, the nurse can discuss the decision but ultimately is to respect the wishes of the victim. As demonstrated in the following clinical example, it is the nurse's responsibility to be concerned about the *victim's concerns* and not what the nurse would like to see done.

CLINICAL EXAMPLE

*Nurse:* Is there some reason you don't want to wait around for the x-rays?

*Victim:* Oh, I'm so worried about my husband.

*Nurse:* (in concerned tone of voice) What has happened that you are so worried about him?

*Victim:* The doctor said he couldn't be with me because he wrecked the car on the way to the hospital. He must have really been upset. I just have to see that he's okay!

*Nurse:* You know, Janet, we can help you see that he's okay and still help you get the care you need as well.

*Victim:* Ah, come on (sarcastic tone)! He's out on that country road! How can you do that?

*Nurse:* The police officer who brought you here can go out and pick him up, bring him safely to be with you here at the hospital.

*Victim:* Oh, I'd be so relieved! I really need to see him and see that he's okay.

*Nurse:* Would you like to talk with the officer about it?

*Victim:* Yes, could I see him for just a minute? Then maybe I can relax and put up with these stupid tests.

In the above clinical example, the rape victim was so upset over her husband's welfare that she was unable to proceed with the rape exam; the victim's primary concern was her husband, not herself at this time. In order to lower the victim's stress level the nurse talked with the rape victim about alternative ways in which the staff could help her ensure her husband's safety as well as get the medical care she needed at this time. The nurse explored the basis of the victim's inability to proceed in completing the tests, listened to the victim, and helped her with her concern, thus enabling completion of the rape examination.

### Being human

The victim needs to see the nurse as a professional person as well as someone who can feel and think as a real person. Being a "real" person with the victim can be communicated through the use of chit-chat, humor, and touch.

*Chit-chat* is defined as "small talk or gossip" in Webster's dictionary. The value of chit-chat in a stressful situation cannot be underestimated. For example, the nurse may find it helpful to talk about the weather, the latest ballgame, or an event on the national news while awaiting the physician. Chit-chat serves as a nice distractor but should *not* be used to excess or to avoid the victim's feelings.

*Humor* also can be used in helping the victim cope, particularly if humor is the victim's style of coping with stressful situations. Webster defines *humor* as "that quality which appeals to a sense of the ludicrous or absurdly incongruous." Sometimes victims who have been raped are able to identify something amusing or comical that helps them gain distance from their intense emotional response to the rape and thereby strengthen their coping with the crisis. It is not unusual for victims to use humor to express anger or for victims to combine responses of anger and humor in resolving a rape experience. For example, one victim said the following about the rapist:

He ran out of the house so fast when he heard my roommate returning home that the idiot left his pants. (Laughing) Can't you just imagine him running down the street in his underwear in the middle of winter. I hope he freezes his balls off!

*Touch* is defined in Webster's dictionary as an act in which "pressure . . . exerted on the skin or mucous membrane is perceived." Physical contact is comforting and reassuring to many victims who have been sexually assaulted. For example, the use of hand-holding helps some victims during highly stressful moments, or an arm around the shoulder with a gentle hug followed by a comforting remark, "I know you're upset. I'm here to help you." It is important for the nurse to assess *each* rape victim for her response to touch and physical proximity. Some people who are highly anxious may perceive any contact as a threat and require increased physical space; other people simply do not relate in that kinesthetic way with other people so the nurse's physical closeness may only increase their sense of discomfort and stress.

### Waiting

One of the most difficult experiences for rape victims in crisis is endless waiting in an emergency department. They often become case numbers on a waiting list and respect for them as human persons is lost in the task of getting a job done efficiently. It takes only a minute or less to explain to people what is happening and, when combined with an empathetic approach, the nurse is armed with the best tool for keeping all parties calm, cool, and collected. For example, the nurse might say: "I'm sorry to keep you waiting. We're still helping the patient with the cardiac condition in the next room. We haven't forgotten you. We'll be with you as soon as possible."

Any delays in completing a prompt physical examination need to be explained to the victim. The nurse intervenes to de-escalate the victim's worry about delays and being forgotten, feelings of being unimportant, and questions about what is happening by explaining to the victim exactly what is creating a delay. When people, whether they be the victim or family members, are given a rationale for a delay, they find waiting for care more tolerable. It is hard to wait for medical care when in a stressful situation, particularly if no reason is given. Many people fear expressing their impatience or concern because they are in need of the professional's help or cooperation. People in distress often view angering the nurse as a threat to their care. *The nurse holds the power* to treat the victim humanely and to expedite rapid attention to her needs. Power is an important concept for the nurse to be aware of in providing care to rape victims. The victim just survived an assault in which power and control were key issues. Therefore it is understandable that the victim may be upset by any interaction that continues to put her in a powerless and helpless position. Further, many victims of rape are not used to questioning people who are in (what they perceive as) authority positions, such as nurses and physicians. Thus a nursing intervention such as explaining a delay helps reduce the victim's stress level because it shows that the nurse believes she is a person worthy of respect. Nursing interventions that convey to another person that they are worthwhile raise that person's level of self-esteem. Increasing a rape victim's self-esteem is critical in her recovery from a rape experience because the rapist attempted to divest her of any sense of self-esteem.

Sometimes professionals have delayed providing prompt care to sexually assaulted victims because of judgmental attitudes or belief in rape myths. When nurses assess that delays in patient care are occurring for no rational cause, the situation can be discussed with the person responsible for delaying the patient care and, if necessary, supervisory staff. Rape crisis center staff sometimes exert pressure on bureaucratic systems to effect change in nonprofessional behaviors—for example, delayed care without cause—and can be contacted to assist the nurse in efforts to work with administration toward quality victim care.

### Anticipatory guidance

Anticipatory guidance is a counseling process in which the nurse helps the victim prepare for a stressful or hazardous event in the near future. The nurse helps the victim identify problematic features of a hazardous situation and offers possible approaches toward solving them.[8] For example, the victim often believes many of the myths about rape. The victim may encounter rejection and be rebuffed by persons one would normally expect to be caring and understanding. It is important, therefore, for the nurse to help the victim develop "emotional innoculation" by discussing rape myths with the patient as these arise in the course of conversation and even to provide her with a written list of rape myths and facts refuting the myths. In talking with a rape victim one nurse discussed (1) how rape affects many victims and (2) the effect of rape myths on the process she goes through in resolving the rape. The nurse said: "You may feel guilty about being raped. It's normal and a stage many women go through. You may have regrets and find yourself saying, 'If only I hadn't . . . (100 different things). That's also a normal stage women go through."

It is important for the nurse to reassure the victim that she has just experienced a traumatic experience, that her response is normal, and that being raped may or may not happen again. The nurse needs to let the victim know that she will not always feel as upset as she does immediately after the assault. In providing anticipatory guidance, the nurse briefly explains that some rape victims experience an intense reaction to the assault with a wide range of feeling responses and emotional stages in healing. (See Chapter 4 for a discussion of rape trauma syndrome.) For example, several nurses talked with rape victims about common responses to rape as follows:

> We can't give you an aspirin and promise you that you'll feel just fine in the morning like we can with some illnesses. You experienced a bad trauma, and it will take time for you to work this through.

· · ·

> You might find yourself getting really angry, furious in fact, if you are not already furious. You might find yourself experiencing absolute RAGE! Feeling intense rage might frighten you since a lot of women are brought up to be gentle and caring. Don't worry about rage, it's a normal response to being raped.

· · ·

> You might not experience any real anger for several months, or until the time of a trial. There's often no more constructive outlet for your anger than the trial prosecution.

· · ·

You might find that you have trouble sleeping on occasion or become afraid to go out of the house. If you start feeling that way, remember, it is a common response but one that is best to get some help with before it becomes more of a problem. Give me a call, or the rape crisis center, if you notice yourself having trouble eating, sleeping, or functioning on the job and in social relationships.

Anticipatory guidance is also used to help victims prepare for the responses of significant others to the rape (see Chapter 5) and in longer-term counseling of victims through the court process (see Chapter 9).

### Social amenities

There are moments when sensitivity to the comfort needs of people will help in a waiting or stressful period and be appreciated as well. For example, the nurse could offer the victim a magazine to read and the company of her family or friends if delays in the exam procedure arise. Although the victim is not to drink fluids that would rinse away the evidence, the family might appreciate the offer of a beverage. Even if the offer is refused, the attitude of caring about the rape victim and her family's comfort has been conveyed, and that is what is important. Victims and families who feel taken care of or cared about are more likely to relax during the examination process. In some settings such social amenities are the responsibility of a unit clerk or volunteer. At times, social amenities can become grounds for potential problems. For example, a physician or police officer may *expect* the nurse to get them coffee when the nursing care priority at that moment is with the victim. Again, empathic comments reflecting awareness are more effective than outright refusal or militant arguments about the rights and role of women in our society. For example:

I know you guys are just dying for a cup of coffee. You've really put in a long night. But Mary Jane needs me right now, and I'm trying to get her ready for the examination. The coffee is made so feel free to help yourself to it.

With the preceding guidelines in mind, the nurse implements various responsibilities in assisting with the medical aspects of the victim's care throughout the rape examination.

## MEDICAL ASPECTS OF RAPE VICTIM NURSING CARE

Medical care of the rape victim is based on an assessment of the victim's identified symptom pattern or disease state. Somatic therapies are the primary mode of treatment. The rape victim is assessed for signs and symptoms of gynecologic trauma, trauma to other parts of the body, and the presence of sperm for evidence collection. Smears and slides are taken to assess whether the victim had (or later contracted) syphilis or gonorrhea. Treatment may consist of prescribing medication to prevent the victim from contracting venereal disease and, in some cases, mild tranquilizers to assist her over the initial phase of psychologic shock. Follow-up care assesses the status of the victim's body systems: circulatory, respiratory, gastrointestinal, genitourinary, mental functioning, and emotional sense of well-being. Medical care focuses on treating diagnosed illnesses or disease states. Medical treatment of the rape victim consists of three phases: (1) the preexamination phase, (2) the examination phase, and (3) the postexamination phase.

## The preexamination phase

Nursing care provided to victims in the immediate aftermath of a rape is directed toward reducing the victim's stress state, and quality nursing care is crucial in meeting that goal. Rape victims enter the medical health care system at a point called the preexamination phase. The *preexamination phase* is defined by the point when the rape victim enters the hospital system and ends at the point when the rape examination begins. Care during the preexamination phase includes: (1) preserving the evidence; (2) consent to treatment; (3) notification of authorities, family or friends, including attention to practical matters; and (4) preplanning for the rape examination. Discussion of each component of the preexamination phase in the medical care of a sexually assaulted victim follows.

### *Preserving the evidence*

Immediately after a rape experience victims are usually intent on reestablishing their safety, obtaining medical care for injuries sustained, and verifying the health status of their body and mind. Prosecuting the assailant may be a remote concern of the victim during the immediate aftermath of a rape. However, the victim may later decide to prosecute the assailant. Therefore it is important that every piece of evidence, however insignificant or seemingly small, be preserved in order that the victim's case be strengthened should she later decide to prosecute the assailant. (Some states, Pennsylvania for example, will permit a victim to prosecute an assailant up to 2 years following a rape.) Nurses can assist rape victims with their immediate crisis and help preserve evidence by sharing with the victim the information presented in Table 6-1.

### *Do's: Things to do after a rape*

When a nurse talks with a victim by phone in the immediate aftermath of a rape, the nurse *calmly* suggests to the victim that she lock doors and windows in order to protect her safety. By ensuring the victim's safety until someone can reach her, the nurse conveys to the victim that she cares about her and helps *the victim* initiate mea-

**Table 6-1. Preserving evidence and coping with a rape experience**

| Do's | Don'ts |
| --- | --- |
| Lock doors and windows | Wash |
| Call the police | Douche |
| Call the rape crisis center | Gargle or rinse mouth |
| Call a friend to be with you | Urinate |
| Wrap up warmly to prevent shock | Defecate |
| Get medical care for injuries and prevention of disease | Change clothes |
| | Eat |
| Know your feelings and responses are okay | Drink |
| | Straighten up the scene |
| | Blame yourself |

sures to reduce her fear and anxiety. If the victim is not in a safe place, the nurse intervenes to help her find a safe place; that may require any number of measures such as contacting a social worker, the police, or rape crisis center for the victim. Thus from the first contact the nurse helps the victim regain control over her life. The nurse advises the victim to wrap up warmly so that energy used because of high psychologic and physiologic post-traumatic stress will not throw her body into a state of shock. Knowing that the assailant is a dangerous person who repeats rape until apprehended, the nurse advises the victim to consider contacting the police so that investigative and arresting procedures can be started. Sometimes victims are so fearful and anxious they welcome the assistance of an advocate from the rape crisis center to help them through this crisis and to explain the many confusing and upsetting events that follow a rape. Therefore the assistance of an advocate is offered to the victim and may even be the first recommendation made by the nurse in an effort to help the victim.

There is no set order or rule for offering the suggestions cited in Table 6-1. The order in which the recommendations are made by the nurse can follow the concerns presented or overlooked by the victim. Usually rape victims are very receptive to obtaining medical care for injuries. Reluctance to seek medical care is often related to issues such as: How do I get to the hospital?, Can someone come get me?, How will I pay for the bill?, or I don't want my parents to know, so how can I get treatment without their knowledge? Finally, nurses reinforce for the victim that whatever feelings or responses she experiences, these are okay because rape is a terrible experience and victims respond in all kinds of ways. It is important that the victim knows from the first contact that the nurse is available to and supportive of her, that the nurse is part of her support network in resolving a crisis precipitated by the rape.

### Don'ts: Things not to do after a rape

In talking with rape victims about the advisability of obtaining medical care for injuries and an evaluation of their health status, nurses inform victims that there are a number of things they can do that would preserve the evidence and help both to identify and convict the assailant. For example, sperm often collect around the teeth; thus it is important not to gargle, eat, or drink. Similarly, evidence of sperm will be lost if the victim washes or showers, douches, urinates, or defecates because swabs are taken of the body in search of evidence of the assailant. Clothing worn by the victim is also collected for evidence of the assailant; thus the nurse advises her to remain in the clothing in which she was assaulted until the police (or designated person) arrives. If the victim cannot stand the thought of staying in the clothing, she needs to at least put each item of clothing in *separate paper* bags to give to the police. The nurse tells the victim to bring the clothing with her to the hospital, where she will get a *signed receipt* for the evidence and thereby protect any possible loss of evidence (see chain of evidence discussed later), or obtain a written, signed receipt for the clothing when she turns them over to the police at her home. And last, but not least, the nurse reminds the victim, "Don't blame yourself. You are not responsible for someone else's violent behavior." Because many victims believe the common myths, they experience a "double whammy:" (1) feelings of guilt and depression to resolve, along with (2) extremely high levels of fear and anxiety from surviving a "brush with death." The victim's stress state is generally quite high in the immediate aftermath of a rape, and nurses can decrease a victim's stress level by refuting rape myths with facts.

### Consent to treatment

The victim of rape has just undergone an experience in which she was humiliated, degraded, physically and psychologically assaulted—all against her will. Therefore it is important and essential to therapeutic care to obtain the victim's consent to the procedures involved in a physical examination and in collection of evidence. Rape victims are helped to regain control over their lives when they become involved in their care by contracting for treatment with consent.

Obtaining written, witnessed, *informed* consent to treatment from the rape victim is mandatory. The nurse explains to the victim each phase of the examination in terms the victim can understand and obtains her consent to *each* of the following phases or procedures:

1. Medical and gynecologic history
2. Physical examination
3. Collection of evidence
4. Photographs of her body and her possessions
5. Release of information to the authorities
6. Any medical treatment rendered[14]

Consent to treatment is a significant procedure because rape victims, by signing consent forms, decide to enter the medical system and assume a new role position, the role of a "patient." Appendix A shows sample consent forms for the medical examination and for photography.

A parent or guardian usually must be contacted for consent to treatment in the case of a minor. In the absence of proper authorization, according to the laws of the state, the physician and examining institution can be held liable.[2] The need for parental consent presents a problem for many adolescents who want an examination and treatment for venereal disease, gonorrhea, and pregnancy but do not want their parents to be informed of the rape. Some adolescents elect to go without treatment rather than inform their parents of the rape. Given the high incidence of rape among adolescents, the absence of alternative provisions for medical treatment poses long-range problems for the health of the youth in the nation: venereal disease, abortion, and psychologic disturbances. Nurses can inform adolescents or rape victims who do not wish to obtain parental consent for treatment about free clinics available for care in the community. Nurses can also work to develop alternatives to care within "traditional" institutions to accommodate the health care needs of adolescents.

Rape victims sometimes confuse consent to treatment with intent to prosecute the assailant. Nurses inform the victim that she does *not have to prosecute* if she signs consent forms for the medical examination and release of evidence. Prosecuting requires completion of a formal complaint with the police and district attorney, which the victim can decide to do at a later date, after she has had time to think about her alternatives. It is necessary, however, to collect evidence in the event that the victim later decides to prosecute and the case comes to trial. The nurse can explain the legal process to the victim and offer the assistance of a volunteer advocate at this time to answer the victim's questions; or the nurse can suggest that the victim refrain from an immediate decision and think about prosecution as a possibility for the future. (The legal process and nursing, and volunteer advocacy are discussed in Chapter 8.)

The nurse explains to a rape victim that she has the right to change her mind at a later date, that the present gathering of evidence will enable the victim to *make* that choice, whereas failure to gather evidence would limit her options later. Similarly, the nurse can explain that if the victim signs the consent form for the release of evidence, the evidence will not be used in any way unless prosecution is decided upon. Should the victim decide to prosecute, the collected evidence is then used to help resolve the case within the judicial system. Although cooperation and coordination with law enforcement agencies is essential, the nurse must ensure that the physical and emotional well-being of the rape victim is not compromised.

In the case of an accused rapist, a consent for each phase of the examination is obtained similar to consent procedures for the rape victim. The accused offender needs to be informed of his right to avoid self-incriminating statements during the examination procedure. In some cases suspects are brought to the emergency room by the police with a court order for an examination. It is important that the medical examiner carefully read the court order to ensure that the examination is properly authorized. If the suspect refuses to sign consent to treatment, the medical examiner may elect to examine the suspect anyway rather than lose valuable evidence of the assault. Examination of the accused without consent is a risky action, however, in terms of the examiner's physical safety and legal liability, and the medical examiner would be wise to obtain legal counsel before proceeding.[4]

By this point in the preexamination phase the nurse will discuss with the victim two aspects of care if these have not already been discussed: (1) the assistance provided by volunteer advocates and (2) a review of her rights as a patient. (See Chapter 8 for a discussion of advocacy and patient rights.) The next step in the preexamination phase consists of helping the victim notify her family, friends, and authorities.

### Notification of authorities, family, and friends

Most states require that sexual assault be reported to the police. However, some hospital settings do offer treatment to victims of rape without reporting the case to the authorities and simply record the presenting problem as something less than rape—for example, traumatic intercourse. Nurses need to become familiar with the regulations for the hospitals in their community and the protocol to be implemented, which usually includes matters such as who to call, when, during what hours, and the contact person.

The victim will usually ask any questions she has throughout the initial interview and physical exam. Areas of concern, not listed according to importance to the victim, often focus on the following issues:

1. Notification of parents or significant others
2. Informing others and relationship with mate (to tell him or not)
3. Rape examination
4. Pregnancy, venereal disease, and gonorrhea
5. Notification of legal authorities
6. Identification of the assailant
7. Prosecution of the assailant and the trial
8. Publicity
9. Religious or spiritual concerns[17]

     *Nurse's role in notifying others.* The nurse helps the victim explore those areas that concern her the most. The nurse's role is to facilitate the victim's problem-solving process, not to give advice or decide for the victim how to handle expressed concerns. When victims are provided with information needed to make decisions and an opportunity to explore feelings or conflicts about them, they are usually able to make self-care decisions.

One of the most difficult concerns for victims to work through is often the matter of informing others about the rape. The nurse intervenes by helping the victim decide who to notify about the rape. *Before* notifying family or friends that the victim is in the emergency department, the nurse always obtains the victim's *consent and participation* in the disclosure process. For example, the nurse might say: "Is there someone I can call to bring you clothes?" or "Is there someone you would like to have here with you that I can call?" or "Shall I tell the person over the phone what has happened, or would you rather I just ask them to come to the emergency department?"

It is not unusual for the victim to be concerned whether or not to tell her husband, boyfriend, or significant other. The victim may ask the nurse what she should do. If so, the nurse discusses the victim's concerns about such a decision. For example, one nurse helped a rape victim decide who to notify by asking her the following questions about her boyfriend:

1. "What kind of relationship do you have with him now?"
2. "You really know him better than I. How do you think he will react?"
3. "What kind of guy do you think he is?" (The victim may say, for example, "He thinks women who get raped deserve it.")

Involving the victim in disclosing the rape to others is a nursing intervention that helps the victim take charge of her life, ensures her privacy, and respects her right of consent in matters that affect her life. Nurses can also offer information about psychiatric–mental health clinical specialists who provide counseling to rape victims, their families, and significant others (since those emotionally close to the victim often also experience a crisis response to the rape).

In addition to informing others about the rape, all victims need a certain amount of *practical information*. The nurse or physician provides the victim with a practical explanation of the medical procedures involved in a rape examination both before and throughout the examination. The explanation given by the nurse also needs to inform the victim of her legal rights (for example, issues related to evidence collection and prosecution, as discussed earlier).

### Preplanning for the rape examination

The last component of the preexamination phase is planning in advance for the rape examination that will follow. An essential part of the rape examination is the use of a rape kit that contains all the essential equipment for such a procedure. Rape kits are available from medical supply companies, or they can be prepared by the hospital central supply service for a nominal cost. (Appendix B presents a list of contents for a rape kit and instructions to follow in assembling a hospital-prepared rape kit.)

Rape kits usually contain everything necessary for the rape examination and therefore offer greater probability that the procedure will be properly implemented. Standard kits include paper bags; name-tag labels for proper identification; equipment for collecting evidence, such as combs, fingernail files, and envelopes; test tubes for collecting blood and saliva samples; glass slides for smears; and in some cases consent forms. Appendix B contains a list of items usually provided in a standard or commercially prepared emergency department rape kit. However, the emergency room needs to be equipped with additional supplies not necessarily contained in commercially prepared rape kits. (These additional supplies are listed in Appendix C.)

With rape kits the medical team is assured that all necessary equipment is at hand and that there will be no need to leave the examining room to look for equipment while the patient waits. It is recommended that nurses examine a rape kit thoroughly prior to using one, becoming familiar with its contents and practicing the rape exam protocol. With practice nurses will become competent and confident in implementing the rape examination procedure.

Having prepared the victim for the examination phase, the nurse stays with the victim and helps her throughout the rape examination, which is discussed next.

### The examination phase*

The particular rape examination conducted depends on the protocol of the hospital in which the nurse is employed. This section discusses one rape examination protocol that meets criteria for evidence to be legally admissible in a rape trial. The examination phase includes the following procedures:

1. Meeting the medical examiner
2. Recording the medical and gynecologic history
3. Description of the assault
4. Physical examination
5. Oral examination
6. Pelvic examination
7. Rectal examination
8. Whole blood sample collection
9. Examination for motile sperm

It is essential that prompt physical treatment be provided to sexually assaulted victims in the emergency department. The victim will need medical care for the following:

1. Treatment of injuries that occurred during the rape
2. Medical evaluation of the victim's physical and mental state of health
3. Collection of crucial evidence that could corroborate the victim's testimony in a court of law
4. Evaluation of the need for preventive or prophylactic treatment for venereal disease or pregnancy and the need for follow-up counseling[14]

Throughout the rape examination the nurse implements crisis intervention techniques and the core qualities of helping relationships (discussed in Chapter 7). Each component of the examination phase is discussed below and should be considered along with what is required by the nurse's particular community or agency of employment. (Appendix D shows a checklist nurses may find helpful in assisting with a rape examination.) Some hospitals also use a wall chart to assist all medical personnel in treating sexually assaulted victims. (Fig. 6-1, p. 197, depicts one such wall chart.) The

---

*Examination of the male patient, accused or victim, is presented following this discussion of the rape examination.

chart is displayed in the emergency department examination room to offer guidance for staff in the treatment of victims and in the collection of evidence.

### Meeting the medical examiner

Traditionally the physician has been responsible for conducting the rape examination, instituting treatment as indicated, and testifying as the expert witness in court. The nurse in the emergency department has been responsible for orienting the victim, assisting the physician with the physical examination, providing health teaching, and activating referrals for follow-up care. Such traditional role responsibilities are now recognized as being ineffective in terms of time, cost, and the quality of care provided to sexually assaulted victims. Therefore community clinics and hospital-based programs have begun identifying those responsibilities in examining sexually assaulted victims that can be assumed by nurse practitioners.

Nurse practitioners conducting a physical examination of sexually assaulted victims are registered nurses who have had additional education and training in pediatrics, adult primary care, gynecology, or family planning and often an internship in the care of sexually assaulted victims. One of the major concerns in having nurse practitioners conduct the rape examination has been whether the court would accept the nurse as an expert witness. In many states the court will accept only the physician as an expert witness; and altering that requirement will necessitate the collaborative efforts of professionals within the judicial system. One state (Wisconsin) that has accepted the nurse practitioner as an expert witness identified the following role responsibilities for nurses as reported by the Family Hospital, Milwaukee, Wisconsin and others[5]:

1. Perform a speculum examination
   a. Position victim comfortably
   b. Explain procedure
   c. Insert speculum
   d. Recognize signs/symptoms of trauma or infection relative to assault
   e. Remove speculum comfortably
2. Do gonorrhea culture
3. Do saline washing
4. Collect all materials appropriate and necessary
5. Recognize symptoms that require a physician's interpretation
6. Document observations

Other responsibilities deemed appropriate to the nurse practitioner in providing care to sexually assaulted victims include:

1. Initial crisis intervention
2. Coordinating management of victim care
3. Health teaching and follow-up after-care, including examination and testing
4. Testifying as an expert witness in court
5. Long-term "follow-up" assessment and counseling of the victim, family, and friends
6. Nursing research[19]

The Family Hospital in Milwaukee, Wisconsin, is one setting where nurse practitioners conduct the physical examination of sexually assaulted victims. The *protocol* developed by the Family Hospital for the use of nurse practitioner skills is as follows.[5]

### NURSE-PRACTITIONER SKILLS POLICY*

1. A nurse who has completed the training and has been certified as having "practitioner skills" may examine a sexual assault victim for evidence of bruises and other trauma, may perform a speculum examination of the vagina and cervix, and may collect all material necessary to complete the legal investigation.
2. All laboratory tests both at the time of initial examination and at follow-up contacts may be performed or ordered.
3. Documentation of observations, laboratory tests performed, and materials collected will be done.
4. The House Physician will be contacted when there is physical trauma that requires immediate medical intervention.
5. If medications are necessary, the nurse will consult by telephone with the SATC [Sexual Assault Treatment Center] Physician on call. This would cover the administration of DES, antibiotics, take-home tranquilizers, take-home analgesics, and tetanus toxoid.
6. Abrasions, contusions, and surface scratches need to be documented on the examination sheet and may be treated by the nurse using first aid techniques such as washing, the application of cold packs, and bandaging.
7. The SATC Physician on call will be consulted by telephone when questions arise which are deemed "beyond normal." For example:
   a. head bruises with evidence of neurological symptoms such as headache
   b. chest bruises and injury with painful respirations
   c. asymmetrical joint swelling
   d. pregnancy or suspicion of existing pregnancy.
8. A nurse with "practitioner skills" will not examine a sexually assaulted victim when anal or vaginal penetration has occurred and
   a. major physical and/or genital trauma has occurred
   b. bleeding from the vagina is present and the victim denies menstruation at this time
   c. victim is extremely tense and uncooperative
   d. children are 13 years old or younger
9. The SATC Secretary will take the physical examination forms signed by the nurse to the Medical Director for his approval and signature on Tuesdays and Fridays. He will then see that this signed form is returned to the SATC Office to be taken to Medical Records for filing in the patient's chart.

   If one of the on-call physicians is consulted by telephone, he will be requested to sign the physical exam form held in Medical Records.

Sexually assaulted victims may be examined by a male doctor. Although most victims report greater concern about the manner in which they are treated than the gender of the examining physician,[12] a male physician may add to the discomfort of some victims. Many women find it unpleasant to have an unknown man touch their body (even in a professional capacity) when they have just been sexually assaulted.[15]

---

*This material is reproduced with the permission of Family Hospital, Milwaukee, Wisconsin.

Similarly the male physician may experience discomfort in examining a sexually assaulted victim. Therefore educational efforts are being directed toward helping physicians become more comfortable in all aspects of care with sexually assaulted victims.[16]

The physical examination subjects the sexually assaulted victim to poking and intrusion, which may symbolize a second rape for some women. The victim may be in physical pain from trauma sustained as a result of the rape, may feel frightened and helpless, and may be quite angry that she is being subjected to the medical care she needs. Thus it is particularly important for the nurse to be caring and sensitive to the sexually assaulted victim's feelings and needs during a rape examination, ensuring that it is not conducted as a "routine procedure."

Principles of competent nursing care during physical and pelvic examinations apply to the conduct of a rape examination as well. For example, when the initial interviewing and testing have been completed and the physician enters the room to conduct the rape examination, the nurse introduces the physician in a manner that treats the victim with respect and personal care. Respect for the victim's dignity, which is particularly important after the humiliation and degradation experienced during a rape, can be conveyed by allowing the victim to be in a sitting position when meeting the medical examiner. For example, the nurse could introduce the medical examiner as follows:

> Miss Smith (or first name if a child or adolescent), this is Nurse_____ (or Doctor_____) who is going to conduct the physical examination that I have been talking about with you. Do you have any questions you want to ask the doctor?

Because a lithotomy position places the victim in a helpless position, it is especially upsetting for some women post-rape, particularly if the medical examiner is a male.

During the physical examination process, nurses convey caring and concern for victims in many ways. It is important for nurses to be attentive to nonverbal cues of distress expressed by sexually assaulted victims, to ask if the victim is in pain, to help the victim relax with the procedure, and to explain every aspect of the physical examination and evidence collection. Frequently the person designated to conduct the rape examination also interviews the victim to obtain a medical and gynecologic history. At times this responsibility is delegated to the nurse or a resident physician. However, because of requirements for legally admissable evidence in court, the history is more often obtained by the medical examiner responsible for the rape examination.

### Obtaining medical and gynecologic history

Obtaining the rape victim's medical history is a delicate task. Often the victim is reluctant to answer many of the questions, which may seem embarrassing to her. Therefore it is necessary for the nurse or medical examiner to first establish rapport and trust with the victim by explaining the reasons for some of the questions asked of her. The nurse or medical examiner needs to be aware that the medical record may be subpoenaed if the victim decides to prosecute the assailant. In all cases the medical information must be recorded objectively and, when possible, in the victim's own words. The importance of the medical record in the courtroom has been well-documented in the literature.[6]

Since some of the information recorded in the sexual assault form can be used by the defense attorney to defame or damage the character of a rape victim, a special form can be used to collect the medical and gynecologic history and restricted to hospital use only. (Appendix E depicts one sexual assault form used for hospital records only.) Use of a separate sexual assault form permits the nurse to do the following:

1. Obtain necessary medical and gynecologic information that may affect the victim's treatment
2. Clarify the nature of observations made in the process of the examination *while*
3. Protecting the victim's right to privacy in personal matters not related to proving that she was raped

A medical examination form includes information about the victim's physical status (blood pressure, temperature, pulse, and respiration) and personal health (allergies to medication, any medication currently being taken, and any preexisting health problems). The medical history assures the examining physician or nurse practitioner that the victim's physical status is stable and that the immediate danger of hemorrhage, shock, or respiratory distress is no longer present.

The *gynecologic history* includes information about the victim's use of contraceptives, pregnancy, abortion, venereal disease, last menstrual period, any recent gynecologic problems, and date and time of last intercourse. The gynecologic history helps the examiner to be astute in collecting evidence during the pelvic examination. Motile sperm remain in the vagina for 6 to 12 hours and in the cervix for as long as 10 days. Therefore if the victim had intercourse several days prior to being raped, the examining physician or nurse practitioner would collect evidence from the vagina and avoid the cervix.[2] Knowledge about the victim's menstrual cycle and use of contraceptives is essential in order for the examiner to discuss pregnancy prevention in relation to the rape. Some victims will want to talk about spiritual concerns, such as the right to life of an unborn fetus, and the nurse intervenes to help the patient with such needs.

Information about recent gynecologic surgery helps the medical examiner differentiate between trauma that has resulted from surgery and trauma caused by the rape. Finally, it is important to distinguish a history of venereal disease from venereal disease contracted from the rapist. Therefore the medical examiner records information regarding tests completed for pregnancy and venereal disease. Since the *medical and gynecologic history* is unrelated to the sexual assault itself, *recording* this information *on a separate form avoids biasing a jury against the victim by the use of information unrelated to the sexual assault charge*. The medical form remains at the hospital with the victim's record and is *not* included with other evidence collection forms.

When the nurse or medical examiner interviews an accused rapist, only a general history of the patient's personal health is obtained (an interesting difference to note). The interviewer asks about allergies to medication, any medications presently being taken, any prior health problems, and any history of syphilis or gonorrhea. Assessment of the patient's history is then used in planning treatment.[4]

### Description of the assault

Emergency department settings differ with respect to who interviews the victim about the nature of the rape assault. When the patient is an accused rapist, questions about the alleged assault are deleted in the examination process because these are deemed to be part of the police and detective legal investigation rather than a medical or nursing responsibility. Furthermore, questions about the assault asked by a medical examiner may only complicate the legal proceedings if confusing facts are elicited and may increase the probability that the medical examiner will be called upon to testify in court.[4]

In some settings the nurse or nurse practitioner asks the victim to describe what happened and records the details of the rape assault; in others the physician may complete this part of the interview. Nurses need to be familiar with the procedure for the setting they are employed in. Some law enforcement agencies prefer that medical staff ask *only* those questions necessary to provide safe medical care because if any discrepancies in the account of the assault are recorded, they will weaken the victim's case in court (if she prosecutes the assailant). It is the job of the police and sexual assault detectives to investigate the case, not the nurse or health professionals.

Important information for the nurse or physician examiner to ask the victim in obtaining a description of the rape includes the following:

1. Date and time of the assault
2. Where the assault took place
3. Nature of physical injury that resulted from the assault
4. Weapons used, or threats of violence or retribution
5. Nature of restraints used
6. Number of assailants and any identifying information
7. Forced acts of fondling; vaginal, anal, or oral intercourse
8. Ejaculation, use of a condom, or sexual dysfunction during the rape
9. Use of drugs or alcohol before, during, or after assault by consent, pressure, or force
10. Any loss of consciousness during the assault
11. Whether the victim scratched the assailant or otherwise injured and scarred him
12. Whether the victim douched, bathed or showered, gargled, urinated, defecated, changed clothes, ate or drank beverages following the rape

Appendix F presents a sample form used in hospitals for recording the victim's description of the sexual assault.

As mentioned earlier, the victim is often embarrassed about describing the rape assault. However, if the nurse or medical examiner introduces the rationale for a question along with a request for information and applies creative listening skills in the interview process (see Chapter 7), it is sometimes easier for the victim to begin to talk about the assault. For example, in asking about acts of oral and anal intercourse, the nurse or medical examiner could say:

> I am going to ask you some questions about specific sexual acts that took place during the rape—for example, whether oral and anal intercourse took place. I am asking you these questions because oral and anal intercourse are the *rule* rather than the exception in rape. Even though it may be embarrassing for you to answer these questions, the information is important for us to know in taking care of you and for the medical record.

Obtaining a description of the assault from the victim has both medical and legal objectives. Asking the victim *where* the assault occurred provides the medical examiner with a clue to investigate a physical injury that might otherwise be overlooked. For example, if the victim was raped on the ground near a car, the medical examiner would look for grease, gravel, dirt, and skin abrasions; if the victim was raped near a wooded area on a road, the medical examiner would look for dirt on her body, splinters of wood, grass, and leaves; if the victim was raped on a beach, evidence of sand would be sought.[2] The *date and time* of the assault help the medical examiner correlate physical findings with the victim's account of the rape. A record of prompt medical care is viewed by attorneys and juries as evidence of a "real" rape rather than a false accusation. It is important to note, however, that interpretations of "prompt complaint" and prompt medical care, or of failure to seek help immediately after a rape, do not take into account the state of shock and crisis that many rape victims experience which contributes to delay in seeking care.

Questions about the nature of the *physical injury* are often obtained by asking where the assault occurred or what happened. A report indicating the *use of weapons* (most frequently a gun or knife) is often accompanied by an account of physical injury because the victim was beaten or cut with the weapon.[9] Threats or intimidation used to obtain the victim's compliance are also considered weapons—although psychologic in nature. Elderly women tend to be severely brutalized during a rape assault both by weapons and physical abuse.[10] A history of cuts, scratches, or bruises (prior to the rape) has to be ascertained to distinguish these markings from physical injury sustained as a result of the rape. By the time of the trial abrasions and bruises usually have healed; thus a history of pre-rape injury distinguishes between the different injuries and can corroborate the victim's allegation of rape in court. Questions about the *number of assailants* will remind the examiner to look for severe physical injuries when there has been more than one assailant. Gang rapes tend to last for hours and become progressively violent as each assailant "outdoes the feat" of the preceding one. Also, in such cases a wider range of evidence may be collected to discriminate sperm and blood antigens of the accused offenders.

Information regarding the *nature of sexual acts forced on the victim*—such as fondling and vaginal, oral, or anal intercourse—offers clues to where the victim may have suffered physical injury and where evidence of sperm can be collected. By asking the victim: "Did he force oral or anal sex on you?" or "Did he force his penis or attempt to force his penis into your mouth (vagina or anus)?", the medical examiner is phrasing the question to suggest that the victim was *not* an active participant in the assault, that the assault was an act against the victim carried out against her will. Because victims who have been subjected to oral and anal sex often find reporting such acts embarrassing, sometimes they will not admit to them. Therefore it is important that oral and anal areas be examined and evidence collected despite the victim's account of the assault. If the victim has been sexually assaulted in the oral cavity, this area must be swabbed (particularly around the teeth and gums because sperm tends to collect there). Most often, however, victims have washed their face, and sperm evidence has been eliminated by the natural flow of saliva or the victim's use of a mouthwash. Similarly, a report of forced anal intercourse indicates the need for swabbing of the area for evidence of sperm as well as examination for trauma. Rapists frequently degrade their victims by ejaculating in their face, hands, thighs, hair, ears, or any body surface believed by the assailant to be degrading. A report of ejaculation on or in *any* body site requires collection of evidence, and the site needs to be checked for further trauma. Occasionally rapists will use a condom, but use of a contraceptive mode is the exception rather than the rule. Rapists have been known to force the victim to douche prior to their departure, both to destroy the evidence of sperm and to degrade the victim. Any acts by the rapist that would destroy evidence of the rape assault, such as forcing the victim to douche or bathe after the rape, are to be recorded on the sexual assault form. Finally, because the rapist frequently tends to be sexually dysfunctional during the rape (see Chapter 3), *the absence of sperm does not mean that the victim was not raped*.[11] If the victim describes the nature of the sexual assault and this information is recorded on the sexual assault forms, then the medical record will often reflect the rapist's sexual dysfunction during the assault and provide corroborating evidence in court. For example, the victim may testify: "He couldn't get an erection until he forced me to fondle him (or until I resisted him)"; "He couldn't come, he went in and out of me for hours and yelled at me for not exciting him enough so he could ejaculate"; or "After beating me he ejaculated on my leg before he got inside me, and then he didn't have anything left, which only made him mad and he beat me more. He said it was all my fault."

*Loss of consciousness* during the assault is evaluated in several ways. Defense attorneys will attempt to assert that the victim did not know what happened and claim, therefore, that the victim is an unreliable witness in bringing forth a rape charge. Medical personnel will attempt to evaluate the victim's consciousness in terms of head injuries sustained during the assault and traumatic stress reactions. Consciousness is also affected by the *use of drugs and alcohol*. In some settings data about drug and alcohol use are deleted from the sexual assault form because the defense attorney will use this information to discredit the victim's testimony and defame her character. Information about drug and alcohol use is important when used to alert the medical examiner to evaluate the victim for toxicity or intoxication. Some victims take tranquilizers or consume alcohol post-rape—for example, to calm down while determining what course of action to take—and are unaware of the damage such acts have on their case in court. Historically, intoxicated victims or victims who have used drugs have received poor care in health care systems because of the many prejudices toward them. It has been our experience, as well as that of others reported in the literature, that many sexually assaulted victims who have been under the influence of alcohol or drugs are disregarded, disrespected, left to wait for hours, disbelieved about having been raped, or otherwise not taken seriously because of the social stigma associated with their alcohol or drug condition. Professionals have been heard to say, for example, "She's just a drunk. Let her dry out and go home. When she's sober, then we'll see what she says; but as far as I'm concerned, she's just loose." Women who have been drinking when they were raped tend not to report rape because they fear (realistically) that their testimony will not be believed; they also tend to have more fear of being blamed or disbelieved and have more feelings of guilt than women who have not been drinking at the time of the rape. Discounting the drug or alcohol condition of the victim ignores the medical problems that these victims may suffer—for example, exposure to the cold, poor circulation, and poor judgment to plan for safety after discharge. Finally, loss of consciousness may be due to *bizarre acts on the part of the rapist*. For example, one rapist chloroformed his victims. The chloroformed victims, usually under the age of 16, awoke in strange places knowing that their body had been assaulted but with no conscious knowledge of the act. Similarly, some rapists will add drugs to the drink of their victims during a social encounter and thereby render the victim helpless. Thus the victim's account of the rape assault is to be taken seriously; she should not be blamed or judged for what happened. The medical examiner's role is to obtain information that will facilitate completion of a competent, comprehensive rape examination, not to judge the victim.

As a final act of force some rapists degrade the victim by inserting a foreign object (for example, a bottle or a bladed instrument) into the woman's vagina. The *insertion of objects* such as knives, bottles, or wood may require surgical attention. If the victim reports having *scratched the assailant*, the medical examiner will be alerted to look for evidence under her fingernails and for scars on the accused assailant. Finally, if the woman has douched, bathed, gargled, urinated, defecated, changed clothes, eaten or drunk beverages, she will have destroyed evidence of the assault by such cleansing behaviors. However, cleansing behaviors, when noted in the record, will emphasize the revolting nature of the assault to the victim in contrast to any "romantic" aspects that the defense attorney may suggest in court. Cleansing behaviors post-rape also serve to explain the absence of evidence of the assault, support the victim's case, and refute accusations of a false charge. When a description of the assault is completed, the victim is then given a physical examination.

### The physical examination

A physical examination is given to sexually assaulted victims to determine the nature and extent of any physical injuries sustained as a result of the rape. The information obtained is used to provide the victim with good medical care and to gather evidence that is documented in case the victim prosecutes the assailant. *The proper collection of medicolegal evidence in the emergency department is a nurse's professional, ethical, and legal responsibility.* When efforts are coordinated between the police, medical personnel, and the courts, conviction rates for reported rapes increase significantly, and the victim receives a high quality of care. The physical examination is an external examination of the body that includes two aspects: (1) the collection of evidence of sexual assault and (2) the examination of the victim for injuries.

#### Collection of evidence

In many settings the nurse does most of the initial evidence collection—for example, pubic hair and head hair combings. It is important for the nurse to explain such procedures to the victim as they are being implemented and to converse with the victim in the following way:

> Some of this may seem odd to you, but I'll tell you why I'm asking you to do this (for example, comb pubic hairs).
>
> (or)
>
> Some of the questions we have to ask may seem very personal and they are, but they are necessary for us to ask in order to help you. For instance, I need to know if you douched once you were by yourself again because . . .

Sexual assault teams and rape centers have found the wall chart (Fig. 6-1) and printed guidelines to be helpful in collecting evidence and in assisting with the rape examination. The guidelines developed by the Interagency Task Force on Rape-Related Services in Pittsburgh, Pennsylvania, for collection of rape evidence are depicted on pp. 198 and 199.

## THE SEXUAL ASSAULT EXAM

APPROACH
- Be nonjudgmental
- Acknowledge victim's psychological trauma
  (emotional shock may be present even if the victim is outwardly calm)
- Before proceeding, explain what will be done and why

WRITTEN INFORMED CONSENT
- Examination and treatment
- Release of evidence

GENERAL HEALTH/GYNECOLOGICAL HISTORY
- Allergies
- Medication

ASSAULT HISTORY
- (Ask only the questions on the sexual assault medical report form)

COLLECT CLOTHING
- Place in separate *paper*, not plastic, bags

GENERAL PHYSICAL EXAMINATION
- Trauma
- Evidence

PELVIC EXAMINATION
- External trauma and evidence
- Warm-water-moistened speculum, NO lubricant
- Specimen collection (use evidence collection instructions)
- Bimanual

ANAL AND ORAL EXAMINATION

VDRL/GC CULTURES

PREGNANCY TEST, IF INDICATED

CHART EXACT TRAUMA SITES AND EVIDENCE COLLECTED

LABEL ALL EVIDENCE

MAINTAIN CHAIN OF EVIDENCE

TREATMENT
- Explain options and implications
- Trauma/VD/pregnancy

WRITTEN AFTERCARE INSTRUCTION/VICTIM HANDBOOK

REFERRALS FOR MEDICAL AND PSYCHOLOGICAL FOLLOW-UP

**Fig. 6-1. The sexual assault examination.**

Courtesy Interagency Task Force on Rape-Related Services of Allegheny County, Pittsburgh, Pa., 1979.

## HOSPITAL COLLECTION OF RAPE EVIDENCE*

**Instructions**

1. All envelopes and bags used in evidence collection should be paper.
2. Do not include urine sample or agar plate. The Crime Lab does not handle these items.
3. Semen fluoresces under ultraviolet light. If available, an ultraviolet light is useful in locating seminal fluid on the patient's body.
4. All containers used in evidence collection should be labeled with patient's name, where material was collected (body origin), initials of collector, and date.
5. If any portions of a rape kit are not used, label such items "*unused*" or do not return them with the specimens.

• • •

1. *Clothing:*
   a. Package each item separately in a paper bag.
   b. If the article of clothing is wet, air dry and then package.
2. *Debris collection:* Collect all obvious debris, including dried seminal fluid, adhering to the patient, and enclose in separate envelopes properly labeled. If debris is wet, dry first, then package.
3. *Collection of foreign/loose hairs:* Collect and package any loose/foreign hairs. A pubic hair combing should be made of the exterior genitalia to collect any foreign pubic hair that could have been transferred at the time of the assault. Comb hairs onto sheet of clean paper, fold paper, and place into properly labeled envelope. Include used comb in envelope.
4. *Standard pubic hairs:* Collect 15-20 hairs. 12 minimum.
   a. Pulled hairs are preferred. It is less uncomfortable for the patient if the hairs are pulled gently in a clump.
   b. If hairs cannot be obtained by pulling, a second and third combing should yield standard hairs, provided that 15-20 hairs are collected. Include used comb in the envelope.
   c. Place standard hairs on clean paper, fold, and put in properly labeled envelope.

*Reprinted with permission of the Interagency County Task Force on Rape-Related Services (300 Ross Street, Pittsburgh, PA 15219), 1979.

5. *Foreign head hairs:* Same procedure as #3 except comb head region.
6. *Standard head hairs:* Collect 15-20 hairs. Pull hair standard from different sections of the head.
7. *Swab specimens:* Use a set of two dry swabs simultaneously for each area and make one smear from each set of swabs. Routinely swab the vagina, anus and mouth. You are also looking for blood, sputum or semen on other parts of the body; swab pertinent area. *After making the smears, the set of two swabs from each area should then be:*
   a. Air dried, and packaged in properly labeled test tube.
   b. Do not submerge the swabs in saline or water at any time.
   c. Include an unused control swab.
8. *Smear specimens:* As listed above make one smear from each pertinent area, air dry and label as to body origin, etc.
9. *Whole blood sample:* 5cc of whole blood of patient. Use a tube with an anti-coagulant.
10. *Saliva sample:* Have the patient deposit saliva on a sterile cloth or gauze pad. Be sure an area about 1″ square is thoroughly wetted. It is important that no one touches the cloth except the patient. Air dry and place in properly labeled envelope.
11. *Fingernail clippings or scrapings.* Fingernail clippings are preferred but scrapings are acceptable. DO NOT DO BOTH.
    a. *Clippings:* Nails should be clipped and placed on clean white paper. Clippings from the right and left hands should be collected separately. The papers should be folded and placed in properly labeled envelopes.
    b. *Scrapings:* Clean/scrape under the nails. Scrapings from the right and left hands should be collected separately. The papers should be folded and placed in properly labeled envelopes.
12. *Physician's report:* Include Medical Report form with the evidence.

*All evidence is to be labeled* with the victim's name, date, the nurse's name, time of collection, the victim's charge number, and *most important*, the *body area* from which the specimen was obtained. (A form being used in hospitals to record collected evidence is shown in Appendix G.) In our experience, sexual assault cases brought to trial have ended in acquittal because a slide was not labeled as to where the specimen was collected from; in such cases the crime lab expert was limited in interpreting the findings when giving testimony during the trial.

*Clothing* provides corroborative evidence in court, and therefore it is not to be discarded. If the victim's clothing is to be confiscated as evidence of the assault, a clean set of clothing will be needed. The victim can take additional clothing to the hospital with her, or family and friends can be asked to bring these items for her. Sometimes the hospital may have arrangements for loaning or distributing clothing to victims in need. (It is important that victims be warmly dressed after a traumatic event because of the potential for physiologic shock; they should not be discharged in the winter without adequate provision for their physical well-being.) Each item of clothing is packaged *separately* in a *paper* bag, *never plastic*. Plastic bags promote molding of seminal stains, which destroys the evidence. If an article of clothing is wet, it is to be *air dried* before being packaged in a paper bag. It is important that the nurse *not* touch the victim's clothing to avoid contamination of the victim's clothing with the nurse's blood-group antigen secretions. Blood-group antigen secretions are analyzed by the crime lab to detect the assailant's blood-group antigen in saliva, perspiration, or semen present. All paper bags containing clothing are to be properly addressed and labeled, with identification information such as the victim's name, the date, and the nurse's initials. Identification of evidence collected begins what is called a *chain of evidence*— that is, a record of who the collected matter belongs to, who did the collection of the evidence, or any exchange of evidence to other authorities. Establishing a chain of evidence applies to all evidence of sexual assault collected (see Appendix G).

If the police have escorted the victim to the hospital, the nurse is to excuse the officers from the examining room while the victim undresses or has portions of her body exposed—for example, during the collection of pubic hairs or examination of the breast for injuries. There is no *legal* reason for a police officer to be present during the physical examination of a sexually assaulted victim. As a professional, the physician, nurse, or practitioner is an expert witness in court for cases brought to trial. However, if the victim is combative, or if an accused rapist is combative during an examination, the medical personnel may request the presence of a police officer for their own protection or may use a security system available through the setting where the examination is being conducted.[2]

*Excretory products* are also part of the evidence collected from victims who have been sexually assaulted. In some settings victims are required to have pubic hair combings and matted semen collected before being permitted to urinate so that evidence will not be destroyed through urination. However, in many settings the victim is permitted to empty her bladder prior to the remainder of the physical examination. A urine sample is taken for pregnancy testing (pregnancy due to intercourse *prior to* the rape) and drug screening. The nurse needs to discourage excessive wiping of the perineum so that the victim will avoid accidental removal of semen or foreign materials that may serve as evidence. Urine samples are labeled with the victim's name and date and then sent to the hospital lab for analysis (analysis for pregnancy and drug screening is not usually completed in analyses conducted by the crime lab in a rape case). Similarly, defecation prior to collection of swabs and smears during the examination is to be discouraged, particularly for anal rape, because evidence may be destroyed.

*Photography* is an essential part of the evidence collection process. It establishes for the record the victim's condition, or that of the accused rapist's, at the time of the examination. Photographs are particularly important as documentation of the extent of injuries sustained as a result of the rape; by the time of the trial injuries that would support the victim's case in court may have healed. *Only black and white film* is to be used. Color photographs are generally not admissible in court because of variations in printing, which the defense attorney will assert make the case appear worse than it actually was and therefore cannot be considered an objective account of the facts. Photographs are usually a police responsibility, not one delegated to hospital staff. However, some settings instruct medical personnel to take photos of the victim, and some instructional media portray medical personnel taking photos of the victim. If possible, the victim is first to be photographed in the clothing worn at the time of the rape assault; then photography of injuries sustained can be completed.

The *collection of debris* is another aspect of evidence collection with rape victims as well as with accused rapists. All materials collected in this process are recorded on a sexual assault form. (see Appendix G). All obvious debris is collected and enclosed in a separate *paper* envelope labeled with the victim's name and the date. If the debris is wet, it is dried prior to packaging. Samples collected include dried seminal stains, fingernail clippings or scrapings, and foreign or loose head hairs and pubic hairs. This material is analyzed by a crime lab (or other designated lab) for the presence of foreign matter that may identify the assailant. *Dried seminal stains* can be removed from the skin by using a swab moistened in saline and gently rubbing the stain from the skin. With the aid of an ultraviolet or Wood's light, seminal stains can be recognized by their brittle scaling and by glistening and slightly yellow areas. Swabs containing seminal stains are to be dried *prior to* being placed in a properly labeled test tube, which is then sealed. The lab analysis examines the swab for semen and acid phosphatase. *Fingernail clippings* are preferable to *fingernail scrapings* because more evidence can be obtained from them; however, scrapings are adequate. It is recommended that only one procedure be done, not both clippings and scrapings; because one method provides adequate evidence. Fingernail scrapings or clippings are checked by the crime lab for foreign material, such as skin and blood from the assailant. If the medical examiner decides to clip the victim's nails, the clipped nails are to be placed on a clean white paper, which is then folded and placed in a properly labeled envelope. Note that a *separate* envelope is used for the right and the left hand. Using a clean white paper helps the lab experts to locate the evidence with ease, as opposed to searching the corners of envelopes for foreign material. If the medical examiner decides to scrape the nails, scrapings are taken from under the nails of the right and the left hand as two separate steps in the procedure. The scrapings for each hand are placed on a separate clean white paper and then put in properly labeled, separate envelopes. If portions of the rape kit remain unused after this procedure, the unused items are usually not sent to the crime lab; if sent, these items are to be marked "unused" so that experts analyzing the debris do not needlessly search for evidence on them.

Collection of *foreign and loose hairs* on the head and pubic regions comprises the final step in the collection of evidence from external portions of the victim's body. *All* loose and foreign hairs are collected with a new, clean, or unused comb. Usually a gentle combing of the head and pubic hairs by the victim is sufficient to dislodge loose hairs. By permitting the victim herself to complete the combing process, the amount of tension and discomfort can be determined; also, in this way the combing process feels less like having something abusive done to oneself again. Loose hairs are collected from the exterior genitalia to find any foreign hairs that might have been transferred from the assailant at the time of the assault. Collected hairs are combed onto a sheet of clean paper, and the paper is folded and placed into a properly labeled envelope *along with the used comb*. The head hairs are combed first and placed in a separate envelope. This is followed by pubic hair combings, which are also placed in a separate envelope. Note that pubic hairs and head hairs are *not* to be combined in the same envelope. When such evidence is being collected, the victim is often more comfortable if the nurse begins with less private parts of the body, such as the head, and proceeds to more intrusive sites, such as the pubic region. Finally, 15 to 20 hair standards are taken separately from the crown of the head and the pubic regions. *Hair standards* are hairs that are pulled out by the roots and analyzed by the crime lab for color and curl in comparison to loose and foreign hairs and to those hairs obtained from the assailant. Hair standards are to be pulled from *different* sections of the head all around the crown because they differ according to the site. Some victims find this procedure painful and may express an additional sense of injury. Although explanations will not minimize the victim's discomfort, offering a rationale can serve to enlist the victim's cooperation and in some cases may activate a healthy anger about the assault. After external evidence of assault has been collected, the victim is then examined for physical injuries. (See Appendix H for a sample form used to record injuries identified in the physical examination of a sexually assaulted victim.)

### Examination of victim for injuries

Examining the victim for injuries includes a complete physical examination. The medical examiner gives particular attention to those sites the victim has indicated as being injured and having soreness or pain. Scratches and bruises prior to the rape are distinguished from those related to the rape. Photographs are taken of injuries visible to the eye (for evidence in court). Attention is given to bruises, punctures, lacerations, abrasions, redness, swelling, fractures, teeth or ligature marks, burns, stains, blood, and foreign material on the body. Observations made are recorded on the sexual assault form (see Appendix H).

It is particularly important for the medical examiner and nurse to pay attention to injuries to the head, neck, and throat because reports indicate that 30 to 60% of reported rape victims sustain severe injuries to these sites.[5] It is also important to thoroughly examine the victim's back and buttock areas because these may have been injured while the victim was forced to lie in a dirt road or alley or was resisting the assailant. If the offender asserts in court that the victim willingly invited sexual advances, evidence of physical injury can refute such an assertion.

Finally, recording observations of the development of the victim's physical stature is important because some victims progress from a prepuberty body structure to a pubescent or mature development before the assailant is brought to trial. For example, we are aware of one case in which an adolescent, now 16 years of age, was gang raped by four men, beaten with an ax, and knifed. Each of the four men required separate trials according to due legal process, and so the victim went through the agony of four separate trials over a 2-year period. One of the assailants appealed the case on a technicality and won the appeal; this resulted in another trial for the rape offense committed 2 years earlier.[15]

Because the medical examiner does not know at the time evidence is being collected how a sexual assault case will develop in the judicial system, it is important to collect evidence comprehensively and accurately. Once the physical examination of the victim is completed, the next step is the oral examination.

### Oral examination

The victim is asked by the medical examiner to deposit saliva on one or more sterile gauze pads or cloths to help determine the victim's secretor status for blood-group antigens. It is important that about a 1-inch surface be thoroughly wetted and that no one touch the cloth except the victim because the evidence would then be contaminated. The sample is to be *air dried* and placed in a properly labeled envelope. Samples of saliva are analyzed by the crime lab to determine if the assailant is a nonsecretor or a secretor. If the victim is a nonsecretor, specific blood-group antigens will not be present in her saliva; and if specific blood-group antigens are found in vaginal secretions when evidence is collected, it is possible that the blood-group antigens from vaginal secretions represent evidence of semen from the victim's assailant and that her vagina is normally absent of such blood-group antigens (since none were found in the victim's saliva). Therefore the saliva sample serves as a specialized tool in identifying the victim's assailant and needs to be carefully and accurately collected.

The victim's oral cavity is swabbed where the gums meet the teeth, and smears (previously described) are made, particularly if fellatio was forced on the victim. A gonorrhea culture is taken and streaked across a Thayer-Martin culture plate. The oral cavity is also inspected for the presence of venereal disease because the disease occurs in the oral cavity as well as other body orifices. Not all victims are aware of the possibility of becoming infected with venereal disease in the oral cavity and need to be informed of the seriousness of the problem as well as the need for follow-up care to check for both syphilis and gonorrhea. Cultures and blood samples taken at the time of the physical examination only indicate the presence of syphilis and gonorrhea *prior* to the assault. Finally, the oral cavity is inspected for evidence of trauma, lacerations, and tenderness.

### Pelvic examination

The pelvic examination consists of an internal examination of the victim's sexual organs to determine the extent of injuries sustained and to collect evidence of the sexual assault. During the pelvic examination attention is given to three aspects of the procedure: (1) nursing care interventions, (2) collection of evidence of sexual assault, and (3) determination of the extent of internal physical injury sustained from the rape. (Appendix I depicts one form used in hospitals to record pelvic injuries and genitourinary trauma sustained in a sexual assault.)

### Nursing care interventions

Throughout the pelvic examination procedure the nurse should extend empathic understanding to the victim, acknowledging that the exam procedure is difficult for some victims after having been sexually assaulted. The nurse needs to inquire about how the victim is feeling about being examined after just being raped. The nurse needs to determine if the victim has ever had a pelvic exam; if the victim has not had a pelvic exam previously, the procedure is to be explained in terms the victim can understand. The medical examiner needs to keep eye contact with the victim while completing the pelvic exam, and the victim is to be draped in a manner that ensures her dignity and self-respect. Draping can be done in a way that permits the medical examiner to maintain eye contact with the victim. Portions of the victim's body that are not being examined are not to be exposed unnecessarily. When it is time for the victim to assume a lithotomy position, the nurse needs to ask whether the victim would like help in getting positioned for the pelvic examination. The victim may be in pain and require assistance in assuming a lithotomy position, or the victim may prefer to make the position adjustment without assistance.

Since the victim may be inflamed in the genital area and quite sore from the assault, the internal pelvic exam will feel more comfortable if the medical examiner uses a *warmed speculum*. Only water is used to lubricate the speculum because prepared lubricants contain chemicals that negatively affect the results of an acid phosphatase test. Using a warmed speculum is a standard procedure in many settings, and it is a very important step in the examination of sexually assaulted victims.

*Muscular tension* during a pelvic examination that follows a sexual assault is quite common. The nurse can assist the victim by encouraging the medical examiner to proceed slowly, avoiding pressure until the victim can relax. If the victim has difficulty relaxing during the exam, the nurse can use deep-breathing exercises to help the victim relax. Throughout the pelvic exam, when the victim is uncomfortable or in pain, the nurse is to inform the medical examiner of the victim's discomfort and the location of the discomfort is to be noted in the medical record. Some victims have difficulty being assertive about their needs, and under stress they may be even less assertive in making the pelvic exam a comfortable procedure.

### Collection of evidence

Following the physical examination the victim is placed in a lithotomy position for (1) the collection of evidence of sexual assault and (2) for examination to determine the extent of injuries sustained internally. The lights in the examining room are turned off, and a Wood's light or another type of ultraviolet light is used to detect the presence of seminal fluid on the body. Examination of the victim's body includes the thighs, perineum, and entire body surface because the assailant does not restrict ejaculation to internal body orifices. Semen will appear with a bluish-white brilliant flourescence, while other body materials, such as urine and feces or pus, assume a less brilliant appearance. If semen is found matted in the body hair, it is clipped, air dried, and placed in an envelope and properly labeled. Evidence of semen is then examined by the crime lab.

Specimens from the oral, anal, and vaginal areas are obtained from the victim by using a set of two dry swabs simultaneously for each area swabbed, with *one* smear made from each set of swabs. (Fig. 6-2 depicts the areas of a woman's body that are

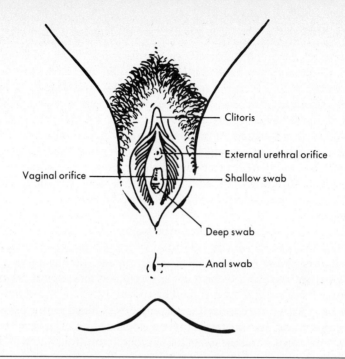

Clitoris

External urethral orifice

Vaginal orifice

Shallow swab

Deep swab

Anal swab

**Fig. 6-2. Areas of a woman's body swabbed for sperm evidence in a rape examination.**

swabbed for sperm evidence in a rape exam.) Swabbing of the mouth for evidence of sperm is done in the area where the gums meet the teeth because sperm seem to collect at that point. (The oral examination was discussed in detail earlier.) The vagina, anus, and mouth are to be swabbed as a routine procedure even if the victim denies being sexually assaulted at one of the given sites. (Recently three young women were raped and forced to perform fellatio. The hospital did not do an oral swab because the women were too embarrassed to inform the medical personnel of the offense.) A circular motion is used to obtain specimens from the entire vaginal area because when a man ejaculates the emission is not uniform. For example, if a man ejaculated onto a piece of paper in 10 different spots, the medical examiner or lab analyst would not find sperm in each of these spots. Thus to obtain a specimen from the vaginal vault a circular motion needs to be used.

Finally, the date and time of prior intercourse (if any) is important information to obtain when completing the medical and gynecologic history. (The victim's report of prior intercourse is to be noted on the medical record.) If the victim engaged in intercourse several hours prior to the rape, sperm will have traveled to the cervix and the medical examiner would want to avoid the cervix when collecting evidence so as not to confuse two blood types (that of the victim's sexual partner prior to the sexual assault and that of the assailant). For cases in which victims have had intercourse prior to a sexual assault, swabbing of the vaginal vault is limited to the lower region, and the report is recorded on the form that remains with the hospital record. These data are necessary for conducting an analysis of swabs, and an omission would be suspect to inquiry. (It is probable that a defense attorney would use the information, if available in the record, to defame the character of an adolescent, single, or divorced woman.) The medical examiner also looks for blood, sputum, or semen on other parts of the body. Pertinent areas evidencing specimens of sexual assault are to be swabbed. After the smears have been made, the set of two swabs from each area are to be (1) air dried and packaged in properly labeled test tubes; (2) not submerged in saline or water at any time; and (3) submitted for analysis, along with a control swab that is used for comparison purposes by the crime lab. If a commercially prepared rape kit is lacking a control swab, the department responsible for ordering the equipment in the nurse's setting needs to request that an additional control swab be included in sets ordered from the company. Rape kits prepared by the hospital can be requisitioned to include a control swab.

The crime lab analyzes swabs from the vaginal vault and from the oral and anal body orifices in a variety of ways and for a variety of purposes, as described below.

1. *Acid phosphatase.* A test is made to determine if acid phosphatase from seminal fluid is present. In a color test the specimen will reflect a bright red color if seminal acid phosphatase is present.
2. *Sperm.* Swabs from collected specimens are examined for the presence of sperm. If seminal acid phosphatase is present (indicated by a bright red color) and/or if sperm are present on the swab, the lab completes an analysis to determine blood and enzyme grouping of the specimen in the event that no sperm are found (some males have had a vasectomy or are azoospermatic).
3. *PGM.* A phosphoglucomutase (PGM) is an enzyme found in vaginal and seminal secretions. In the general population there are three common PGM patterns. A PGM test is done to determine the patterns of the victim and the assailant. If the victim and the assailant should differ in their PGM patterns, this would make identification of the assailant an easier task.
4. *Smear specimens.* Specimens are obtained from the oral, anal, and vaginal areas of the victim and analyzed for evidence of spermatozoa. One smear is made from each of the pertinent areas. Smear specimens are to be air dried, labeled as to body origin, and identified (as specified earlier).

### Inspection to determine internal injury

Once specimens used to determine evidence of sexual assault have been collected, the medical examiner conducts an internal pelvic exam to ascertain the presence of injury. Areas examined include the vulva area, the hymen, the vaginal wall, the uterus, and the rectum. Prior to entering the vaginal vault, the examiner inspects the genitourinary area for evidence of trauma, and the findings are recorded on the sexual assault form.

The vulva area is subject to injury from the trauma of forced intercourse and is more likely to be injured in pediatric and elderly victims than in other adults. The condition of the hymen is to be reported on the sexual assault form. Frequently the defense attorney will attempt to use the medical examiner's statements to ascertain the legitimacy of the victim's allegation of rape. One of four objective statements can be made by the medical examiner to report the condition of the hymen: "(1) the hymen is present, intact and free of evidence of trauma; (2) the hymen is present, intact, and shows old scarring; (3) the hymen is present and recently ruptured; or (4) the hymen is absent."[2] Bleeding or fresh blood clots are commonly present if the hymen has been ruptured recently.

Lacerations of the vaginal wall and the posterior fornix are to be noted in the pelvic examination. Adult women frequently sustain lacerations higher in the vagina, while younger victims generally evidence trauma closer to the introitus. Deep lacerations may need to be evaluated by a surgeon or pediatric specialist (in the case of younger victims). The condition of the cervix is to be described in terms of parity, menstruation, trauma, tears, bleeding, edema, abrasion, and tenderness. A bimanual pelvic examination is conducted next to check for tenderness or trauma, lacerations and tears.[2]

After the vagina and the cervix have been inspected, some examiners complete an aspiration of vaginal contents. This procedure varies from state to state and county to county. The nurse needs to be familiar with the procedure for the setting where she is employed. Some crime labs do not examine vaginally aspirated contents and do not wish to receive such evidence. Some crime lab experts assert that if swabs and all prior evidence are properly collected there is no need to aspirate vaginal contents. Lab analysts who recommend not analyzing vaginally aspirated contents assert that such specimens tend to breed yeasts and bacteria that can give false identities in blood groupings and show no PGM enzyme activity. Lab experts give the same explanation for refusal to analyze aspirated rectal washings. If the nurse's work setting requires vaginal contents to be aspirated, the procedure described below is generally followed.

The pelvic examination is then completed with the procedures followed in a routine examination. A Papanicolaou (PAP) smear is completed for medical purposes and also to check for the presence of sperm (which may be in the cervix if the assault

---

### PROCEDURE FOR ASPIRATION OF VAGINAL VAULT CONTENTS

1. Secretions in the vaginal vault are aspirated with 5 to 10 ml normal saline.
2. Aspirated contents are placed in a sterile container.
3. The secretions are examined for motile sperm, acid phosphatase, blood-group antigens, and, on occasion, a sperm precipitin test to detect if sperm was of human origin.
4. If the victim reports consensual intercourse with a partner prior to the rape, the cervix needs to be avoided in aspirating vaginal contents because sperm will remain in the cervical mucosa for several days. Thus only the lower vaginal vault is aspirated.

occurred several days prior to the examination). A culture for gonorrhea (GC) is taken after aspiration of vaginal contents; however, agar plates are usually analyzed by the hospital or a community-based lab, not by a highly specialized crime lab. For a gonorrhea culture secretions from the cervix are obtained and streaked onto a Thayer-Martin culture plate without delay. In completing a routine pelvic examination attention is given to the uterus to ascertain pregnancies or tumors existing prior to the assault, adnexal masses or tenderness, and rectal masses or tenderness.[2]

### Rectal examination

After the pelvic examination is completed, the rectal area is inspected for trauma and evidence of sexual assault. (Many women are too embarrassed to report anal sexual assaults.) The medical examiner examines the internal and external rectal areas for trauma, being careful not to cross-contaminate vaginal and rectal specimens in the examination process. In completing a rectal examination two procedures are implemented: (1) genitourinary trauma is diagramed and described and (2) a gonorrhea (GC) culture from the rectal area is taken and immediately streaked on a Thayer-Martin culture plate. Agar plates are usually analyzed by the hospital lab and the results are used for follow-up care. Victims may also be given a rectal washing, depending on the setting where the rape examination is conducted. Rectal washings are implemented only after the rectal area has been examined for trauma and a gonorrhea culture has been taken. In a rectal washing the rectal vault is washed with 10 ml of normal saline injected into the anus, which is aspirated after 5 to 10 minutes. The aspirated contents are preserved in a sterile, properly labeled container and saved for sperm analysis and/or acid phosphatase tests. In some settings if the victim has reported no anal intercourse, the medical examiner may elect to omit the rectal examination, particularly since there is disagreement among crime lab experts as to its validity.

### Whole blood sample collection

The physical examination is nearly complete when blood samples are drawn. It is sometimes reassuring to the victim to let her know that the procedure is almost over. The physical examination is a long, tedious, and detailed procedure; it may last as long as 2 hours, not counting the time the victim may have waited in the emergency department. Therefore the victim is usually quite fatigued by the time blood is drawn. A brief moment of empathic listening to the victim's feelings will enable her to cooperate more smoothly with the medical examiner in completing this phase of the examination. The victim will also be inclined to depart from the physical examination feeling that the professional staff genuinely cared about her well-being throughout the entire process.

Whole blood samples in the amount of 5 cc are drawn for drug and alcohol screening, blood typing, Venereal Disease Research Laboratories (VDRL) testing for syphilis, and in some cases pregnancy testing. Blood for pregnancy testing is usually not sent to the crime lab for expert analysis; pregnancy testing is usually done by a hospital laboratory or delegated agency. An anticoagulant is used with the specimens to prevent coagulation of the blood sample. It is important that an alcohol swab *not* be used at the puncture site for cleansing because the swab would destroy evidence of the sexual assault. A blood analysis can be completed with 5 cc of blood; larger specimens are usually unnecessary for the rape examination and medical care tests.

### Examination for motile sperm

The final phase of the physical examination is completed following an examination of specimens for the presence of motile sperm. States and counties in the nation vary with respect to whether they require, or even want, hospital personnel to complete an examination for motile sperm. Some crime labs consider this examination a very subjective test; they prefer that only experts complete the test or that the test not be done. Other settings want medical examiners to examine wet mounts for the presence of motile sperm, which may be lost if one waited several days for the forensic pathologist to complete the examination. Nurses need to know the requirements of the specific setting where they are employed regarding the examination for motile sperm. If a wet-mount examination is conducted, the results need to be recorded on the sexual assault form. (Appendix J depicts one form being used in hospitals to record the presence of absence of motile sperm and tests conducted on specimens.)

The presence of sperm upon a wet mount is determined by the appearance of a light blue color when stained with a drop of Sedi-Stain, a commercial stain. It is *important that specimens be examined immediately* after a physical assessment of the victim because motile sperm are extremely sensitive to air and do not survive long. The presence of motile sperm is a good indicator that intercourse has transpired recently and serves as evidence corroborating the victim's case in court.

### Examination of the male patient: victim or accused

A male patient can be either a rape victim or an accused rapist. If the patient is an *adult male rape victim*, it is important to discuss the fact that erections occur during a rape assault. Many men wonder about having had an erection during the rape and often silently feel doubts about their sexuality and worry about being homosexual. They are too embarrassed to ask about the erection they experienced and relax only after they are given factual information. For example, the nurse could tell the patient,

> It's not unusual in cases of anal rape for a man to get an erection. What it means is that there has been stimulation of the prostate gland; it's a physiologic reaction. It doesn't mean you enjoyed it or that you are a homosexual. It's a normal body response to stimulation.

A male often shows rage and anger in response to being sexually assaulted even though he may feel a lot of fear inside. A male may not show his fear except through his rage, which he has been socialized to view as an acceptable outlet for fear. It is not uncommon for a male rape victim to throw or destroy property, or sometimes to beat people up, or try to assault a person nearby in the emergency department in expressing both fear and rage. The nurse needs to view aggressive behavior in perspective to the situation that prompted the aggressiveness and not label or diagnose the man as psychotic.

For a male rape victim, examination of the victim is similar in all respects to that of the female victim except that the pelvic exam is omitted and greater attention is given to the male genitalia and rectal area. Since males usually resist assailants with considerable force, the male victim is also quite likely to suffer considerable physical trauma, particularly about the head, neck, back, and flanks.[3] Because forced oral and anal intercourse are the rule rather than the exception in sexual assault, attention needs to

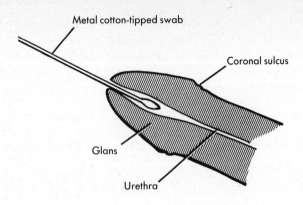

**Fig. 6-3. Metal cotton-tipped swabs used to collect samples from ure-thra.**

be given to injuries sustained in the mouth and anal areas. The frenulum at the base of the lower lip needs to be inspected to determine that it is intact. Local swelling of the pharynx or lacerations, contusions, and exudates of the pharynx may require treatment. The male genitalia are to be inspected for trauma and rectal fissures, bites, and lacerations. Samples are to be collected from the urethra by using a metal cotton-tipped swab that is inserted 2 to 3 centimeters into the urethra (see Fig. 6-3). The sample is then mixed immediately with a drop of saline and examined under a microscope to determine the presence of trichomonads. A digital rectal examination is generally conducted to determine rectal bleeding, tumors, edema, or fissures. If the rectal area is highly sensitive because of trauma, a rectal aspiration can alternately be obtained for an acid phosphatase test. Evidence of sexual assault can be found from an analysis of swabs containing fecal matter or lubricant, which may contain spermatoza or semen. The male victim has no need of a pregnancy test; however, testing for venereal disease and gonorrhea are completed and treatment provided as needed (discussed later). Tests for motile sperm may or may not be conducted depending on the setting. The male victim receives the same follow-up care as the female victim in terms of health teaching about syphilis and gonorrhea and counseling. It is helpful to inform the male victim that male advocates or counselors are available—through the rape crisis center, the counseling services offered through the hospital, or community or prison system programs.[3]

Although women are sometimes accused of being accomplices in rape cases or of raping male victims, it is rare that nurses will provide care to female offenders. More often nurses will provide care to males accused of rape. It is important for nurses to remember that *the suspect is only an accused offender,* not yet found guilty of the charges, *and deserves the same respect provided to any patient* seeking care. Further, many rapists have a history of sexual or physical abuse as children and of poor relationships with men, women, and authority figures (see Chapter 2). Therefore when nurses respond to accused rapists with disrespect and judgmental attitudes, the interpersonal psychodynamic problems of the offender are only perpetuated. The examination of accused rapists is the first point of entry into potential therapeutic treatment, so it is paramount that it be conducted in a nonjudgmental, professional manner.

With an accused rapist, collection of evidence and the medical examination both follow the same general procedure as with a victim—except that a description of the assault is omitted. Consent to treatment is obtained and followed by a general medical history. This examination is best guided by information from the police, which is particularly helpful in observing for signs of injury inflicted by the victim (for example, scratches, bruises, or bites) that may lend corroborating evidence to the case in court. The male rape victim is given a physical examination to determine the presence of injuries and to provide treatment as necessary. Clothing is collected for analysis of evidence of the assault along with debris adhering to the body; foreign pubic and head hairs, which may be from the victim; standard head and pubic hairs, which facilitate identification procedures; and smears and swabs of specimens. Particular attention is given to the penis for the presence of vaginal epithelium, fecal matter, or lubricant, which may adhere around the coronal suculus; it is collected with a moistened cotton swab. Saliva samples are taken to determine the accused assailant's secretor status, and whole blood samples are drawn for alcohol and drug screening. Finally, a chain of evidence (discussed later) is established by persons responsible for the collection or exchange of evidence to the authorities.[3]

### Closing the examination phase

The drawing of blood samples and the examination of wet mounts for motile sperm are the last steps in the examination phase. The victim is then helped off the examination table, permitted to shower and clean up, and given fresh clothing to wear. The victim may also appreciate other gestures of attention to her well-being, such as a snack, a cup of coffee, hot chocolate or juice, and a warm blanket—along with the presence of her family or friends. The victim often needs to be given or appreciates time to rest before completing the next phase of treatment, the postexamination phase. While the victim is preparing for the postexamination phase, the physician and nurse need to complete the medical record form by checking to see that it contains a complete documentation of the history, the examination, and any treatment rendered. The medical record form needs to explicitly state the medical examiner's findings, conclusions, and diagnosis. The medical record is not to contain the subjective opinions of the medical examiner or nurse about whether the victim was raped. Rather it is the responsibility of the professional staff to report *objective* findings and observations from the medical examination.

## The postexamination phase

The postexamination phase of the rape examination begins with completion of the preceding examination phase and includes (1) establishing a chain of evidence, (2) health teaching, (3) after-care referrals, (4) paying the bill and obtaining compensation, and (5) explaining the legal process and assistance provided by advocates.

### Establishing a chain of evidence

In the judicial system the collection of evidence and medical examination of sexually assaulted victims is regarded as seriously as a homicide case. The collected evidence is analyzed by crime lab experts familiar with analyses used to identify assailants in cases of violent assault such as rape and murder. Therefore it is extremely important that the evidence be properly collected, not contaminated or mixed up in the process, properly labeled and identified, and that each person responsible for handling evidentiary material sign for the release or exchange of collected evidence.

The chain of evidence is greater than the exchange of collected evidence. The chain of evidence begins with the victim's entry into treatment with the signed consent for treatment and release of information. It involves the presence of the nurse and/or volunteer advocate throughout the medical examination. The evidence is further chained by labeling identification of each specimen and the signing of release of specimens for analysis by pathologists or crime lab experts. Some settings provide a locked box where specimens are kept until they can be picked up—for example, if the victim is examined in the middle of the night and the lab is closed or the police sexual assault specialty squad is off duty until the morning hours.[18] Less concern is focused on who signs the form for the exchange of collected evidence than the fact that a *person needs to be designated for the responsibility*. Often the designated person is a head nurse or a supervisory or administrative level employee. A description of technicalities in a chain of evidence procedure follows.

Technically the chain of evidence requires that a receipt for the release of evidence to the police must be signed by the hospital employee *and* the police officer for all items exchanged, (such as laboratory specimens and clothing). (Appendix O depicts one form used in hospitals to record receipt for the release of evidence.)

Items listed on the sexual assault forms (see Appendixes A, F, G, H, I, and J) are sent to the crime lab for analysis. In addition, some institutions request the urine sample for drug screening; others do not. The nurse needs to be familiar with the requirements for the setting where she is employed. Finally, it is critically important that the medical examiner's report or the physician's report accompany the evidence to the crime lab. The report is to contain a description of the examiner's findings and any treatment rendered. The report needs to be *legible,* clear, and concise because it is used in the trial; illegible reports have been misread at trials, thus jeopardizing the victim's case.[7]

### Health teaching

The victim of rape needs to be informed about preventive health care needs. A victim's preventive health care needs post-rape include (1) testing for both veneral disease (gonorrhea and syphilis) and pregnancy on follow-up appointments; and (2) crisis intervention and counseling to facilitate the victim's psychologic adaptation to the stress induced from the rape experience. Two guidelines are followed in providing preventive care to rape victims in the postexamination phase: (1) prophylactic treatment for gonorrhea and syphilis needs to be considered in all cases of sexual assault unless contraindicated; and (2) treatment for the prevention of pregnancy needs to be considered for all rape victims unless contraindicated (as for male or elderly victims). A discussion of preventive and prophylactic treatment of a rape victim follows.

### Pregnancy prevention

Current literature indicates that only about 5% of women who are raped become pregnant from the rape. The nurse or medical examiner can help the victim determine the need for pregnancy prevention through active measures such as diethylstilbestrol (DES), menstrual extraction, abortion, or careful surveillance of a missed period. Most routine pregnancy tests are not valid until the victim is 4 weeks pregnant (or 41 days after the last menstrual period). However, a serum blood test called BIOCEPT-G can detect a pregnancy 6 to 10 days post-intercourse and alleviate the worries of many rape victims more rapidly than the commonly used urine test. However, BIOCEPT-G is not 100% accurate; it has given false positive results on occasion.

In the event that pregnancy does result from a rape, a woman has two options to consider: (1) carrying the child to full-term or (2) abortion through one of several means. If the woman decides to carry the child to full term, counseling is recommended to help her adapt to an unwanted pregnancy. Some women who carry the child to term decide to release the child for adoption; in such cases, preventive mental health counseling is recommended. Whatever the woman decides to do about a pregnancy, supportive counseling should be available to her through the rape crisis center or a community agency.

A woman who decides to have an abortion can elect one of several methods: (1) intrauterine devices, (2) menstrual regulation or an early abortion, or (3) diethylstilbestrol (DES). A woman electing to abort a pregnancy resulting from rape needs to be informed of the dangers, precautions, side effects, cost, and nature of the method decided upon; that is, the woman needs to decide on a method of abortion only after being fully informed about the method and after giving informed consent to the procedure. The commonly used methods for aborting a pregnancy resulting from rape are discussed below.

*Intrauterine devices.* An intrauterine device (IUD) is a synthetic mechanical device or instrument inserted into the uterus to prevent a pregnancy. An IUD can prevent pregnancy if it is inserted within 5 days of the rape. One of two intrauterine devices are used: the Copper 7 or Progesterone T. Both devices have been found to have a 98% effectiveness rate.[5] However, intrauterine devices are uncomfortable for some women, causing cramping and pain. Other women, who are frightened of the devices because of reports about their causing uterine ruptures, remove or do not use an IUD and elect an alternate method of abortion.

*Menstrual regulation or early abortion.* Menstrual regulation is a procedure in which the contents of the uterus are drawn out through a cannula (thin plastic tubing) into a hand-held syringe. This procedure does not involve a dilation or widening of the cervix and is reported to have a 99% effectiveness rate. Menstrual regulation takes only a few minutes, but the victim may experience mild to severe cramping. *Early abortion,* or vacuum-suction abortion, involves a dilation of the cervix. In this procedure the contents of the uterus are drawn out through a mechanical suction device that is attached to a machine. A vacuum-suction abortion takes about 7 to 10 minutes, and the victim feels cramping from the procedure. The time frame and cost factors often influence the victim's choice in selecting one method over the other. The time frame and approximate cost factors for 1982 are depicted in Table 6-2. Current costs will reflect changes resulting from inflation and discontinued federal programs that assisted disadvantaged persons.

The advantage of a menstrual extraction, beyond the element of cost, is that the procedure is less traumatic—both physically and emotionally—for the victim. The earlier the abortion is performed, the safer and easier the procedure is for the woman.

**Table 6-2. Time variables and cost factors in menstrual regulation and early abortion**

| Time variables | Approximate costs* | | |
| --- | --- | --- | --- |
| | Planned parenthood | Hospital | Outpatient clinic |
| **Menstrual regulation** (menstrual induction or menstrual extraction) | | | |
| Performed from 17-20 days after a late menstrual period<br>Usually done in a doctor's office<br>Symptoms of pregnancy but no positive pregnancy test is required<br>Considered safer than DES | Not a service | $700 to $1,000 | $150 to $200 |
| **Early abortion** | | | |
| Done 8-10 weeks pregnant<br>Some dilation<br>Performed in clinic<br>Positive pregnancy test is required | $180 in 6-12 weeks; *after* 12 weeks referred to hospital | $700 to $1,000 | $250 to $300 |
| **Abortion** | | | |
| 10-12 weeks pregnant<br>Vacuum-suction abortion and dilation<br>Performed in clinic<br>Positive pregnancy test is required | $180 in 6-12 weeks; *after* 12 weeks referred to hospital | $700 to $1,000 | $250 to $300 |
| **DES** | | | |
| Advised if in mid-menstrual cycle<br>Given in ER and by prescription<br>Effective in 3-5 days<br>Dose: 25 mg b.i.d. x 5 days<br>No positive pregnancy test required | Not usually offered | $5 | $5 |
| **IUD** | | | |
| Not usually a recommended treatment<br>Performed in physician's office or clinic<br>No positive pregnancy test required | $60 | | $60 |

*Cost will vary depending on current inflation rates and federal programs available or discontinued.

Although no documentation is readily available, some clinics report that menstrual regulation has a high failure rate because the procedure is done so early in the pregnancy that the fertilized egg is often missed and not extracted. Further, hormones released during states of extreme fear may stimulate ovulation in some women, sometimes resulting in an unsuspected pregnancy. However, calculations of the risk of pregnancy are based on the victim's report about her current menstrual cycle; unsuspected stressors are not taken into account when assessing the victim's risk for pregnancy resulting from rape.[14] If a woman has an unsuccessful or ineffective menstrual extraction, she must return for an abortion procedure if she elects not to continue the pregnancy. As a precaution, any woman who elects a menstrual regulation procedure needs to return for a follow-up pregnancy test 2 weeks later.

Physicians protect themselves legally when performing abortion procedures, and abortion laws are subject to change. Thus physicians often require a positive pregnancy test prior to performing abortion procedures to protect themselves from later accusations of conducting unnecessary surgery. If a physician does not require proof of pregnancy to perform an abortion, this information usually has been passed along by word of mouth among women in the community, or the physician may be a close friend of the family. The laws that govern menstrual extraction vary from state to state. For example, some states permit a menstrual extraction with a negative pregnancy test, whereas in the state of Pennsylvania a positive pregnancy test is required.[14]

*Diethylstilbestrol (DES, Stilphostrol)*. DES, also known as the "morning after" pill, is a synthetic estrogen given to women after intercourse to prevent pregnancy. It has been prescribed to treat amenorrhea, primary ovarian failure resulting from estrogen deficiency, female hypogonadism, drying up of breast milk, uterine bleeding, and menopausal symptoms, and also as an antimiscarrige agent.[13]

In 1970 the literature began reporting a rare cancer of the vagina in daughters of women given DES therapy. The effects of DES on the female fetus, as reported in the literature, include clear cell carcinoma of the vagina, cancer, mis-shapen uteri, and impaired ability to carry a pregnancy to term; on the male fetus, the effects include abnormal semen and penile and anatomic lesions of the genital tract, but no apparent reduced fertility or testicular cancer has yet been reported. Since the 1970s, when early reports about DES appeared in the literature, 22% of daughters identified as born to women given DES therapy in a sample of 250 women have died, and an untold number of women are unaware of their medical history are not yet accounted for.[13] If a woman has taken DES and becomes pregnant (which is rare since the drug is 98% effective), the woman needs to reassess whether she wants to carry the child to term—given the known carcinogenic effects of the drug on the fetus.

Because of the high risks associated with DES therapy, many professionals recommend an early abortion or menstrual extraction post-rape rather than DES, particularly since the risk of pregnancy post-rape is considered low, according to statistics on *reported* rapes. The options for pregnancy prevention must be weighed *by the woman* after she has been completely informed of the risk factors. Several crisis centers have reported that it is not unusual for women to be given DES without being informed about the nature of the drug, its high risk factors, and its side effects. (Our experience as medical advocates corroborates that finding.) Essentially, DES is best regarded as an emergency measure and prescribed only when (1) the woman has been fully informed about DES and (2) the woman has learned about the other options for unprotected intercourse. If a woman decides to take DES, she should be provided with information about the drug (dosage, side effects, unusual symptoms, and contraindications) as depicted on p. 216.

*It is unlawful and unethical to withhold information about DES from a victim.* If a woman takes DES and is 2 weeks late in a menstrual period, a pregnancy test needs to be done. Follow-up care must be provided at 2-, 3-, and 6-week intervals to women taking DES.[2] At this time there is no evidence that a short course of DES therapy causes long-term harmful effects to the woman herself; according to current research reports, it is the fetus that is adversely affected.

## DRUG DATA ON DIETHYLSTILBESTROL (DES)*

1. *Dosage.* 25 mg pills.
2. *Frequency.* Twice a day for 5 days.
   Initial dose needs to be taken within 25 hours of the unprotected intercourse and no later than 72 hours following unprotected intercourse.
3. *Side effects.* 7 out of 10 women report one or more symptoms as follows:
   a. Severe nausea and vomiting which usually subside in 2 to 3 days
   b. Headaches
   c. Menstrual irregularities
   d. Breast tenderness
4. *Unusual symptoms.* Any of the following symptoms needs to be reported:
   a. Severe leg pain (which could be due to a blood clot in a leg vein)
   b. Severe headache or sudden blurred vision (may be due to a blood clot in the brain)
   c. Chest pain or shortness of breath (may be due to a blood clot in the lungs)
5. *Effectiveness control.* The drug will *not work if* the patient is unable to keep the drug down, so an antinauseant drug such as Compazine may be needed to control *vomiting*.
6. *Contraindications.* Women having any of the following conditions are advised not to take the drug due to the high risk factors associated with DES:
   a. A current condition of pregnancy
   b. Known tumors of the breast or reproductive organs
   c. A strong family history of cancerous tumors
   d. A history of thrombophlebitis (blood clots in the vein)

*Resources: Glover, D., and others: Diethylstilbestrol in the treatment of rape victims, West. J. Med. **125**:331, 1976; Pittsburgh Action Against Rape: Training manual, Pittsburgh, Pa., 1979; Burgess, A., and Holmstrom, L.L.: Rape: crisis and recovery, Bowie, Md., 1979, Robert J. Brady Co.

### Gonorrhea and syphilis

A woman may contact and incubate gonorrhea and/or syphilis and show no visible symptoms for a long period of time. *Gonorrhea* is a bacteria (gonococcus) contracted by direct transfer from one person to another during very close physical contact, such as vaginal, oral-genital, or anal intercourse. Because the organism dies within a few seconds outside the human body, it is almost impossible to contract gonorrhea through other modes of contact, such as toilet seats, bath linens, or dishes.

*Syphilis* is a microscopic organism (treponema pallidum) that causes a disease called venereal syphilis. The organism is sensitive to the environment and dies outside the human body. It is nearly impossible to contract syphilis except through vaginal, oral-genital, or anal intercourse.

Treatment of gonorrhea and syphilis requires strict adherence to a regime of pre-scribed medications. The drugs and dosages for gonorrhea are not the same as those prescribed for syphilis; therefore careful adherence to the regime is important. Also, it takes time for symptoms of venereal disease (gonorrhea and syphilis) to develop, and some medical practitioners prescribe preventive treatment *just in case* the victim devel-ops the condition. Such preventive measures are highly recommended because many rape victims dislike returning for follow-up care. For example, the victim may be in an adjustment phase when she prefers to forget the assault and get on with her life or she may fail to understand the importance of follow-up care. Some women may be unaware that they have contracted gonorrhea and/or syphilis until the symptoms develop in their partner. Finally, professionals are not always clear about the need to return for follow-up testing to ascertain the presence or absence of venereal disease. For example, nurses have been observed to say to victims, "Don't worry about it, honey. It's all taken care of. I sent the tests to the lab, and if there's any problem we will call you."[15] This type of communication to the victim may be misunderstood as total clearance from concern about venereal diseases; yet, in fact, testing at the time of the rape exam only indicates whether the victim had either of the diseases prior to the rape. Thus it is important for the nurse to emphasize that the victim must return in *2 weeks* for tests for gonorrhea and in *4 to 6 weeks* for tests for syphilis. If the medical examiner elects to give the victim a preventive dose of medication for venereal disease, 4.8 million units of aqueous procaine penicillin is administered because this drug is effec-tive in treating both gonorrhea and incubating syphilis. However, this measure is *not* being used routinely in VD clinics and is not recommended by the Center for Disease Control (CDC).

Because of the importance of health teaching with sexual assault victims, hospitals have begun to develop treatment protocols to assist the professional staff in providing competent patient care. A treatment and follow-up protocol provides professional staff with a complete, easy-to-follow guideline that summarizes the important care to be implemented. The Rape Crisis Service of Planned Parenthood of Rochester and Monroe County in New York has developed a treatment and follow-up protocol that has been modified and reprinted here (see Appendix K). Medical examination of sexually assaulted victims is a very detailed and comprehensive procedure. (See Appen-dix P for a summary of the key points in the medical examination of a rape vic-tim.)

### After-care referrals

The plan for after-care is agreed upon by the victim, the physician or nurse practitioner, and others involved in the treatment process (such as the crisis counselor). *Written after-care instructions* are reviewed verbally with the victim and *given to the victim to take home* (see Appendix M); non-English instructions are provided if indicated. The after-care protocol developed by the Santa Monica Hospital Medical Center has been modified and reprinted here (see Appendix N). Settings that have developed a protocol for examining sexually assaulted victims have developed written follow-up care plans that are completed by the medical or nursing staff and given to the victim at the time of discharge. (Appendixes K, M, and N depict follow-up care forms being used in hospitals for sexually assaulted victims.)

The crisis intervention counselor or staff member giving medical after-care instructions to the victim needs to inform the victim about the normal feelings and reactions experienced by many victims of sexual assault (see Chapter 4). The Santa Monica Hospital Medical Center recommends the following instructions for rape victims:

1. Discuss the physical symptoms she may notice the days or weeks to come. Also give her written instructions concerning her medications and their side effects. Don't assume that she'll absorb your oral instructions; patients under stress seldom do.
2. Commonly experienced victim reactions are explained, such as flashbacks, anxiety, and other psychosexual distress.
3. It is emphasized that these are a "normal" reaction to the trauma of sexual assault.
4. Alternative ways of coping with these reactions are identified and explored with the victim, including talking about the feelings with supportive others or seeking supportive counseling from the hospital's crisis intervention counselor or other community agencies.
5. Give her a phone number to call if she has any questions or if any alarming symptoms appear after leaving the premises.[1,5]

Before discharging the victim, the nurse or crisis counselor needs to see that arrangements are made to ensure that the victim has a safe place to go and transportation to get there. If the victim was raped at home, she may prefer not to return there. Often the rape crisis center or volunteer advocate knows of alternate resources for accommodating women in distress on a temporary basis and can be of great assistance in arranging for a safe shelter. The following guidelines for the victim's safety were developed by the Santa Monica Hospital Medical Center and are reprinted in a modified text here.

1. Consider overnight hospital admission if the victim has severe emotional difficulties and no suitable accommodations for the next 24 to 48 hours.
2. Help arrange transportation. The victim will have no money if she was robbed as well as raped, and she may have come to the emergency room without friends or family. See if the hospital or nearby crisis center will assume transportation costs.
3. It is desirable for the victim to leave the facility with someone, such as a friend, relative, or advocate.

4. Some victims may not wish to return home in a police car; an unmarked police car may be requested, or a crisis or advocacy agency may provide assistance with transportation.[1,5]

### Paying the bill and compensation

A rape victim needs to be informed of the cost of her care and the avenues for compensation. Fee schedules vary depending on the health care setting and can be quite costly to the victim. Often victims consider these costs as "insult added to injury." Most states now have laws providing for victim compensation for unreimbursed medical expenses, loss of wages or support resulting from injuries, and mental suffering resulting from the rape. A rape victim may also sue for punitive damages—that is, monetary reimbursement from the convicted rapist as punishment for the crime. The nurse, registration clerk, or volunteer advocate needs to be aware of, and inform the rape victim about, eligibility guidelines for compensation in the victim's state of residence. Generally, compensation eligibility criteria include the following conditions:*

1. The incident was reported to the police within 72 hours
2. The victim has unreimbursable medical expenses, or
3. The victim suffered an unreimbursable loss of income or support for at least two continuous weeks
4. The victim's combined unreimbursable expenses exceed $100.00
5. The victim did nothing to provoke the incident
6. The victim's claim is filed within one year from the date of the incident
7. The victim cooperated fully with the law enforcement agencies
8. No relationship existed between the victim and the offender

Note that rape myths are operating within these criteria (see 5 and 8 above).

The victim should be given written instructions that provide her with information about how claims are investigated; where to obtain forms for filing a claim (for example, the hospital, police office, courthouse, or crisis center—including the street addresses and phone numbers of these agencies); where to mail these forms; and the length of time it takes to process them. The victim also needs to be advised about the following matters:

1. Information and receipts needed for private insurance
2. Special aid to victims of violent crime that may be available through state or local agencies
3. Medicaid procedures
4. Portion of expenses borne by law enforcement agencies

See Appendix L for a list of resources and services available to sexual assault victims.

### The legal process and victim advocacy

A rape victim may also file a civil suit for compensation from her convicted rapist. To do so, the victim must bring a civil suit against the offender and supply her own

---

*Reprinted with permission of the Interagency Task Force on Rape-Related Services: A handbook for victims, 1979 (200 Ross Street, Pittsburgh PA 15219).

personal attorney. In a civil suit the burden of proof is not as great as in a criminal suit, and juries are more likely to convict on assault charges than for a crime misperceived as a sexually motivated act.[14] (The legal process and advocacy are discussed in Chapters 8 and 9.)

## SUMMARY

Hospital care of the rape victim is discussed within the framework of the medical aspects of care, which emphasizes illnesses or disease processes that affect rape victims. This chapter divides hospital care of rape victims into three distinct phases: (1) the preexamination phase, (2) the examination phase, and (3) the postexamination phase. The *preexamination phase* begins when the rape victim seeks medical care in a hospital setting, clinic, or physician's office. During the preexamination phase the rape victim signs a form granting consent to treatment and enters the role position of "patient." Rape victims have a right to an accurate, comprehensive rape examination and collection of evidence, confidentiality, and self-determination in their care. Nurses discuss the rights of patients at this time and offer alternatives to care if the victim so requests. Guidelines for nursing interventions throughout the rape examination, and particularly during the preexamination phase, emphasize technical and interpersonal interventions that respect the dignity of the victim and facilitate effective relationships among professionals, the victim, and the victim's family or significant others.

The *examination phase* begins with closure of the preexamination phase and includes inspection to determine injuries sustained and collection of evidence. In some settings nurse practitioners conduct the rape examination; however, most settings accept only the testimony of a physician as the expert witness in judicial proceedings. Regardless of who examines the victim, it is important that the medical examiner be introduced in a manner that respects the victim's dignity and condition of stress. Prior to a physical examination the nurse or medical examiner obtains the victim's medical and gynecologic history. Since information obtained can be used to defame the victim's character in court proceedings, it is recommended that medical and gynecologic data unrelated to the rape be recorded on a separate form that is retained in the hospital record and not sent with evidence collected. The initial interview also includes a description of the assault by the victim about what transpired prior to, during, and after the rape. The victim's account of the rape provides evidence that is used in court, in conjunction with medical evidence from the physical examination, that corroborates the allegation of rape. The victim is then examined for the presence of evidence from the assailant (such as foreign hairs and semen) on the external body surface, and specimens are collected following procedures that will ensure preservation and admissability in court. During the pelvic examination nurses intervene to assist with the examination process. They ensure the victim's comfort, explain procedures, and answer questions. Nurses also facilitate the victim's coping with stressful feelings such as anxiety about body integrity and embarrassment. The victim is inspected to determine the presence of internal injuries, which (if present) are treated. All victims are to receive rectal and oral examinations with a collection of evidence because oral and anal assaults are the rule rather than the exception in rape. Whole blood samples are drawn for analysis of drug and alcohol toxicity, venereal disease, and in some cases pregnancy testing. The male victim is examined in the same manner as the female victim except that the pelvic exam is omitted and attention is given to male genitalia and the rectal area. Male victims are often subjected to considerable violence because many men resist the assailant and as a result suffer severe physical injury. Finally, some settings examine collected evidence for the presence of motile sperm, while other settings prefer to leave the evidence to crime lab experts to analyze.

The *postexamination phase* begins when the rape examination is completed. It includes the provision of health teaching to rape victims about venereal disease, gonorrhea, pregnancy, and care of injuries or trauma sustained as a result of the rape. Nurses emphasize the importance of follow-up care and provide victims with a resource list for after-care for medical and psychologic needs. Victims find it helpful to have follow-up care instructions in writing because of poor recall resulting from high stress levels at the time medical care is obtained. Many rape victims are unaware of the availability of compensation to assist them in paying for emergency services, for emotional injuries sustained that may temporarily interfere with their ability to work, and appreciate written information about how to apply for compensation. The final step of the examination process consists of an interview with the police once the victim's physical status is stable and the evidence has been collected. It is recommended that a nurse or volunteer advocate be present with the victim for the interview process. At this time the victim usually confronts a decision about whether or not to prosecute the assailant, which then sets in motion the legal process involved in prosecuting a rapist. There are many reasons that victims choose not to prosecute assailants. (A detailed discussion of the judicial process is presented in Chapters 8 and 9.)

A rape examination is a tedious and detailed procedure that can last for several hours. The manner in which professional staff treat the victim aids or impedes the victim's resolution of the rape experience as a crisis in her life. Rape victims have a right to expect that professionals complete an accurate, comprehensive rape examination, collect evidence in a manner that ensures its preservation and admissability in judicial proceedings, record their findings in a legible manner using objective statements, and testify in court if called to do so. The professional who fails to carry out these responsibilities may, according to Burgess and Laszlo, "be failing an individual just at the moment when he is most needed."[7]

## Learning activities

### EXERCISE 1. Noel questionnaire on medical care of rape victims*

*Directions:* The questionnaire is designed to assess the reader's knowledge about the protocol for a rape examination and nursing actions during an examination. Place a check by a response for each statement. Check your responses with the answer key at the end of the Learning Activities.

---

*Edited and reprinted with permission of the author; Noel, N.: *Emergency room nurses' knowledge of a specified protocol for the immediate care of rape victims,* unpublished master's thesis, December 1979, University of Pittsburgh School of Nursing.

I. When you treat a victim of rape who arrives at the emergency room, which of the following steps should be completed?

**True      False**

1. Provide the victim with a private room.
2. Notify the police or the proper authorities (according to policy of the agency).
3. Permit the police officer in the examination room during the exam.
4. Insure that someone is with the victim at all times during the hospital procedure.
5. Insure that the victim gets an explanation of the medical and evidence-gathering procedures.
6. Use a rape kit or specially prepared gynecology tray.
7. Assess the victim's psychological response to the assault.
8. Document any cuts, scratches, and bruises.
9. Obtain consent from the victim for photographs.
10. Place the fingernail scrapings in one paper envelope.
11. Insure use of a KY-jelly moistened speculum.
12. Examine the mouth for extragenital trauma.
13. Place each item of clothing in a separate plastic bag.
14. Collect obvious debris adhering to the victim and place it in a separate plastic envelope properly labelled.
15. Take pubic hair combings with an available comb.
16. Place comb used for hair combings in same envelope with the sample hairs.
17. Insure that head hairs are pulled from the temporal area.
18. Write a description of the vulvar trauma.
19. Record the condition of the hymen.
20. Use a Wood's light to determine genital trauma.
21. Use a set of two dry swabs simultaneously when obtaining specimens.

| True | False | |
|------|-------|---|
| ____ | ____ | 22. Make one smear from each set of swabs. |
| ____ | ____ | 23. Discard extra unused swabs. |
| ____ | ____ | 24. Insure prophylactic treatment for VD. |
| ____ | ____ | 25. Insure a tetanus toxoid. |
| ____ | ____ | 26. Insure prophylactic treatment for pregnancy with victim's consent when indicated. |
| ____ | ____ | 27. Provide the victim with information on her health care needs after leaving the hospital. |
| ____ | ____ | 28. Recommend gonorrhea testing two weeks after assault. |
| ____ | ____ | 29. Recommend syphilis testing six weeks after assault. |
| ____ | ____ | 30. Recommend pregnancy testing within ten days of missed period. |
| ____ | ____ | 31. Instruct the victim to call the physician or clinic if she experiences signs of infection such as fever, pain, sores, discharge, etc. |
| ____ | ____ | 32. Instruct victim to call the physician or clinic if she experiences urinary symptoms such as pain or frequent and difficult urination. |

II. When you treat a victim of rape who arrives at the emergency room, which of the following information should be obtained from the victim?

| True | False | |
|------|-------|---|
| ____ | ____ | 33. A consent for examination. |
| ____ | ____ | 34. An objective medical history in the patient's own words. |
| ____ | ____ | 35. Types of pre-existing health problems. |
| ____ | ____ | 36. The time and place of the assault. |
| ____ | ____ | 37. The nature of the physical acts. |
| ____ | ____ | 38. A description of the sexual acts. |
| ____ | ____ | 39. A statement on whether she has bathed. |
| ____ | ____ | 40. A statement about whether the assailant inserted any foreign objects into the vagina, mouth, or rectum. |
| ____ | ____ | 41. Use of a weapon. |
| ____ | ____ | 42. A statement on whether there was struggling. |
| ____ | ____ | 43. Present feelings about the assault. |
| ____ | ____ | 44. Use of threats by the assailant. |
| ____ | ____ | 45. Last menstrual period. |

|   True  |  False  | |
|---------|---------|---|
| _____ | _____ | 46. History of gynecologic surgery. |
| _____ | _____ | 47. Previous genital disease. |
| _____ | _____ | 48. Site on the body where rapist ejaculated. |
| _____ | _____ | 49. Level of consciousness (conscious/unconscious) during the assault. |

III. When you are following procedures for the gathering of evidence, which of the following steps should be completed?

|   True  |  False  | |
|---------|---------|---|
| _____ | _____ | 50. Initiate a chain of evidence form. |
| _____ | _____ | 51. Place a swab from the vaginal pool in a test tube containing saline. |
| _____ | _____ | 52. Send the pregnancy test to the crime lab. |
| _____ | _____ | 53. Send the gonorrhea culture to the crime lab. |
| _____ | _____ | 54. Send results of the acid phosphatase test to the crime lab. |
| _____ | _____ | 55. Send fingernail scrapings to the crime lab in one envelope. |
| _____ | _____ | 56. Obtain a saliva sample on an available gauze pad. |
| _____ | _____ | 57. Place the wet gauze saliva sample in a properly labeled envelope. |
| _____ | _____ | 58. Send a medical report form with the evidence. |
| _____ | _____ | 59. Insure everything is labeled with the victim's name, date, your initials, and the body area. |
| _____ | _____ | 60. Insure a signed receipt for the hospital record for what the lab received, when, and to whom given. |
| _____ | _____ | 61. Obtain a receipt from the police for the transfer of any evidence. |

IV. Different counties in the nation vary in the recording of a victim's psychological response on the treatment form. Some counties find such data facilitative as corroborative evidence, while others find it to be detrimental to the case. Of the following items, indicate which characteristics would be recorded on the treatment form in your setting.

| True | False | |
|------|-------|---|
| ____ | ____ | 62. Rationality of thought. |
| ____ | ____ | 63. Rationality of behavior. |
| ____ | ____ | 64. Ability to make decisions. |
| ____ | ____ | 65. Fluctuation between rational and irrational thought. |
| ____ | ____ | 66. Fluctuation between rational and irrational behavior. |
| ____ | ____ | 67. Signs of emotional trauma. |
| ____ | ____ | 68. An expressive (crying, hostile, tense, smiling) verbal style. |
| ____ | ____ | 69. A controlled (calm, composed, subdued) verbal style. |
| ____ | ____ | 70. Symptoms of emotional trauma. |
| ____ | ____ | 71. The range and variety of emotional responses the victim has in response to the assault. |

## EXERCISE 2. Audiovisual reinforcement of learning

*Directions:*

1. Observe one of the films listed below in the learning resource center or in the classroom. (It is recommended that this exercise be carried out in small groups or in the classroom to allow for discussion.) See Appendix U for information describing the film and where it can be ordered.
2. After viewing the film, discuss the questions listed below.

*Films for observation (see Appendix U):*

A. The Rape Examination
B. Treating the Sexual Assault Victim
C. If It Happens to You

*Discussion questions:*

1. What do you think of the nurse's interventions? Were they effective? If so, why?
2. What do you think about the interventions made by the other health team professionals? Were they effective? If so, why?
3. Was the portrayal of how evidence should be collected (to meet standards of legal admissability into court) accurate or correct? Did you notice any errors in how the procedure was carried out? If so, what were these?
4. Was the portrayal of providing sensitive and competent care to a rape victim realistic? Explain your reply.
5. Could a rape examination modeled after the one portrayed in the film be implemented in your work setting? If not, what are the impediments in the system that would need to be changed? How could you begin to make these changes?

## EXERCISE 3. Rape examination

*Directions.* Study the protocol for implementing a rape exam using the guide in Appendix P. The study guide accompanies the film *The Rape Examination* and will reinforce your learning. Make corrections on the study guide if certain practices differ in your state of residence or agency of employment.

### Answer key* to Noel questionnaire†

| Test item | Category[1] | Answer key[2] | Test item | Category | Answer key |
|---|---|---|---|---|---|
| 1. | P | T | 36. | L-M-P | T |
| 2. | L | T | 37. | L-M-P | T |
| 3. | M-L-P | F | 38. | M-L-P | F |
| 4. | P | T | 39. | M-L | T |
| 5. | P-M | T | 40. | M-L | T |
| 6. | M-L | T | 41. | M-L | T |
| 7. | P-L | T | 42. | L | F |
| 8. | M-L | T | 43. | P-L | T |
| 9. | L | T | 44. | P-L | T |
| 10. | L | F | 45. | M | T |
| 11. | ML | F | 46. | M | T |
| 12. | M-L | T | 47. | M | T |
| 13. | L | F | 48. | M-L | T |
| 14. | L | F | 49. | M-L | T |
| 15. | L-M | F | 50. | L-M | T |
| 16. | L | T | 51. | L | F |
| 17. | L | F | 52. | M-L | F |
| 18. | M-L | T | 53. | M-L | F |
| 19. | M-L | T | 54. | M-L | F |
| 20. | M-L | F | 55. | L | F |
| 21. | M-L | T | 56. | L | F |
| 22. | L | T | 57. | L | F |
| 23. | L | T | 58. | L-M | T |
| 24. | M | T | 59. | L | T |
| 25. | M | T | 60. | L-M | T |
| 26. | M | T | 61. | L-M | T |
| 27. | M-P | T | 62. | P | * |
| 28. | M-P | T | 63. | P | * |
| 29. | M | T | 64. | P | * |
| 30. | M-P | T | 65. | P | * |
| 31. | M | T | 66. | P | * |
| 32. | M | T | 67. | P | * |
| 33. | M-L | T | 68. | P | * |
| 34. | M-L | T | 69. | P | * |
| 35. | M | T | 70. | P | * |
| | | | 71. | P | * |

*Answers depend on nurse's state of residence.
†Category: P = Psychological aspects; M = Medical aspects; L = Legal aspects; O = Other aspects. The answer key was scored according to in-service education conducted by the Interagency Task Force on Rape-Related Services and the Allegheny County Sexual Assault Forms, Pittsburgh, Pa.

# REFERENCES

1. Abaranel, G., and Klein, S.: Hospital-based treatment of the sexual assault patient, Santa Monica, Calif., 1979, Sexual Assault Treatment Center.
2. Braen, G.R.: Physical assessment and emergency medical management for adult victims of sexual assault. In Warner, C., editor: Rape and sexual assault: management and intervention, Germantown, Md., 1980, Aspen Systems Corp.
3. Braen, G.R.: The male rape victim: examination and management. In Warner, C., editor: Rape and sexual assault: management and intervention, Germantown, Md., 1980, Aspen Systems Corp.
4. Braen, G.R.: Examination of the accused: the heterosexual and homosexual rapist. In Warner, C., Editor: Rape and sexual assault: management and intervention, Germantown, Md., 1980, Aspen Systems Corp.
5. Burgess, A.W., and Holmstrom, L.L.: Rape: crisis and recovery, Bowie, Md., 1979, Robert J. Brady Co.
6. Burgess, A.W., and Laszlo, A.: Courtroom use of hospital records in sexual assault cases, Am. J. Nurs. **1**:64, 1977.
7. Burgess, A.W., and Laszlo, A.: The professional as a court witness, J.E.N. **2**(2):25-30, March-April 1976.
8. Grace, H., Layton, J., and Camilleri, D.: Mental health nursing: a sociopsychological approach, Dubuque, Iowa, 1977, Wm. C. Brown Publishing Co.
9. Groth, A.N., with Birnbaum, J.: Men who rape, New York, 1979, Plenum Press.
10. Groth, A.N.: The older rape victim and her assailant, J. Geriatr. Psychiatry, Oct.-Nov.:203, 1977-78.
11. Groth, A.N., and Burgess, A.W.: Sexual dysfunction during rape, New Engl. J. Med. **10**:764, 1977.
12. Holmstrom, L.L., and Burgess, A.W.: The victim of rape: institutional reactions, New York, 1978, John Wiley & Sons, Inc.
13. Marieskind, H.: Women in the health system: patients, providers, and programs, St. Louis, 1980, The C.V. Mosby Co.
14. Pittsburgh Action Against Rape: Training manual, Pittsburgh, Pa., 1979, Pittsburgh Action Against Rape and personal communications of staff, particularly P. Hayes.
15. Pride, A.: Personal communication, April 1981, Pittsburgh Action Against Rape, administrator.
16. Silverman, D.: First do no more harm: female rape victims and the male counselor, Am. J. Orthopsychiatry **47**:91, 1977.
17. Sutherland, S., and Scherl, D.: Crisis intervention with victims of rape, Soc. Work **17**:34, 1972.
18. Terzian, J., and Martin, B.: Rape cases: is your test handling fail safe? In Halper, S., editor: Rape: helping the victim, Oradell, N.J., 1978, Medical Economics Company Book Division.
19. Warner, C., and Robbins, J.: Dimensions in planning: a blueprint for action. In Warner, C., editor: Rape and sexual assault: management and intervention, Germantown, Md., 1980, Aspen Systems Corp.

## ADDITIONAL REFERENCES

Abrams, N.: A contrary view of the nurse as patient advocate, Nurs. Forum **3:**258, 1978.

Belden, L.: Why women do not report sexual assault, Aegis: magazine on ending violence against women **1:**5, Winter-Spring 1980.

Bowen, M.: The use of family theory in clinical practice, Compr. Psychiatry **7:**345, 1966.

Brown, B., and others: Nurse-practitioner skills in rape victim care. In Protocol of the Family Hospital, Milwaukee, Wis., 1979, Family Hospital Sexual Assault Treatment Center.

Brown, B., and others: Nurse-practitioner skills policy. In Protocol of the Family Hospital, Milwaukee, Wis., 1979, Family Hospital Sexual Assault Treatment Center.

Burgess, A.W., and Holmstrom, L.L.: Rape: victims of crisis, Bowie, Md., 1974, Robert J. Brady Co.

Chapman, J., and Chapman, H.: Behavior and health care: a humanistic helping process, St. Louis, 1975, The C.V. Mosby Co.

Christy, T.: New privileges . . . new challenges . . . new responsibilities, Nurs. '73 **11:**8, 1973.

Cleveland Rape Crisis Center: Birth control for victims of rape. In Rape resource, Cleveland, Ohio, 1979, The Center.

Curtin, L.: The nurse as advocate: a philosophical foundation for nursing, Adv. Nurs. Sci. **1:**1, 1979.

Dock, L., and Stewart, I.: A short history of nursing, New York, 1925, G.P. Putnam's Sons.

Donahue, M.: The nurse: a patient advocate? Nurs. Forum **2:**143, 1978.

Gambrell, L., and Wilson, R.: Focusing on the strengths of children, Belmont, Calif., 1973, Lear Siegler/Fearon.

Garver, N.: What violence is, The Nation **6:**817, 1968.

Glover, D., and others: Diethylstilbestrol in the treatment of rape victims, West. J. Med. **125:**331, 1976.

Gustafson, J., and Laney, J.: On being responsible, New York, 1968, Harper & Row, Publishers.

Handbook for victims, Pittsburgh, Pa., 1979, Interagency Task Force on Rape-Related Services of Allegheny County.

Hoover, H.: On the uncommon man. In Address upon the American road: 1948-1950, Stanford, Calif., 1951, Stanford University Press.

Kahn, A., Kamerman, S., and McGowan, B.: Child advocacy report on a national baseline study, New York, 1972, Columbia University School of Social Work.

Kalkman, M.: Models of psychiatric treatment. In Kalkman, M., and Davis, A.: New dimensions in mental health-psychiatric nursing, New York, 1974, McGraw-Hill Book Co.

Katz, S., and Mazur, M.A.: Understanding the rape victim: a synthesis of research findings, New York, 1979, John Wiley & Sons, Inc.

Kjervik, D.: The stress of sexism on the mental health of women. In Kjervik, D., and Martinsion, I., editors: Women in stress: a nursing perspective, New York, 1979, Appleton-Century-Crofts.

Lange, A., and Jakubowski, P.: Responsibile assertive behavior: cognitive/behavioral procedures for trainers, Champaign, Ill., 1976, Research Press.

Lazare, A.: Hidden conceptual models in clinical psychiatry, New Engl. J. Med. **288**:345, 1973.

Protocol for examination of rape victims, Pittsburgh, Pa., 1979, Interagency Task Force on Rape-Related Services of Allegheny County.

Meyer, K., and Meyer, F.F., Jr.: Split roles in performance appraisal, Harvard Bus. Rev. **1**:123, Jan.-Feb. 1965.

Nowakowski, L.: A new look at client advocacy. In Hall, J.E., and Weaver, B.R., editors: Distributive nursing practice: a systems approach to community nursing, Philadelphia, 1977, J.B. Lippincott.

Price, S., Catlin, G., and Cruthis, D.: Protocol on preventing pregnancy and venereal disease, Rochester, N.Y., 1979, Rape Crisis Service of Planned Parenthood of Rochester and Monroe County, New York.

Rosenbaum, C., and Beebe, J.: Psychiatric treatment: crisis/clinic/consultation, New York, 1975, McGraw-Hill Book Co.

Schiff, A.: A statistical evaluation of rape, Forensic Sci. **2**:339, 1973.

Stevens, D.: Personal communication, Feb. 1981, Sexual Assault Center, Harborview Medical Center, Seattle, Wash.

Stevens, D., and Ousley, N.: Sequelae of chemically-involved sexual assault, Harborview Medical Center, 1981, Seattle, Wash.

Topalis, M., and Aguilera, D.C.: Psychiatric nursing, ed. 7, St. Louis, 1978, The C.V. Mosby Co.

## ANNOTATED SUGGESTED READINGS

Braen, G.R.: The rape examination (monograph), 1978, Division of Emergency Medicine, University of Kentucky College of Medicine. Available from Professional Relations Department, Abbott Laboratories, Abbott Park, North Chicago, IL. Fee $.50.

This monograph provides a written text that accompanies the film *The Rape Examination*. It is a comprehensive discussion of the medicolegal examination that follows sexual assault. The film reinforces and complements the reading.

Burgess, A.W., and Holmstrom, L.L.: The rape victim in the emergency ward, Am. J. Nurs. **10**:1741, 1973.

This article is an excellent synopsis of what happens to a rape victim as she is swept along in care systems. The victim's psychologic responses are poignantly illustrated. Details of the medical process and evidence collection are provided, along with nursing implications and the use of crisis centers in immediate and follow-up care.

Burgess, A.W., and Holmstrom, L.L.: Accountability: a right of the rape victim, J. Psychiatr. Nurs. **13**(3):11 May-June 1975.

The authors define accountability and focus on two aspects: defining one's role and explaining the services to be provided. They describe reactions of victims to police, hospital staff, and counselors. The authors also make a comparison of victims' reactions to three professional groups. They state that victims want explanations from professionals about role expectations and want procedures to be accurately implemented.

Burgess, A.W., and Laszlo, A.T.: Courtroom use of hospital records in sexual assault cases, Am. J. Nurs. **1**:64, 1977.

This article discusses the use of medical records to prosecute rapists and the role of health care professionals as witnesses in legal proceedings. Collection of evidence—particularly the objective, factual recording of signs and symptoms of emotional and physical trauma—is presented. A sample patient record assessment and formulation form is illustrated.

Bush, M.A., and Kjervik, D.: The nurse's self-image. In Kjervik, D., and Martinson, I., editors: Women in stress: a nursing perspective, New York, 1979, Appleton-Century-Crofts.

The authors discuss the historical roots through which women and nurses have systematically learned not to value themselves but to have a poor self-concept and sense of self-worth. They describe nurses' values and attitudes as affecting the care they give to patients, their degree of assertiveness, and tension among interdisciplinary health team members.

Fogel, C., and Woods, N.: Health care of women: a nursing perspective, St. Louis, 1981, The C.V. Mosby Co.

This text provides nurses with an overview of topics and issues that influence women's health in contemporary society. Unit 1 addresses the importance of the nurse's awareness of prevalent health problems that affect women. Unit 2 focuses on promotion and maintenance of health with women. Unit 3 addresses problems that commonly affect women (such as violence, sexual dysfunctions, and pregnancy). Unit 4 emphasizes the promotion and maintenance of women's health over the life cycle. The text is an excellent resource for all clinicians and students.

Foley, T.S.: Counseling the victim of rape. In Stuart, G., and Sundeen., S., editors: Principles and practice of psychiatric nursing, ed. 2, St. Louis, 1983, The C.V. Mosby Co.

This chapter discusses the medical examination of the victim of rape. The author offers nursing intervention guidelines and introduces a limited presentation on collecting medicolegal evidence.

Freibert, P., and Bridwell, M.W.: An intervention model for rape and unwanted pregnancy, Counseling psychologist **6:**50, 1976.

The authors present the analytic grief process as one framework for understanding and helping a woman who is working through feelings about pregnancy resulting from rape. They describe their philosophical orientation and related counseling interventions.

Halpern, S.: Rape—helping the victim: a treatment manual. Oradell, N.J., 1978, Medical Economics Company Book Division.

This text addresses: the victim's immediate needs; the arrival at the emergency room; the medical history; the medical examination and collection of evidence; venereal disease and pregnancy information for the victim; and exit procedures. The book is a helpful reference resource.

Herman, S.J.: Becoming assertive: a guide for nurses, New York, 1978, D. Van Nostrand Co.

The first part of this book discusses the background and history of assertiveness training. The author defines terms and gives sample work situations to use, a bill of interpersonal rights, assertiveness communication skills, and a self-help unit on assertiveness instruction. In the second part the author begins with caring assertions that foster rapport in working relationships and then presents a discussion of assertiveness in terms of patient advocacy.

Holmstrom, L.L., and Burgess, A.W.: The hospital as healer and detective. In Holmstrom, L.L., and Burgess, A.W., editors: The victim of rape: institutional reactions, New York, 1978, John Wiley & Sons.

The authors describe how rape victims confront and endure institutional processes in hospital emergency departments. Two contradictory staff tasks presented are: (1) provision of therapeutic medical care and (2) collection of legal evidence. Discussion focuses on the staff's conflicting duties; attitudes and behavior; the victim's perception of the hospital; tasks, hospital protocol, and violation of the body; victims kept in ignorance; victims depersonalized by the system; lack of privacy; recording of information; and specialization and professional isolation.

Magee, J.: The pelvic examination: a view from the other end of the table. In Halpern, S.: Rape—helping the victim: a treatment manual, Oradell, N.J., 1978, Medical Economics Company Book Division.

A female gynecologist presents a sensitive discussion of ways to make the pelvic examination more comfortable for a woman through a style of care that conveys a sense of respect and involves the woman in her own welfare. Nurses can recommend to physicians the suggested care approaches when assisting with rape examinations.

Silverman, D.: First do no more harm: female rape victims and the male counselor, Am. J. Orthopsychiatry **47:**91, 1977.

The author sensitively describes the difficulties involved when men are responsible for aiding female victims of rape. This article explains the misconceptions and responses that may interfere with the well-meaning efforts of male counselors. The author discusses the approaches men commonly employ to handle their feelings and offers alternate approaches that are more helpful to the victim. Nurses may find this article useful in working with male physicians in emergency room settings.

Welch, M.S.: Rape and the trauma of inadequate care, Prism **9:**17, 1975.

The author describes many of the concerns of the rape victim. It discusses many ways of making the examination and treatment process more humane and sensitive to the woman's needs. This article is helpful in developing sensitive nursing interventions with victims.

Woods, N.F., and Luke, C.: Sexuality and abortion. In Woods, N.: Human sexuality in health and illness, ed. 2, St. Louis, 1979, The C.V. Mosby Co.

Pregnancy and abortion are major concerns for victims of rape. Abortion forces nurses to reexamine their beliefs, values, and attitudes; thus the issue needs to be investigated in terms of the woman's psychologic adaptation and biologic problems. The authors address (1) sexual antecedents of abortion, (2) a review of sexual sequelae of abortion, (3) feelings that the woman and the professional work through at the time of, and subsequent to, a decision to obtain an abortion, and (4) the professional's role in helping a woman who has an abortion and her partner to make a positive sexual adjustment.

## CHAPTER 7

# Basic counseling and crisis intervention

My life has changed since that night. In the beginning, the days were rough—long and hard. The nights were worse, endless and filled with nightmares. In time, however, the bad days grew further and further apart, and the happy days returned.

Anonymous victim. In Interagency Task Force on Rape-Related Services: *A handbook for victims*, p. 13.

## CHAPTER OUTLINE

**Core qualities of helping relationships**
  Accurate empathy
  Nonpossessive warmth
  Respect
**Crisis theory**
  Types of crises
  Development of a crisis

Resolution of a crisis
**Crisis theory and rape victim responses**
  Assessment of a crisis state
  Crisis intervention model
**Crisis theory and family response**

**Telephone crisis counseling**
**Creative listening**
  Self-exploration
  Self-understanding
  Action
**Summary**

## LEARNING OBJECTIVES

After reading this chapter the student will be able to:

1 Describe three core qualities of helping relationships essential to effective counseling of rape victims

2 Relate the development and resolution of a crisis to rape victim responses

3 List six areas of assessment in the mental status examination

4 Apply the crisis intervention model to rape victim situations

5 List ten objectives of telephone crisis counseling

6 Describe crisis reactions of families of rape victims

7 Identify three phases of the creative listening model in counseling rape victims

An important role for many professional nurses involves counseling rape victims who need emotional support after the rape event. Professionally skilled nurses who counsel these victims have the responsibility of developing a sound knowledge base for directing and guiding their counseling techniques in clinical practice. Rape victims look to nurses for direction, guidance, and emotional support.

How do nurses counsel rape victims? Are there basic guidelines for counseling these victims? Nurses skilled in counseling practice use many models and theoretic bases in their professional work. This chapter presents two models that provide nurses with basic guidelines for helping rape victims: the crisis intervention model and the creative listening model.

Crisis theory provides nurses with an understanding of how a crisis state develops in a rape victim's response to the assault. Not only do crises develop according to designated phases, but their resolution also follows a predictable course. The crisis intervention model provides nurses with guidelines for helping rape victims and their families work through the crisis resolution process. The model can also be effectively applied to telephone counseling of rape victims.

Another basic counseling technique, creative listening (sometimes referred to as active listening), provides nurses with fundamental guidelines for developing effective helping relationships with rape victims. This model guides nurses to respond empathically to the feelings of rape victims in helping them decide for themselves what to do about their situation. Nurses skilled in counseling practice can easily incorporate the creative listening model in their work.

Regardless of a professional nurse's level of education, the progress of clients in counseling is related to three dimensions of the counseling relationship called *core qualities*. When present at high levels in the relationship, core qualities promote client growth. When present at low levels, these qualities lead to deterioration in the counseling relationship and a lack of client progress.

## CORE QUALITIES OF HELPING RELATIONSHIPS

Three core qualities in counseling are (1) accurate empathy, (2) nonpossessive warmth, and (3) respect. Each of these qualities is discussed in detail in the section that follows.

### Accurate empathy

The first essential quality is *accurate empathy,* which is defined as the ability to perceive and communicate accurately and with sensitivity the feelings, thoughts, and experiences of the client. Accurate empathy involves subjectivity to the extent that nurses have the capacity to participate in a victim's feelings or ideas. Yet it also involves objectivity to the extent that nurses differentiate their own experiences from those of the victim. In other words, nurses who have accurate empathy recognize their own separateness from rape victims.

*Sympathy* is a quality that is characterized by feeling sorry for a rape victim. (Table 7-1 illustrates the differences between accurate empathy and sympathy.) Sympathy involves subjectivity to the point that nurses do not differentiate their own feelings from the victim's feelings and experiences. Sympathetic nurses may even experience

**Table 7-1. Accurate empathy vs sympathy**

| Accurate empathy | Sympathy |
| --- | --- |
| Perceptions are mainly objective | Perceptions are subjective |
| Some subjective, less intense feelings | All subjective, very intense feelings |
| Aware of client's thoughts, feelings, and experiences | Experiences client's thoughts, feelings, and experiences |
| Separateness from client is recognized | No separateness from client |
| Focus is on the client | Focus is on the nurse |
| Shows sensitivity | Shows little concern |
| Feels concern and wants to help | Feels sorry for and wants to console |
| Constructive to nurse-client relationship | Destructive to nurse-client relationship |

the same intensity of feelings as rape victims. Listening and focusing on rape events or post-rape experiences as though the rape happened to them, sympathetic nurses show little concern for or understanding of what a rape victim is experiencing. The following example demonstrates that some nurses have difficulty providing care that reflects accurate empathy.

### CLINICAL EXAMPLE

Mrs. Ray, a 67-year-old widow, lived alone in her own home following the death of her husband 5 years previously. She had one son who lived out of state. Upon the death of her husband, the son had encouraged Mrs. Ray to live with him and his wife, but Mrs. Ray had declined the offer saying she preferred to remain in her own home.

One night as she was sleeping, Mrs. Ray was suddenly awakened by a man who was on top of her in her bed. The man held his hand over Mrs. Ray's mouth and a knife at her throat. He whispered, "Not a sound or you'll be dead, lady!" The man then raped Mrs. Ray and forced her to have oral sex. Mrs. Ray could not believe that the rape was happening and felt that she had no recourse but to comply with the man's demands. Mrs. Ray feared for her life! After what seemed like hours, the man left the home, but before leaving he hit Mrs. Ray across the face and stated, "You'll be stupid, lady, if you tell anyone about this!"

Mrs. Ray was in a state of shock. It took her 10 or 15 minutes before she was able to move. Realizing that she was physically injured as a result of the trauma, Mrs. Ray decided she had better go to a hospital for help. She called a neighbor who helped her get to the hospital. The neighbor provided support to Mrs. Ray until they reached the emergency department.

In the emergency department, Mrs. Ray was nonverbal. Her only response was to shake her head and say, "I can't believe this happened. I can't believe this happened." Jan, a staff nurse, had taken care of younger women but never an older rape victim. Jan's perception was that older women are asexual, and therefore she could not quite understand Mrs. Ray's severe shock state after the trauma. Jan commented to another nurse, "I can't understand why Mrs. Ray is taking this so hard. If she were younger, she would really have something to be shook about!"

Jan's co-worker, Mary, herself an older woman, quickly identified with Mrs. Ray. Mary said to the younger nurse (Jan), "Oh, the poor dear! You can't possibly understand what Mrs. Ray is going through. If I were raped, I would feel overwhelmed and helpless. After all, she's all alone and frightened. Let me take care of her—I feel sorry for her!"

Overhearing the conversation, a third nurse, Michelle, offered to take the case assignment. Michelle also realized that older women are especially traumatized physically by a rape assault because of the beginning of advanced tissue atrophy. Michelle responded to Mrs. Ray by stating, "I can understand that this has been a shocking and painful experience for you."

The clinical example above demonstrates three different nursing approaches. The first staff nurse (Jan) lacked the ability to perceive the rape victim's feelings of shock and disbelief. The second nurse (Mary), unable to differentiate what she would feel from the feelings of the rape victim, showed sympathy for the victim. The third nurse (Michelle) demonstrated accurate empathy by perceiving the victim's emotional and physical discomfort and sensitively communicating to the victim that she understood those feelings.

### Nonpossessive warmth

A second core quality is *nonpossessive warmth*, which is defined as an emotional intensity that signals to a rape victim that the nurse cares about her. Nurses who possess this quality have integrated the attitudes of acceptance and high regard for victims. Nonpossessive warmth is conveyed to rape victims by two styles of nursing care: (1) nonverbal behaviors (usually the mode for communicating warmth) and (2) verbal statements. Examples of nonverbal communications of nonpossessive warmth are tones of voice, gestures, body postures, and length of silences. The following example shows how rape victims sense a nurse's real attitudes by the congruency between what the nurse says and what the nurse does.

CLINICAL EXAMPLE

When Carol, a 32-year-old rape victim, entered the emergency department, she sensed that no one really cared about her. Physicians and nurses were bustling around in what looked like a frenzy of activity. No one gave Carol attention because other emergencies were obviously getting priority. Sitting alone in the examination room, Carol started to cry. When Dennis, the staff nurse, passed by the room, he observed Carol's sad, dejected mood. Knowing Carol was a rape victim, Dennis hesitated to approach Carol. Being a male, Dennis did not want to increase Carol's fears by moving in too close. Standing in the doorway, Dennis said, "I sense that you're having a rough time. Can I help you any?" Startled, Carol looked at Dennis and noticed his reassurring smile and concerned manner. Carol was not frightened; instead she felt relief that Dennis showed some concern for her situation. Carol responded, "I guess I'm not really an emergency . . . but I didn't know where else to go!" Dennis replied, "You've come to the best place for care. Right now the emergency department is receiving car accident victims. That's why we're so busy." Reassured that she was not being rejected, Carol managed a smile. She said, "That's what I thought was happening, but I wasn't sure. Thanks for telling me. . . . Thanks for caring."

The clinical example above illustrates that nonpossessive warmth is conveyed by both verbal and nonverbal communication techniques. Through these techniques the rape victim senses that the nurse cares about her. Even a brief interaction can communicate genuine concern for the victim. Counseling relationships involve a longer time and a deeper intensity in the nurse-client relationship. However, even during brief interactions, rape victims quickly sense nurses who genuinely care and have the quality of nonpossessive warmth.

## Respect

Respect is the third core quality in a helping relationship. *Respect* is defined as special regard for the value and worth of a person. Nurses who respect rape victims accept victims as they are, rather than demanding that they be the way someone else would like them to be. Victims who sense respect from nurses feel valued as persons. Respectful nurses have a high regard for the rights of rape victims to act in accordance with their personal perceptions and values. Victims who feel respected also feel free to be themselves. The following clinical example demonstrates how one nurse combined respect with the other core qualities of accurate empathy and nonpossessive warmth.

### CLINICAL EXAMPLE

Winnie is a 23-year-old rape victim who met with Terri, a nurse who was volunteering at a rape counseling center. After introducing herself, Winnie shared a brief description of her situation. Winnie had been riding along a bike trail in a park area near her home. Stopping for a drink of water, she was grabbed from behind by an overpowering man. Winnie felt something sharp in her back. The man directed her to walk into the park, saying, "I have a knife and I'll slice you up!" Complying with his demand, Winnie walked deeper into the park away from the bike trail. Holding a knife to her throat, the man raped Winnie and threatened to leave her dead. While begging the man not to kill her, Winnie heard voices nearby and, taking a chance, she screamed for help. Frightened, the man ran away. Two bikers found Winnie and offered to take her to a nearby hospital. Needing time to sort out her thoughts, she declined the offer of assistance. Still terrified, shocked, and somewhat embarrassed, Winnie biked home and, going in the back door, slipped up to her bedroom unobserved. One hour after the rape, Winnie called the rape hotline for help and talked with Terri, the nurse on call. Winnie did not want to tell her parents for she feared that her parents would feel humiliated.

Terri listened patiently as Winnie gave an account of the rape incident. Terri used a quiet, reassuring tone of voice to convey a concerned, caring attitude. She also used intermittent verbal messages to indicate acceptance and high regard for Winnie. Terri's verbal statements included:

"It must have been terribly frightening for you."

"It's upsetting when you go through such a horrible attack."

"I'd like to help you through this rough time."

"It helps sometimes to tell someone about all the awful things that happened."

"You're worried about upsetting your parents. Let's talk more about that."

The rape victim in the clinical example above sought counseling help because she could not tell her parents about the experience. Using the core qualities of accurate empathy, nonpossessive warmth, and respect, the nurse counselor (Terri) directed counseling skills toward working through Winnie's concerns.

Nurses use the core qualities of helping relationships in assisting rape victims to progress in counseling. Nurses promote client growth through the therapeutic use of self by being someone who:

1. Accepts and respects the victim as a person
2. Listens in a nonjudgmental manner
3. Accurately perceives and understands the victim's thoughts, feelings, and perceptions
4. Is willing and professionally trained to help the victim through her personal crisis

Because rape is a crisis event for most victims, the following section describes how crisis states both develop and are resolved according to predictable courses. Application of the crisis intervention model to the nursing care of rape victims and their families is emphasized.

## CRISIS THEORY

Caplan defines a crisis as "an upset in a steady state when a person faces an obstacle to important life goals that is, for a time, insurmountable through utilization of customary methods of problem-solving. A period of disorganization ensues, a period of upset, during which many abortive attempts at solution are made."[4] For most rape victims a crisis follows the traumatic event. However, *a crisis does not have to follow a rape.* Some victims have adequate resources to handle the impact of rape and therefore may not experience a crisis. But if the stress of the rape overwhelms victims and they are unable to handle their responses with customary coping patterns, a crisis results.

**Table 7-2. Crisis development**

| Crisis phase | Responses |
|---|---|
| 1. Tension rises | Impaired reasoning |
| | Emotionally anxious |
| | Fearful, angry, guilty |
| | Perception is narrowed |
| | Cognitions are rigid |
| 2. Lack of success in coping | Rise in emotional tension |
| | Increased intensity of response |
| | High anxiety level |
| 3. Emergency problem-solving | Uses every resource available |
| | Uses unusual or new means |
| | May redefine or change goals to avoid crisis |
| 4. Disorganization | Internal strength lacking |
| | Social support lacking |
| | Problem is unresolved |
| | Unbearable degree of tension and anxiety |

## Types of crises

It is important for nurses to distinguish between two types of crises: developmental and situational. A *developmental (or maturational) crisis* occurs as a normal process of growth and development. Each person goes through major transition states that challenge the steady state. Generally, the person experiences a high level of anxiety during this transition and may be aware of increased feelings of disequilibrium. Major developmental or maturational crises occur during periods of great psychologic, social, and physical change, such as puberty, young adulthood, and marriage. These are times when people make a transition from old roles, tasks, and responsibilities to new ones.

The second type of crisis is a *situational crisis*, which occurs as a result of some unanticipated traumatic event. Since the event is unforeseen, the person is generally not prepared to handle it. The stressful event threatens the person's sense of biologic, psychologic, or social integrity, resulting in disequilibrium and loss of control. Common situational crises include the death of a loved one, divorce, loss of a job, diagnosis of a chronic or fatal illness, and disasters (such as fire or flood).

## Development of a crisis

The highly *subjective nature* of crisis experiences cannot be overestimated. What may be a crisis for one person is not a crisis for another person. Table 7-2 illustrates the development of a crisis.

A crisis develops over a period of time that is unique to each individual. However, there are identifiable phases of crisis development that result in a crisis state. Crises usually follow four developmental phases:

1. Initial rise in tension occurs as habitual problem-solving techniques are tried.
2. There is a lack of success in coping and restoring homeostasis with the usual coping mechanisms. The stress continues and more discomfort is felt.
3. A further increase in stress acts as a powerful internal stimulus. The person mobilizes internal and external resources to solve the problem and reduce the painful state of anxiety.
4. If the problem continues and can neither be solved nor avoided, tension increases and a major disorganization and/or disintegration of personality occurs.[1,4]

A full-blown crisis can be avoided at any phase of development if the rape victim constructively copes with the anxiety. A victim gains support from other persons who help with the coping process. The means of avoiding a crisis is specific to the individual and depends on personality structure, life circumstances, and support networks.

Many crises develop from the *interaction* of developmental and situational variables. The rape victim is assessed both for her developmental status and her situational state. The following example demonstrates how a traumatic event that occurs during a developmental transition can increase the likelihood of an intense physical, emotional, and social response.

### CLINICAL EXAMPLE

Mary, age 19, just left home for her first year of college. Her father, mother, and brother helped her find an apartment. Mary moved in several days before the term and planned to set up housekeeping. She was excited but a little scared. This was her first experience in living away from home.

The second evening Mary answered a knock on her front door. Two young men introduced themselves as her neighbors and welcomed Mary to the apartment building. Mary invited them in for a cup of coffee. As Mary prepared the coffee, one young man entered the kitchen and grabbed her. Mary tried to scream, but he had his hands over her mouth. As the young man raped Mary, the other man kept a watch at the front door.

Later that day Mary went to the emergency room of the local hospital. She was in a shock state and badly bruised. She could not respond to the nurse's directions. She kept mumbling: "What will my family think?" "I'll have to go home." "I really blew it."

The above example illustrates a rape occurring during a developmental transition. The victim (Mary) was struggling with maturational conflicts of independence and self-reliance. The situational crisis of rape, occuring at this time in Mary's life, increased the likelihood that Mary would have intense physical, psychologic, or social disturbances after the rape. (See Chapter 4 for a complete discussion of developmental stressors.)

**Table 7-3. Phases of crisis resolution***

| Crisis phase | Response |
|---|---|
| Anticipatory phase | Sense of impending danger, threat, or change is felt. |
| Impact phase | Major disorganization occurs. Characteristics are disorientation and distractability. Present moment is time frame and phase may last hours.<br>Observer may notice that individual does not search for lost object or reminiscence. |
| Recoil/turmoil phase | Feelings of rage, anxiety, guilt, and depression emerge.<br>Thoughts are ambiguous and uncertain. Direction appears detached.<br>Search behavior consists of perplexed scanning.<br>Time frame is days later and perspective is oriented to past.<br>Evidence of struggle to work with aid of personal capacities and outside assistance appears. |
| Adjustment phase | Occurs weeks later. Perspective is toward future and feelings of hope.<br>Able to engage in problem-solving again.<br>Search behavior consists of exploration.<br>Direction is toward search for new objects.<br>Post-traumatic detachment from those who give guidance and assistance is noted. |
| Reconstruction phase | Occurs months later.<br>Differs from adjustment by reattachment and search behavior that now consists of testing. |

*Sources: Aguilera, D.C., and Messick, J.M.: Crisis intervention: theory and methodology, ed. 4, St. Louis, 1981, The C.V. Mosby Co.; Burgess, A.W., and Holmstrom, L.L.: Rape trauma syndrome, Am. J. Psychiatry **131**:981, 1974.

### Resolution of a crisis

Not only does a crisis develop along designated phases, but a crisis is *resolved* according to a predictable course. The person in crisis cannot tolerate a state of psychologic turmoil for an extended period. The acute emotional upset generally lasts from a few days to a few weeks. If the person is still in crisis after this period, the individual expresses a need for resolution of the problem: "I give up! I can't take this any longer! Please help me, I can't stand it!"

There are several phases to crisis resolution. The general phases are presented in Table 7-3. Rape victims are usually in a state of emotional upset and nurses understand that their crisis will resolve following a predictable course.

Several outcomes are possible in a crisis:

1. The person can return to a precrisis state. This happens when problem-solving skills are effective.
2. The person can grow from the crisis experience. This happens when *new* resources or problem-solving skills are developed.
3. The person can handle intolerable tension by lapsing into neurotic or psychotic patterns of behavior. This can happen when people have distorted perceptions, withdraw, become suspicious or depressed, drink excessively, or abuse drugs.

## CRISIS THEORY AND RAPE VICTIM RESPONSES

Rape victims are highly prone to develop crises because of the disturbing and violent nature of rape. Nurses have a professional responsibility to assess rape victims to determine whether they are experiencing a crisis state. If their assessments indicate a crisis state, nurses plan and initiate interventions that help rape victims cope with their crisis experience. The following section emphasizes two important functions of the professional nurse who works with rape victims: (1) assessment of a crisis state and (2) crisis intervention. Crisis intervention has two goals: (1) to help the person return to a precrisis state and (2) if possible, to help the person grow and become stronger as a result of the crisis. Nurses need to recognize that crises can result in positive outcomes. With appropriate support, persons generally cope with crises. Growth can, and often does, occur amidst the pain and turmoil of stressful events.

### Assessment of a crisis state

Chapter 6 emphasized the importance of a thorough physical assessment of rape victims prior to the delivery of medical treatment. Likewise, a thorough *assessment of mental status* of rape victims is essential prior to crisis intervention.

Crisis states are clinically similar to stress reactions (described in Chapter 4). Both theoretic models are used in making nursing assessments of rape victims. Professional nurses decide which theoretic model best applies to a particular clinical setting. Regardless of the model, the accuracy of assessments of mental status *prior to* nursing interventions cannot be overemphasized.

When a victim reports having been sexually assaulted, her emotional status is to be assessed in terms of her current crisis state and post-traumatic stress response. The victim did not seek care for a psychiatric evaluation, and a severe response to rape, in itself (without other evidence), is insufficient reason for labeling the victim as "mentally ill." However, it is important to assess the victim's mental status and add this information to the medical record. Thus the medical record will reflect both physical and emotional signs and symptoms of rape trauma and can be used in court to support the victim's case. Knowledge of the mental status examination provides a base for assessing the nature of a victim's emotional distress. A general outline for this examination is as follows:

*General appearance and behavior*—physical health, hygiene, dress, and manner. Includes attitude, posture, mannerisms, and facial expressions.

*Consciousness awareness*—the state of awareness of the patient. Includes orientation to time, place, and person; ability to focus on a subject theme or event; self-awareness and suggestability; and sleep patterns.

*Affectivity and mood*—the emotional feeling tone that accompanies an idea; mood is a sustained and prevailing emotional set. Includes depression, elation, anxiety, fear, apathy, mood swings, and aggression; style can be controlled or expressive.

*Motor behavior*—the activity level and motor response. Includes goal-directed activity, inactivity, hyperactivity, and underactivity (psychomotor retardation).

*Thought content*—flow of ideas, associations, and symbols. Includes what the persons says, style of thoughts, and perceptual disturbances.

*Intellectual functioning*—The capacity for rational or intelligent thought. Includes memory, judgment, general knowledge, ability to abstract, insight (the act of seeing into a situation), and intelligence.

The mental status exam provides information on observable aspects of a person's psychologic abilities in functioning. Assessment of a victim's mental status is a continuous process that begins with the victim's contact with a health system for treatment and continues throughout the treatment process.

Most rape victims respond to the rape experience within normal limits of a mental status exam and do not attempt suicide. However, systematic data do show that women who have a history of serious psychologic difficulties have a more severe response to rape and are more vulnerable to psychologic problems in resolving the rape experience. Serious psychologic difficulties include suicide attempts, suicidal ideation (thoughts), and psychosis (not being in contact with reality). Table 7-4 presents several high-risk factors in assessing the suicide potential of a victim. Although the characteristics listed in the table were derived from studies of persons expressing suicide intent and those attempting and/or completing suicide, the high-risk factors are not absolute; nor are they the only elements to be taken into account by professional nurses. Nurses responsible for assessing a victim's suicide risk are encouraged to pursue further readings on suicide intervention.[3,5]

A victim's psychologic state (mental status) post-rape usually corresponds to her phase of crisis in resolving the rape. Table 7-5 presents a clinical example of a rape victim's psychologic responses (mental status) and relates these responses to crisis theory (crisis phase). As demonstrated in the table, the victim did not seek psychiatric care after the rape but did seek medical care and treatment. This victim was referred for short-term counseling because of emotional signs and symptoms of rape trauma (fear, self-blame, and anger). At no time was this victim assessed by the nurse as being suicidal. In the adjustment phase the victim resumed her normal activities and showed

Table 7-4. High-risk factors in assessing suicide potential

| Factor | Characteristic |
|---|---|
| Age | Middle and older age |
| | Incidence increases with age for white males only |
| | Adolescents |
| Sex | Men (70%), women (30%) |
| Family status | Separated, divorced, widowed |
| | Recent loss |
| | Lack of supportive network/resources |
| | Social isolation |
| Race | White, American Indian, urban blacks |
| Religion | Protestant |
| Profession | Competitive and/or demanding of interpersonal giving, e.g., nurses, doctors, lawyers, policemen, housekeepers |
| Employment status | Unemployed |
| Geographic location | |
|   Local | Transitional and slum urban areas; renters |
|   National | West Coast (especially San Francisco) |
| Health | Poor health or physical illness |
| | Depression |
| | Alcohol or drug abuse |
| | Unexplained change in behavior |
| Personality styles | Impulsive personality |
| | Compulsive personality (especially if combined with erosion of gratifying life-style) |
| | Risk-taking personality |
| Suicide plan | Suicidal thoughts explicit |
| | Lethal potential in degree of intent and/or chosen method |
| | Availability of means |
| | Plan communicated to others |
| | Sophistication of the client |
| Chronic predisposing psychiatric conditions | Past suicidal history (single most important prognosticator of suicidal potential) |
| | Depression (especially when depression is improving/remitting) |
| | Manic-depressive disease (especially the depressive phase) |

Sources: Hoff, L.A.: People in crisis: understanding and helping, Menlo Park, Calif., 1978, Addison-Wesley Publishing Co.; Rosenbaum, C.P., and Beebe, J.E.: Psychiatric treatment: crisis/clinic/consultation, New York, 1975, McGraw-Hill Book Co., pp. 19-41.

improvement of her mental status. Finally the victim resolved her crisis. The outcome was a growth experience—she felt stronger and had new problem-solving skills.

## Crisis intervention model

The immediate needs of rape victims are met first. Usually the medical emergency needs are readily identified, and structured nursing care can be administered. (See Chapter 6 for specific nursing interventions within a medical system.)

Useful guidelines for nursing interventions with rape victims in crisis states include the following:

1. Creative listening
2. Empathic understanding
3. Helping victims gain a realistic perception of the rape event

**Table 7-5. Rape victim response phases**

| Crisis phase | Mental status |
| --- | --- |
| Anticipatory phase | Neat in dress; good hygiene. Does not feel safe in the parking garage alone at night after shopping; fearful. |
| Impact phase | Rape occurs—victim is confused about whether she should tell anyone or get medical care. She crawls into her car, locks the doors, and does nothing. She is stunned, slightly disoriented, and fearful. Appears disheveled. Activity is not goal directed. |
| Recoil/turmoil phase | Victim seeks medical care. During the physical exam she searches her mind for what she would have done to cause the rape or could have done differently to prevent it. She is furious with the assailant but cannot face him, and that makes her even more angry. No suicidal ideation. She wonders how she can ever discharge her rage. She is referred to a nurse-counselor who plans to help her resolve these feelings. |
| Adjustment phase | Victim resumes her normal life-style and work responsibilities. She is optimistic that this will not ruin her relationship with other men in the future. She is trying out new social activities and finding friends she never knew to be real friends. She expresses that she does not feel the need to continue with counseling. |
| Reconstruction phase | Victim tries out new behaviors learned in counseling. She feels like a stronger person as a result of this experience. She is more assertive and values herself. |

4. Helping rape victims gain a sense of control over their crisis experience
5. Helping victims explore ways of coping
6. Linking rape victims to supportive social networks

Through *creative listening* nurses demonstrate attention and concern for victims who have been hurt deeply. Rape victims need to feel deserving of help. Their ability to cope with their crisis increases when nurses communicate to victims that they are worthwhile persons.

The technique of *empathic understanding* encourages the open expression of victims' feelings. Nurses who accept victims encourage expression of intense feelings of anger, grief, frustration, helplessness, and hopelessness. Nurses can help victims recognize that intense or negative feelings are appropriate responses after a shocking, stressful rape experience.

Perception of the event involves how the rape victim thinks, feels, and acts about the rape.[1] What does the rape mean to the victim? How does she see its effect on her present behaviors and future life? Is she perceiving the rape realistically, or does she distort its meaning?

Nurses *help rape victims gain control of their crisis* by aiding them in understanding and accepting the fact that they are not to blame for their rape. Self-care decisions can be made only after victims are able to work through feelings of self-blame. Victims are encouraged to examine the total situation, including their own behavior. Such a review process helps victims gain an understanding of the rape instead of experiencing self-depreciation and guilt. Victims learn to evaluate the evidence for their assumptions and make appropriate conclusions. With a clear perspective of the event and their responses, victims can free energy for better problem-solving in relation to self-care needs.

Most rape victims have the innate *ability to cope* with a rape crisis, but many need support and reassurance throughout the coping process. Nurses can explore a victim's typical ways of coping with stress to determine if the victim can use those coping mechanisms in resolving the rape experience.[1] Some rape victims need to explore alternate responses and learn new coping skills.

A powerful means of resolving a crisis is the establishment or reestablishment of interpersonal contacts with significant people who are supportive to a victim's needs.[1] *Supportive people* may be mates, spouses, family members, friends, or neighbors. These meaningful relationships can be explored, and the significant persons can be summoned to provide emotional support to the rape victim. Nurses can also assist rape victims in identifying the social resources in their community that are currently available to provide important means of crisis resolution—for example, rape crisis centers, police systems, or medical care systems. Nurses can actively link rape victims with social resources in their community.

The following clinical example demonstrates how a nurse assessed a victim's crisis state and then applied goal-directed nursing interventions to help the victim cope with the stressful situation.

### CLINICAL EXAMPLE

Cheryl is a 24-year-old single woman who is completing her master's degree in the social sciences. She has been traveling about the city to different agencies, interviewing the directors to see if they would participate in her research project. Cheryl finally got her research questionnaire from her typist. She dropped it off with the night supervisor so that the director would have it to read first thing in the morning.

Cheryl stated that as she left the agency two men jumped out of the bushes. One man grabbed her around the neck and mouth and put a knife to her throat, while the other man blindfolded her. They forced her into a car and drove to a nearby park where they raped her. One man would help restrain her while the other one raped her, and then they reversed roles. They laughed at her and made obscene, vulgar remarks. They left her nude in the park and drove off with her car, which they later abandoned. Cheryl pulled herself together and was able to flag down a taxi driver who took her to the emergency department (ED).

Cheryl told the nurse, "I can't believe that this really happened. It's far too crazy to be real." She reported feeling simply glad to be alive and not too badly harmed. Cheryl said she was sure other victims had been treated worse and survived, and that the nurse probably had other patients in the ED that needed care more than she. Cheryl reassured the nurse that she would be alright. She had not had much sleep because she had been working hard on her research, and the accumulated exhaustion was obvious. Cheryl told the nurse not to worry, that she was used to taking care of herself and was "just kind of numb." Cheryl said she was particularly upset because she had lost her virginity and that she had been "saving herself for marriage someday." She wondered how this would affect her future relationships with men, but she acted confident that she would work through her feelings.

Using crisis theory, the nurse in the above clinical example recognized and assessed the following facts:

1. Cheryl was experiencing the impact phase of crisis resolution, which is characterized by shock and disbelief, reliving the event, and feelings of loss (virginity, control over her life).
2. Cheryl was trying to gain some control of her life after a traumatic event that she realistically perceived as life threatening.
3. Cheryl did not identify or request the support of any person during this period.
4. Cheryl's adaptive coping mechanisms included outward adjustment maneuvers of independence, self-reliance, and minimization (denial) of the impact and disruption caused by the assault.

The nurse's planned interventions during Cheryl's crisis were designed to strengthen the factors that facilitate crisis resolution (perception of event and coping mechanism) and to explore the factors that impede crisis resolution (situational supports). The nurse talked with Cheryl about rape as a violent crime, not a sexually motivated act. The nurse pointed out that Cheryl was assaulted by a stranger, not a man she trusted or loved in a relationship. After validating that Cheryl was coping by trying to regain control over her life, the nurse cautioned her that presentation of herself as a strong, capable person could be a way of masking and defending against an underlying sense of trauma that could surface later. Prior to Cheryl's discharge from the emergency department, the nurse helped her identify persons who could be helpful and supportive to her at this time and, with Cheryl's consent, summoned these persons to be with her. The nurse also recommended follow-up care to prevent long-term psychologic disturbances and provided Cheryl with written information about where counseling could be obtained.

## CRISIS THEORY AND FAMILY RESPONSE

It is not unusual for family members of rape victims to come to an emergency department or health center. The crisis experienced by rape victims reverberates throughout the family system. Since the family is the predominant long-term support system for many rape victims, nursing intervention with family members influences rape victim responses and can often reduce a sense of disruption in the family system. Family members react with a variety of responses and influence the rape victim's ultimate resolution of the crisis. (See Chapter 5 for a more detailed discussion of family response.)

A rape awakens each family member to different problems as the feelings of crisis mount to a peak. The stress may be defined differently for each member, but each one is experiencing a change that results in a temporary state of disequilibrium. For example, one member of the family may experience the rape as a loss, while another may experience it as a threat to safety. Regardless of individual reactions, familial methods of problem-solving begin to work as the family looks for ways to resolve the crisis.

Family members' responses to rape as a crisis are similar to how they handle other crises; however, families report specific responses to rape as follows:

1. Acute period (immediate emotional reaction)
   a. React more to the sexual than the violent aspect of the rape
   b. Feel resentment and anger toward the victim, expressed with difficulty and often indirectly or subtly

    c. Tend to view the rape victim as their property, linked with a shared sense of personal devaluation and shame

    d. Reevaluate a previous relationship with the rape victim

    e. Feel a sense of shock, rage, helplessness, and physical revulsion paralleling the victim's affective responses

    f. Think of violent retribution toward the rapist on the victim's behalf

    g. Patronize and overprotect the victim

    h. Insist on keeping the rape a secret to protect the family

    i. Use distractive tactics to keep the victim occupied, as if to undo the effects of the rape

    j. Feel the need to blame someone, either the assailant, the victim, or themselves

2. Long-term period

    a. Confront the sexuality of the victim

    b. Experience communication difficulties

    c. Feel continued anxiety and high level of familial tension

Families have healthy and unhealthy responses to rape. Healthy family responses are caring, concern, and support for rape victims. Healthy families direct anger at the attacker and show the ability to give emotional support to victims. Unhealthy family responses include blame and anger directed at the victim or other family members. Unhealthy family members are concerned about the family's welfare rather than the victim's. For example, family members may say, "What will other people think of us?" Unhealthy families are unable to give the victim support because the family's needs exceed those of the victim.

Nurses can intervene with the families of rape victims and assist with an ultimate resolution of the rape crisis. The goals of crisis intervention for families of rape victims include:

1. Helping the family to openly express their immediate feelings in response to the rape

2. Assisting the family in being supportive of and reassuring to the victim

3. Helping the family work through immediate practical matters and initiate problem-solving techniques

Nurses prepare ahead for family contact by a mental review of goal-directed questions such as the following:

1. How much history taking is needed? Nurses are aware that the here-and-now may be the only thing that is necessary in crisis resolution.

2. How does the family define the problem?

3. How intact is the family system? Who are the present family members? Who are the absent family members? Why are they absent?

4. What is the degree of anxiety in the family system?

5. What alternatives are being planned for to help the rape victim?

6. Is the family capable of following through on recommendations?

### CLINICAL EXAMPLE

Eileen, a 20-year-old college student, is a rape victim whose family has just arrived at the hospital. Eileen's family is stunned and feels responsible for her harm. They are revolted by the fact that their daughter is "no longer a virgin" and insist that she keep the rape a secret to protect others from knowing. Recognizing the family's immediate phase of response, the nurse intervenes in the following ways:

1. Acknowledges that the immediate response of many people is to view rape as a sexual act when in reality it is a violent, aggressive act.
2. Suggests that the staff and Eileen really could use the family's help and that this is one time when the family could really help their daughter.
3. Acknowledges that most parents feel guilty and responsible but that in reality they are not responsible for the rape.

When she returns home, Eileen becomes a recluse. She is afraid to go anywhere alone or even with her college friends. Eileen refuses to go for counseling, and her parents have tried to keep her busy with activities, escorting her wherever she wants to go. Eileen's parents are concerned and seek out the nurse at the hospital to help them with the situation. When Eileen's parents go to the nurse for counseling, the nurse intervenes in the following ways:

1. Helps the parents see that this is a post-traumatic or recoil phase of Eileen's experience in resolving her crisis.
2. Reinforces that it is Eileen's decision if and when to seek counseling; that the parents' role is to remain available and supportive.
3. Discusses their feelings of helplessness, their use of distraction tactics, and their overprotective behavior as their means of adapting to the stress.
4. Suggests that keeping the rape a secret is really destructive because it adds tension to family relationships.
5. Explores alternative ways of handling the situation.

In the above clinical example the nurse acknowledges the immediate responses of the rape victim and the victim's family. The family shows typical immediate emotional responses to rape by reacting more to the sexual than the violent aspect of the act. The nurse uses the techniques of crisis intervention by helping the family members openly express their immediate feelings and responses to the rape which are helplessness, distraction tactics, and overprotective behaviors. Keeping the rape a secret in the family is an unhealthy response that adds tension to the family system. Helping the family be supportive and reassuring to the victim, the nurse then assists the family in working through immediate problem-solving techniques to explore alternative ways of handling the situation.

Most family systems can be supportive to rape victims and can reduce the victim's sense of disruption by assisting victims with the ultimate resolution of their crisis. Nurses can initiate follow-up contacts with rape victims and their families to evaluate crisis resolution. Arrangements for follow-up are made at the beginning of service. Rape victims and their families are given time to try out proposed solutions to problems. Follow-up contact ensures that rape victims are not cut off from a support network. Nurses do not reenter rape victims' lives or family systems unless follow-up contact indicates a need for further support or nursing intervention. (See Chapter 5 for a more detailed discussion of nursing interventions with families.)

Not all rape victims or family members come into emergency departments or rape

centers. Many victims seek help by calling local telephone emergency services.
following section explores ways nurses can offer assistance to rape victims through
telephone counseling. Once again, nurses use crisis intervention techniques to assist
callers in resolving their crisis states.

## TELEPHONE CRISIS COUNSELING

Many rape victims seek help by calling into local telephone hot-line services. A
counselor is generally available to offer assistance on a 24-hour basis. The objectives of
telephone crisis counseling include:

1. To be honest and genuinely interested in helping. This will facilitate rapport
   between the counselor and the caller.
2. To assess a problem situation. This includes indentifying and clarifying the
   problem.
3. To be aware of and respect the caller's responsibility to herself and the decisions she makes. To stress the caller's strengths.
4. To be accepting, objective, and nonjudgmental. To encourage expression of
   feelings.
5. To assist the caller in putting things into perspective by helping her focus on
   her needs and to be aware of her alternatives and resources, including her own
   emotional strengths.
6. To listen carefully to what the caller has to say, allowing her to tell her story
   her own way and to ventilate her feelings.
7. To reassure the caller and offer her emotional support along with assistance
   and guidance.
8. To provide pertinent information to the caller regarding her problem.
9. To refer the caller to the appropriate service that can best meet her needs. This
   also includes making concrete plan for follow-up care.
10. Reinforcement of a mutually agreed-upon plan. The nurse offers to be avail-
    able to the caller if she wants to talk again.[7]

Guidelines for telephone interviewing with rape victims are given on pp. 250-253.
Rape victims rarely answer all the questions listed in the table even though the data are
critically important. However, the guidelines provide areas and content for inquiry to
nurses who provide telephone crisis counseling. Rape victims are likely to answer the
questions more fully once they arrive at the emergency department, where they can be
given support and comfort. The nurse uses clinical judgment in determining which
questions to ask and how much depth to go into over the phone. Generally, four areas
of inquiry are emphasized as having priority: (1) Are you safe? (2) How are you
feeling? (3) Do you want medical care? (4) What can I do to help you right now?

Nurses who take crisis calls write a report of each conversation because many
callers telephone several times before feeling safe enough to initiate action or personal
contact. Through written reports information is available to nurses or counselors who
take subsequent calls from the same rape victim. The following clinical example demonstrates how one nurse helped a victim who sought help through a crisis hot line.

### CLINICAL EXAMPLE

Mary, a 60-year-old married woman, was working as a cook at a Girl Scout
camp. One evening while she was cleaning up, she was attacked by the night

guard. Mary started to scream, but the man shoved a dirty rag into her mouth. At first Mary resisted, but that only seemed to make the assault more violent, and the man repeatedly threatened to kill her if she did not submit. The night guard dragged Mary to an isolated hillside, ripped off her clothes, and forced sexual relations on her. When Mary managed to escape, she ran into the local town and, in a state of shock, called the local rape crisis center's hot line and spoke to a nurse working as a volunteer. Mary wanted to know what to do next.

In assessing the crisis the nurse's objectives were to help Mary in the following ways:

1. To connect present feelings of self-blame and the facts with the rape incident
2. To resolve the situation Mary identified as needing help with
3. To provide Mary with alternatives and ultimately to support the way Mary decided to handle the situation

The nurse's initial response to Mary in the crisis call included:

1. Suggesting that she report the incident to the police
2. Inquiring if she was hurt and how she was feeling at that time
3. Finding out if she was in a safe place or needed transportation
4. Encouraging her to go to the hospital for medical care

> Three days later Mary called the nurse again. She was feeling angry, was in tears, and complained about the quality of care she had received at the hospital. Mary stated that she had lacerations and bruises that were ignored, and she felt embarrassed that she did not know if the man had ejaculated. She said she was told that she was physically okay and was sent home with no clear plans for follow-up care. Mary reported that she had cleaned up and douched at home.

The nurse acknowledged Mary's feelings of disappointment and anger about the care she had received. The nurse asked if tests for venereal disease had been done. Mary indicated that the testing had been completed. Then Mary continued the conversation as follows:

> Mary blamed herself for the rape and had little support following the incident. Her alcoholic husband said he had had enough and was "splitting the scene." Feeling unable to return to work, Mary planned to move home with her family in the Midwest in hopes of forgetting the assault. She thought she would try to handle the situation by herself. After sharing her sense of burden Mary wondered if she was "crazy."

In assessing Mary's status the nurse determined that Mary was experiencing the phase of turmoil in her crisis resolution. Mary also had life-stage developmental concerns involving her husband. The nurse strongly recommended that Mary come into the rape crisis center so someone could help her work through her problems.

Rape victims generally call a telephone hot line because they (or significant others) recognize that "something is wrong." Nurses who help them use clinical judgment in determining priority areas for inquiry, provide pertinent information to callers, and refer callers to services that can meet their needs. The crisis hot line is often the victim's first step in getting needed professional help.

*Text continued on p. 254.*

## TELEPHONE INTERVIEWING GUIDELINES
## WITH VICTIMS OF RAPE

Date _____ Time _____

### General information

Introduction: Hello. This is _____ from _____
How can I help you?
*Name of victim/caller _____
*Phone number calling from _____
*Address or general area _____
Location/neighborhood of assault _____
Why in the area _____
*When did assault occur (date, time)? _____
*Are you in a safe place? _____
*Are you hurt? _____
*How are you feeling now? _____
Time between assault and call to crisis line _____

### Demographic data

Age of victim_____
Race and sex of victim _____
Marital status _____
Description of assailant:
Who did it? _____
Age _____
Race and sex _____
Acquainted with
victim _____
Describe relationship:

### Crisis status

Perception of the
event _____
Response to the
event _____
Situational supports _____
Coping mechanisms _____

### Type of assault

____ Rape
____ Attempted Rape
____ Involuntary deviate
sexual intercourse
____ Indecent assault
____ Sexual assault of a
minor
____ Other degrading
acts
Describe:
____ Use of weapon
Type:
____ Struggle by victim
Feelings now
about that
____ Threats (describe)
Verbal ____
Physical ____

Adapted from Pittsburgh Action Against Rape: Crisis call-form, 211 S. Oakland Ave.,
Pittsburgh, PA 15213, and Burgess, A.W., and Holmstrom, L.L.: Crisis and coun-
seling requests of rape victims, Nurs. Res. **23**:198, May-June, 1974.
*Priority data

### Services requested and questions to consider

*1. Medical intervention (hospital): Has the victim had a medical examination? Encourage going to the emergency department for treatment of injuries and collection of evidence pending decision to prosecute.

   a. **If not examined:** If she does not want to go to the hospital, does she know about the importance of testing for VD, GC, pregnancy now and later? Is she injured other than the sexual assault? What supportive network is available to her? Does she want/need an advocate to accompany her to a shelter/care facility? Give her information about the local hospital procedure and what to expect, her rights.

   b. **If examined:** How did she get to the hospital? What did she expect would be done for her at the hospital? Were tests for VD, GC, pregnancy done? Did she change clothes or clean up before going to the hospital? Was medical evidence collected (what, where)? Was she treated for lacerations, abrasions, bruises? Is she on any medications or DES? Specify these. Does she know their side effects and risks involved? Is she having any medical problems? Was follow-up care discussed/planned? How does she feel she was treated by the health professionals? What is her reaction to this experience? Did she decide to obtain help or did someone else pressure her to seek help?

   c. **Abuse:** Is there evidence of physical abuse to a child or elderly person or battered wife syndrome? Describe the data. Has the evidence been reported to the police, hospital and/or Child Welfare?

2. Shelter and transportation intervention: Does she need emergency transportation?

  From _____ to _____ Date _____

  Time _____ Does she need emergency shelter? _____

  Contributing factors _____

---

*Priority data                                                         *Continued.*

Length of time requested _____

Accompanied (children) or alone _____

Economic/financial concerns (describe) _____

3. Police and legal intervention: Has she reported to the police?
   a. **If not reported:** Does she want to report? Does she want the report kept anonymous? Does she want to press charges? Does she want to talk about the pros and cons of not reporting/reporting? What feelings/factors are contributing to a no-report decision? Does she know about victim compensation-restitution (that she can be compensated for unpaid medical expenses if she reports the crime within 72 hours)?
   b. **If reported:** Does she understand the legal procedure and what to expect at the preliminary hearing, pretrial, trial? Is she aware of the possibility of a trial postponement and of a not-guilty verdict? To whom did she report (which police station and name of officer taking the report)? Was a report taken? Was she encouraged or discouraged from prosecuting? What is happening with the police follow-up at this time? Is she aware of the procedures necessary to identify the assailant? Has the assailant been picked up by the police? Is the assailant in jail, out on bond? Is she being harrassed or threatened by him or others? Describe. Does she have any intent to retaliate against the assailant? Name of officer arresting the assailant and police station(s) he is assigned to? Who is the district attorney? How does she feel the police treated her? What is her reaction to the experience of reporting?

4. Psychological intervention
   a. **The victim:** How did she feel at the time of the assault? And now? Does she feel the rape was her fault? Does she believe in the myths? Which ones and their impact on her as noted by _____. Does she perceive anyone as able to assist her? Did she go or not go to the police/hospital as a result of outside pressure/advice? Is she ambivalent regarding what to do? Describe. Is she seeking others' opinions? (Whose? What content? What action taken?) Was she or the assailant affected by the use of alcohol and/or drugs? (What ingested? When? Amount? By which party? Feelings about this?) Is she unable to verbalize her needs? Is she psychotic? Mentally retarded? History of social difficulties? History of physical difficulties? Hospitalized or under a physician's care now or

previously? Mental status is (describe). What is the most painful part to recall/discuss? Has she been raped before? Is this her first sexual experience? What is her usual sexual style? What does this sexual assault mean to her? How did she react to sexual acts demanded (feelings, behaviors [e.g., compliance, resistance])?

b. **Family and friends:** Who are her friends, relatives? Where do they live? Quality and frequency of contacts? Persons most and least in touch with? Does she have a therapist, minister? Does she attend any women's groups, any rap sessions? Does she want to talk with other victims of rape? Can she rely on her support systems if she wants to talk about the rape? Will they listen? How will she feel if they don't or reject her? How is her church community a support system for her? Has she decided to talk about the incident? (Discuss pros/cons of doing so and with whom—she is the best judge of her situation.) Who knows about the assault? Describe their response. Do family/friends want to talk with a counselor, or does she want a counselor to talk with them? Is the family responding with (1) caring for the victim's welfare, empathy, support, anger directed at the assailant, ability to give to the victim or (2) blaming the victim, caring for their own welfare (e.g., what others will think), recriminations, anger directed at the victim, blaming themselves?

5. Narrative summary

&ast;**Services requested**
    \_\_\_\_\_ Medical
    \_\_\_\_\_ Police/legal
    \_\_\_\_\_ Shelter
    \_\_\_\_\_ Transportation
    \_\_\_\_\_ Advocate
    \_\_\_\_\_ Counseling (specify type)
    \_\_\_\_\_ Other

**Nursing diagnosis** _____
**Plans** _____
**Contacts made** (e.g., police, hospital, name of person/agency)
**Referrals made or suggested** _____
**Follow-up indicated and type** _____

**Self-evaluation**

Describe feelings about the call, personal reactions, influence of biases/myths. List additional information/training that would help improve services. Delineate learning needs.

Rape victims who seek counseling want to do something about themselves or their situation. While implementing the core qualities of accurate empathy, nonpossessive warmth, and respect, many nurses use *creative listening* (also known as *active listening*) to guide victims through the counseling process. The next section discusses the creative listening model as it applies to the counseling of rape victims.

## CREATIVE LISTENING

Creative listening is a technique that nurses use in helping rape victims. Its underlying philosophy is self-care. A philosophy of self-care holds that people are capable of (1) deciding for themselves what they want to do about a situation and (2) being self-directive in determining and responding to the events in their lives. However, for nurses it often seems unnatural to use the creative listening model. This is so because many nurses have been taught to give advice, provide information, or tell someone what is in his or her "best interest."

Creative listening is a method by which nurses listen and empathically respond to the feelings of rape victims. While being aware of their own thoughts, feelings, and behaviors, nurses remain genuinely interested in helping rape victims with *their* concerns. Creative listening facilitates the process of building a victim-centered counseling relationship. As rape victims explore their feelings and perceptions in relation to their situation or stressors, they can achieve self-understanding.

How is creative listening characterized? Nurses use the core qualities of counseling and listen carefully to the feelings that a rape victim relates. As the nurse begins to *identify the specific feelings* that a rape victim is expressing, the nurse searches and ponders: what word or words represent the expressed feeling or situation? Then the nurse decides on the *intensity level of the feeling* (high, moderate, or low) and selects synonymous *feeling-words*. Feeling-words are chosen to match the victim's feelings and their level of intensity. As the nurse begins to use feeling-words that meaningfully reflect the rape victim's feelings, the nurse demonstrates a genuine understanding of what the victim is trying to say. A victim can agree or disagree with a nurse's perceptions and will usually tell the nurse whether they are accurate. If a rape victim's feelings are validated, progress in counseling is facilitated. If a victim's feelings are not validated, the nurse needs to listen more carefully to the victim's responses and reapply creative listening techniques. The process of creative listening thus enables the nurse and the victim to arrive at a mutual understanding of the nature of the victim's problems, experiences, feelings, and cognitive responses. Further, creative listening enables the nurse to collect data essential for a nursing assessment while empathically listening and responding to the victim in a way that conveys genuine concern.

Often rape victims have difficulty being specific and labeling the feelings that they are experiencing. Common rape victim feelings, as expressed through statements, include:

1. *I am scared to death:* "He nearly killed me." "I could be dead." "I thought I'd never see daylight again." "I hope I don't go crazy." Fear results in victims experiencing high levels of stress that can precipitate stress-related illnesses.
2. *I am to blame* (guilty): "I should have known better." "I should have acted

differently." Self-blaming statements lead to depression, and thus it is important for the nurse to intervene in faulty logic processes.

3. *I am humiliated:* "I feel embarrassed, ashamed." "I keep feelings and things like the rape to myself." When a victim feels humiliated, the rape may go unreported; the victim often keeps the assault a secret or confides in emotionally close persons who are sworn to secrecy.

4. *I need help:* "I am anxious and frightened." "I need to talk to someone." "I wish others would help me out for awhile until I get over this." "I feel awful asking for help but I can't help it." Reaching out for help is a behavior nurses encourage in applying principles of crisis intervention with rape victims (for example, the use of support systems).[2]

Table 7-6 presents a feeling-word vocabulary list that helps nurses identify a victim's feelings. The list offers a wide range of synonymous words for expressing feelings. Victims often report feeling: frightened for their life (anxious/scary); blame for the rape (guilt/shame) and therefore worthless (low self-esteem/victimized); uncertain about how to handle the rape and subsequent matters such as notifying family or police (confused); and enraged about what has happened to them (upset/angry). However, there is no uniform feeling response to rape because each victim is a unique person with a special set of circumstances. Further, the feeling state expressed by the victim also depends on what issues she may be confronting (such as whether she is to blame for the rape or feelings about a not-guilty verdict) and where the victim is in the process of resolving the rape (for example, impact phase or adjustment phase). Therefore the creative listening process is particularly useful to nurses because it directs them to *listen* and respond empathically to what a rape victim is reporting, not pigeonhole a rape victim into a phase of response or a feeling state.

The following clinical example demonstrates how a nurse can select feeling words to help a rape victim express her feelings.

### CLINICAL EXAMPLE

*Victim:* (face flushed) Listen! I'm just trying to give my point of view!
*Nurse:* It's frustrating to try to explain what you went through.
*Victim:* Yeah. I also feel ashamed about what happened.
*Nurse:* It's difficult to talk about the rape when you think you're to blame.

In the above example the nurse's words match the victim's feelings of frustration and self-blame. The victim agrees with the nurse's perception and is therefore able to continue expressing her concern. Nurses are sometimes frightened of matching the emotional level of rape victims they are listening to. Many nurses are taught not to allow their own feelings to enter into patient care. However, there is a difference between one's own feelings and empathy for the victim. Reflective feeling statements are not planned. Nurses reflect what they believe a rape victim is experiencing. A rape victim needs to be heard, to be listened to, to ventilate and to feel understood as she shares intense feelings with a professional, empathic nurse. When emotional levels are matched, the high or intense emotional levels decline because the rape victim knows

**Table 7-6. Feeling-word vocabulary list**

| Anxious/scary | Upset/angry | Guilt/shame | Low image/victimized |
|---|---|---|---|
| Afraid | Aggravated | Ashamed | Awkward |
| Apprehensive | Agitated | Blamed | Dejected |
| Distracted | Annoyed | Burdened | Dumb |
| Edgy | Appalled | Condemned | Embarrassed |
| Flustered | Dissatisfied | Crummy | Inadequate |
| Frightened | Distraught | Depressed | Ignorant |
| Horrible | Disturbed | Despair | Incompetent |
| Impatient | Disgusted | Dirty | Inferior |
| Jittery | Enraged | Foolish | Insecure |
| Jumpy | Exasperated | Gullible | Intimidated |
| Panicked | Frustrated | Hopeless | Manipulated |
| Petrified | Furious | Miserable | Mistreated |
| Precarious | Hassled | Naughty | Misunderstood |
| Pressured | Hate | Pained | Picked on |
| Restless | Infuriated | Rejected | Powerless |
| Startled | Irritated | Regretful | Put down |
| Tense | Mad | Remorse | Put upon |
| Threatened | Outraged | Rotten | Ridiculous |
| Uneasy | Pained | Shattered | Sick |
| Unsettled | Pissed-off | Sneaky | Stupid |
| Worried | Rage | Tormented | Ugly |
|  | Resentful | Unhappy | Unimportant |
|  | Threatened | Wicked | Unloved |
|  | Turned-off |  | Used |
|  | Uptight |  | Worthless |

| Tired | Alone | Confused | Coping/forceful |
|---|---|---|---|
| Drained | Alienated | Bewildered | Adamant |
| Disorganized | Abandoned | Disoriented | Assertive |
| Empty | Empty | Divided | Bold |
| Exhausted | Homesick | Forgetful | Capable |
| Helpless | Isolated | Hesitant | Challenged |
| Listless | Left-out | Hysterical | Competitive |
| Lethargic | Lonely | Mixed-up | Confident |
| Numb | Longing | Perplexed | Defiant |
| Quiet | Lost | Puzzled | Determined |
| Useless | Neglected | Scattered | Dominated |
| Vulnerable | Forgotten | Stumped | Domineering |
| Weak | Unloved | Stunned | Driven |
| Weary | Unneeded | Torn | Productive |
|  | Unwanted | Uncertain | Righteous |
|  |  | Unsure | Strong |
|  |  |  | Stubborn |
|  |  |  | Sure |
|  |  |  | Tenacious |
|  |  |  | Together |
|  |  |  | Unafraid |

Adapted from Pittsburgh Action Against Rape: Training manual, Pittsburgh, Pa., 1979. Reprinted with permission.

she does not have to continue trying to convince the nurse of situations, feelings, and concerns.

Important principles related to creative listening that are especially helpful to remember when counseling rape victims include the following:

1. The nurse must have a deep sense of trust in a victim's ability to ultimately solve her own problems and faith *in the counseling process,* remembering that the purpose of creative listening is to facilitate solution finding—a process that might take days, weeks, even months.
2. The nurse must be able to *genuinely accept* the feelings expressed by the victim, however different they may be from those the nurse thinks the victim "should" have. A victim frees herself from troublesome feelings when these feelings can be openly expressed, examined, and explored.
3. The nurse must understand that the victim's feelings are often transitory. They exist only *as of the moment.* Creative listening helps a victim move from one momentary feeling to another; feelings are thereby defused, dissipated, and released.
4. Creative listening *keeps responsibility with the victim* for analyzing and solving her problems. It facilitates problem-solving by promoting "talking it out," "thinking out loud," and "working it through."[4]

While counseling rape victims, nurses apply core qualities and creative listening techniques to specific goal-directed, client-centered relationships. The goal of this counseling is to facilitate a therapeutic change process by which rape victims work through their thoughts, feelings, and values related to the rape experience or conflictual areas emerging after the experience. Professional nurse counselors help rape victims through three phases: (1) self-exploration, (2) self-understanding, and (3) action. Figure 7-1 illustrates the creative listening process of counseling.

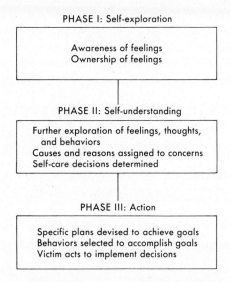

PHASE I: Self-exploration

Awareness of feelings
Ownership of feelings

PHASE II: Self-understanding

Further exploration of feelings, thoughts, and behaviors
Causes and reasons assigned to concerns
Self-care decisions determined

PHASE III: Action

Specific plans devised to achieve goals
Behaviors selected to accomplish goals
Victim acts to implement decisions

**Fig. 7-1. Creative listening counseling model.**

### Self-exploration

The first phase in the counseling process is self-exploration, which is defined by awareness and ownership of feelings.[6] Rape victims need to become aware of their feelings before they can understand them. Ownership of feelings means that a rape victim has immediate and free access to her feelings, expresses them in a genuine way, and is able to identify the source of her feelings.

Nurses understand that many rape victims do not begin the counseling process by immediately sharing their real feelings, issues, or problems. In order to help victims become aware of and own their feelings, it is *essential* that *trusting* relationships be built between rape victims and nurses. The first counseling task of nurses is to facilitate self-exploration by building trust between the nurse and the rape victim.

How do professional nurse counselors build a trusting relationship with rape victims? Three important core qualities of helping relationships essential for building trust are: accurate empathy, nonpossessive warmth, and respect. When a rape victim senses the presence of these core qualities, she is more comfortable in her interactions with the nurse. Trust is established when the nurse listens to, understands, and communicates an understanding of a rape victim's feelings.

In the *self-exploration phase,* presenting problems and their ramifications are explored in all their depth by identifying feelings, thoughts, and behaviors.[6] The best nursing approach at this point in the counseling process is nondirective—with the primary focus of nursing interventions being empathic responses to the victim's feelings. For example, the rape itself may be of minor significance for some women, and some other issue (such as sexuality or male-female relationships) may be more important to the victim to explore. The nurse needs to avoid assuming that what the *nurse* thinks is "the problem" is "the problem" or concern for the rape victim. A professional nurse lets the rape victim identify her current concerns and follows the victim's cues or lead.

Two nondirective responses that facilitate self-exploration are (1) reflecting responses and (2) enhancing responses. *Reflecting responses* express the same effect and meaning of a statement, while *enhancing responses* express additional effect and meaning of a statement.[6] Both types of responses express empathy and understanding of a rape victim's feelings.

*Reflecting responses* of the nurse, in reaction to the expressed feelings of a victim, are essentially interchangeable with those of the victim in that the response expresses essentially the same effect and meaning conveyed by the victim. The nurse responds so as to neither subtract from nor add to the expressions of the victim. Reflecting responses do not respond to how a rape victim really feels beneath expressed surface feelings. (Refer to Table 7-6 for a list of feeling-words to use for reflecting responses.)

#### CLINICAL EXAMPLE: REFLECTING RESPONSE

*Victim:* Yeah, since the rape I think I get a little hurt when boys don't want to go out with me, but I usually get over it.

*Nurse:* (*Reflecting*) It sounds like you feel frustrated and angry because when you try to find a close relationship, you get hurt.

The preceding clinical example illustrates the nurse's reflection of the victim's affect and meaning. Often a reflecting response, especially at the beginning of an interaction, is less threatening and therefore more facilitating in helping a rape victim get in touch with her feelings.

*Enhancing responses* communicate a fuller awareness of what a victim is experiencing. They *add* to the expressions of victims and go beyond expressed surface feelings. Involving more risk on the part of the nurse, enhancing responses add to the expressions of a victim in such a way as to help the victim express deeper feelings. In the process of ongoing, deep exploration of feelings, the nurse communicates a full awareness of what the victim is experiencing.

### CLINICAL EXAMPLE: ENHANCING RESPONSE

*Victim:* It really hurts me when my folks don't listen and keep asking me to go talk to the pastor at church when I don't want to. My folks make me feel so insignificant and small when they repeatedly do that.

*Nurse:* *(Enhancing)* You're feeling hurt and rejected when your parents don't listen to you, and right now you can't bear to feel that again.

*Victim:* Exactly. I need people to accept me just like I am right now. Why don't they do that?

In the above clinical example, the nurse communicates an understanding of the victim's feelings of rejection and intolerance of painful interactions, although neither feeling has been explicitly related by the victim. The nurse recognizes the feelings from the victim's responses and risks a deeper expression of hypothesized feeling states.

### CLINICAL EXAMPLE

Nancy, a 22-year-old college student, came into the health center and stated that she had been raped last week by her best girlfriend's husband (Alan). Nancy reported that she came to town to visit the couple and was sleeping on their living room couch when Alan woke her up. At first Nancy could not decide if she was dreaming or if the assault was real. Alan had a knife and threatened to "cut her up bad" if she did not comply with his demands for sex. Alan also warned Nancy against reporting the rape, stating he "knew where to track her down for revenge."

While talking with a nurse at the college counseling center, Nancy began to cry, saying that she was still in a state of shock and disbelief that the rape had happened to her, especially by someone she knew and had trusted. Nancy could not decide whether to tell her girlfriend: Would it ruin their relationship? Would the girlfriend believe her or perhaps think she seduced her husband? Should she prosecute Alan? What would prosecuting Alan do to her girlfriend's marriage? What would prosecuting Alan do to her friendship with her girlfriend? Should she tell her family? What if she got pregnant? Nancy asked if the nurse could tell her what to do—she felt *so* confused!

Mary, the nurse at the health center, assessed Nancy to be in a crisis state resulting from the rape. Mary decided to facilitate Nancy's regaining control over her life. To do so the nurse reflected the feelings she heard from Nancy. During the next half-hour the nurse's verbal interventions, based on counseling principles, included the following:

| Nurse's technique | Principle |
|---|---|
| "I know you're confused right now. You've been through a frightening experience." | Empathy; reflecting response Identifying feelings |
| "I'm here to help you sort out what you need and want to do." | Reassurance, nonpossessive warmth Identifies victim's confusion |
| "Is there someone that you know who will understand what happened?" | Nondirective response |
| "Tell me about your family." | Recognizes victim's ambivalence about family |
| "Should I get in touch with someone in your family?" | Nondirective approach |
| "You know your girlfriend better than I do. What kind of relationship do you have with her?" | Helps victim gain control of situation by taking responsibility for disclosing the rape to others |
| "How important is it to you if telling your girlfriend about the rape ruins your friendship?" | Helps victim assess relationship with girlfriend and result of telling her about the rape |
| "Do you want to talk about what you would do if you became pregnant from the rape?" | Allows for self-decision Supportive approach |

The above clinical example illustrates the core qualities of accurate empathy (feeling *for* the victim, but not feeling the same as the victim does) and nonpossessive warmth (concern and caring). During her interactions with the victim the nurse used reflecting responses to help the rape victim get in touch with her feelings of confusion. The nurse knew that unless the victim identified her feelings she could not grow in the counseling process. Recognizing the victim's concern about telling others of the rape, the nurse used a nondirective response to explore the victim's relationship with her girlfriend and family support. The victim's relationship with her girlfriend became a primary focus in the initial counseling phase of self-exploration. Another victim concern, pregnancy, was also identified, and the nurse offered the victim an opening to discuss this issue.

### Self-understanding

In phase two of the counseling process, called *self-understanding*, identified feelings, thoughts, and behaviors are clarified. Victims assign causes or reasons to each concern.[6] In this phase the nurse assists the victim in making some sense out of the "pieces of the puzzle" by making many nonspecific thoughts and feelings more concrete. When the victim understands the reasons behind her concerns, she is better able to decide what actions will resolve her difficulties. A specific plan of action, which is both reasonable and attainable, can then be decided upon by the victim.

Nurses are more active and direct in their interventions during the self-understanding phase. As professionals, nurses have been taught how to help rape victims with their concerns. They understand that solutions must come from the victims themselves and that victims are usually realistic about their situations and experiences. Nurses help victims regain control over their lives by resisting the urge to prescribe solutions to their problems. The goal of counseling is to help rape victims make independent, not dependent, decisions about their lives. Making independent decisions and regaining control over one's life can be achieved through self-understanding and self-initiated decision-making. The phase of self-understanding is illustrated in a continuation of the preceding clinical example, as follows:

CLINICAL EXAMPLE

Mary (the nurse) helped Nancy move through to the second phase of counseling, self-understanding. Mary helped the victim identify two concerns that she needed to explore: (1) telling others about the rape (girlfriend, family) and (2) what to do if she was pregnant. During this phase Mary offered Nancy continued support through the following techniques:

| Nurse's technique | Principle |
|---|---|
| "How do you think your girlfriend would react? | Making feelings more concrete |
| "Are you concerned that your family will react in a nonsupportive way?" | Reflecting response |
| "Is there someone in your family who could help you now?" | Allowing for self-care decision |
| "You can get medical care—it is available here—and it is in your interest to see that your body is okay." | Sharing information |
| "Do you want health counseling about pregnancy prevention?" | Allowing for self-care decision |

The above clinical example illustrates the nurse's goal-directed statements, which were planned to help the victim (Nancy) develop self-understanding about her expressed concerns. The rape victim needed to examine her relationships with her girlfriend and her family. The nurse explored many questions: What exactly are Nancy's concerns? Does Nancy fear that her girlfriend or family will not believe her? Are Nancy's fears or concerns realistic? Through the nurse's use of the creative listening process, Nancy developed a clearer understanding of her feelings before making any decisions or taking any action. Nancy came to understand that she was deeply hurt by what had happened because her trust in her friends had been severely violated. Nancy further understood that not informing her family of the rape was related to her own inability to cope with their sense of hurt and trauma. She felt that she could share the experience with them in the near future but not at this time. Nancy realized that she was not ready to be pregnant and raise a child, and the thought of being pregnant by her best friend's husband both repulsed her and violated her moral code. She also understood that it would take time to rework the relationship with her girlfriend, that Alan's rape was a separate matter but that it complicated the friendship with her girlfriend.

Rape victims come to understand that nurses cannot make decisions for them. Nurses assist in the process of decision-making, but rape victims live with the consequences of their decisions. Having to make self-care decisions is not always an easy task. Figure 7-2 illustrates some of the complexities involved in a rape victim's self-care

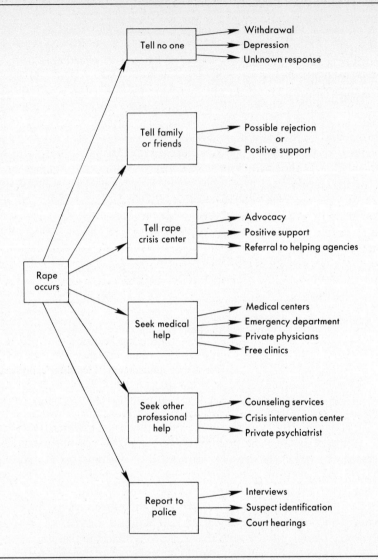

**Fig. 7-2. Victim decisions following a rape.**

Adapted from First night flow chart: victim decisions following a sexual assault. In Harrisburg Area Rape Crisis Center training manual, Harrisburg, Pa., 1977.

decisions. One or more steps in the decision-making process (as illustrated) are generally the target of discussion in the self-understanding phase of counseling. Rape victims have realistic concerns about decision-making. The decisions a rape victim makes (e.g., who to tell) often have profound repercussions (e.g., marital conflict or divorce) and may require long-term resolution (e.g., prosecution of assailant or counseling to resolve depression). Nurses have an important role in supporting and guiding victims through the difficult task of regaining direction and control over their lives.

### Action

In phase three of the counseling process, called *action,* rape victims decide what they will do to accomplish their decisions. Specific plans are devised from concrete and relevant information (for example, medical care or advocacy).[6] Through creative listening nurses act on the philosophy that a rape victim's decision is *her* choice. Nurses demonstrate objectivity and self-control by keeping their own agendas, needs, or desires (for example, wanting the victim to have evidence collected) out of the counseling process.

The action phase is largely determined by the victim's behaviors. Although the victim was unable to control the occurrence of the rape event, the nurse emphasizes that the victim does have control over present and future events, such as the way she thinks about the rape and her behavior following the rape. For example, a sexually assaulted woman exerts control by pressing charges against her assailant. Action decisions of victims also include working on a crisis hot line to help other rape victims; joining consciousness-raising women's groups; or taking self-defense courses. Behaviors selected in the action phase of counseling are directed toward helping the victim regain a sense of control over her life. This phase is illustrated in a continuation of the clinical example discussed previously (with rape victim Nancy).

CLINICAL EXAMPLE

Nancy decided to talk with her sister because she felt emotionally close to her. The sister lived in a nearby town, so Nancy called her. Nancy's sister said that she would visit Nancy immediately. Her sister expressed concern and provided Nancy with positive emotional support. During the next several days Nancy got a complete physical exam and treatment necessary for preventing pregnancy and venereal disease. She also decided to tell her girlfriend about the rape. Nancy continued to see the nurse in counseling because she wanted to work through her thoughts and feelings about prosecuting Alan.

The rape victim in the above example has reached the action phase of the counseling process. The nurse is supporting the victim in exploring feelings about her decision. In addition, the nurse remains available and supportive to the rape victim as she resolves her concerns related to the rape event.

Rape victims proceed through the three phases of counseling at various rates. Most victims progress through the action phase within 4 to 6 weeks after the rape event. Those who do not progress through the phases and who seem to be having a difficult adjustment usually need longer-term counseling. Victims who take action to prosecute the rapist sometimes use longer-term counseling to support their emotional well-being while carrying out their decision. (See Chapter 9 for a discussion of counseling victims through the court process.)

### SUMMARY

Because rape is a violent, sexual assault, many rape victims have post-rape experiences of intense anxiety and disorganization commonly called a crisis state. Nurses who have an understanding of crisis theory and crisis intervention techniques assist rape victims and their families with resolution of physical, emotional, or social crises.

Generally a situational crisis, rape is an unanticipated and traumatic event. Most victims are not prepared to handle the rape or the disequilibrium and loss of control that follow rape. If rape occurs during a major transition in growth and development, rape victims experience greater physical psychologic, or social disruption in their lives. Nurses use situational and developmental frameworks to assess the likelihood of intense post-rape responses of rape victims.

A crisis develops and resolves along designated phases and over periods of time that are unique for each rape victim. Nursing goals of crisis intervention are directed at assessing the phases of crisis development and crisis resolution and at planning nursing interventions to assist rape victims in a healthy resolution of their crisis. Nursing interventions are directed at strengthening factors that facilitate crisis resolution: (1) perception of the event, (2) situational support, and (3) coping mechanisms. Strengths or weaknesses in any one of these factors affect crisis development and crisis resolution. Principles of nursing care in crisis intervention include: active listening; empathic understanding; helping rape victims gain control of their crisis; helping victims explore ways of coping; and helping rape victims establish or reestablish significant, supportive social networks.

Many rape victims in crisis will use a telephone hot-line service for help in crisis resolution. Professional nurses listen carefully to rape victim callers, offer emotional support, and provide pertinent information and referral for follow-up care.

Many families of rape victims experience crisis after a rape. Familial responses can be healthy and facilitate crisis resolution; or they can be unhealthy and impede crisis resolution. Assessing family members' ability to support rape victims, professional nurses intervene by helping family members to express responses that are supportive to rape victims and to develop their own problem-solving techniques. Follow-up contact ensures rape victims and families that support remains available throughout the period of crisis resolution.

The counseling process of creative listening enables nurses to identify a victim's thoughts, feelings, and behaviors by reflecting feeling words that communicate to a rape victim that she is being heard and understood. Nurses use creative listening skills to help a rape victim through three phases of a counseling process: self-exploration, self-understanding, and action. In self-exploration a rape victim gets in touch with feelings, identifies the source of feelings, and owns identified feelings. Reflecting and enhancing responses of the nurse facilitate a victim's self-explorations. In the self-understanding phase a rape victim clarifies the causes or reasons for her reactions and responses after the rape event. Nonspecific feelings are concretized, resulting in a realistic appraisal of situations and concerns by the victim. At this time nurses use more direct responses and share information to help a rape victim with self-care decisions.

In the action phase a rape victim decides precisely what behaviors she will engage in or which plans she will initiate to overcome her problems or concerns. Nurses reinforce the fact that a rape victim does have control over her present and future behaviors. Available as a support to rape victims, nurses help victims discuss thoughts, feelings, and behaviors related to self-care decisions.

Most rape victims have adequate skills to cope with their crisis. With professional nursing support, victims can resolve a crisis state within a short period after a rape. Healthier post-rape outcomes include a return to a precrisis state of physical, psychologic, and social well-being and growth from the rape experience, such as learning new resources and developing new problem-solving skills.

## Learning activities

### EXERCISE 1. Responding to victims in crisis

*Directions:* Read each of the situations below. Identify the crisis factors that you assess to be affecting the victim's equilibrium. Then develop your response to intervene in the crisis as though you were talking to the victim.

### Situations: Victim to nurse

1. "My boyfriend won't have anything to do with me now. I should've lied. I hope, for him, he realizes what he's lost. I wish I could change his mind."

   Crisis factors: _____

   Nurse response: _____

   _____

2. "I haven't been afraid before. This is so ridiculous, but I can't help it. I can't sleep and don't know what to do to calm down. I hear every little noise in the house."

   Crisis factors: _____

   Nurse response: _____

   _____

3. "The guy's wife keeps calling me on the phone and harassing me. She says to drop the charges or I'll ruin his career. He's got four kids to feed and has been a good Christian. She wants to know why I keep making 'trouble' and am insensitive to her. Then she hangs up and rings back. When I answer she hangs up, and she repeats that for about an hour a couple times a day. I'm a nervous wreck and can't get any peace of mind."

   Crisis factors: _____

   Nurse response: _____

   _____

4. "I had to wait two hours to be examined at the hospital. The police were arguing over whether I was at the right hospital or

should go somewhere else. I just felt miserable and only wanted someone to take care of me, I didn't care where."

Crisis factors: _____

Nurse response: _____

_____

5. "My sister said it shouldn't bother me so bad. After all, I'm not a virgin. But she didn't live through the filthy assault. How can she put it on such a basic level?"

Crisis factors: _____

Nurse response: _____

_____

## EXERCISE 2. Telephone interviewing

The following case illustration is a telephone call received by a nurse at a rape crisis center. After reviewing the case, complete the assigned activities.

*Victim:* I don't know why I'm calling you. I guess I don't know what to do.

*Nurse:* You're feeling confused about something that happened to you tonight and don't know what to do?

*Victim:* Yes. I had an incident with my ex-husband tonight, and I don't want to report it.

*Nurse:* Do you want to tell me what happened and see if together we can figure something out?

*Victim:* Well, I don't know . . . Well, tonight he raped me and beat me up. But I don't want to report it because I don't want him to go to jail or to ruin his career. What *can* I do?

*Nurse:* (Thinking how incongruous it is that he has harmed her and yet she wants to protect him) Well, what would you like to have happen?

*Victim:* I just want him to leave me alone. I don't want him to come back and do it again. How do I stop him?

*Nurse:* There are a number of things you can do. You can report the incident to a magistrate and have a warrant issued to keep him off your premises; you can report the incident directly to the police and have them assist you with the legal process; or you can obtain medical care and at that time explore your rights in an interview with the police, while still retaining your right not to prosecute the crime.

*Victim:* Well, I don't know what to do. I want to think about it. I don't want him to go to jail. I just want to stop it from happening again and take care of myself also.

(*Pause*)

| | |
|---|---|
| *Nurse:* | You care about his welfare and for your own welfare. Have you thought about getting a physical exam to be sure that you are okay physically? |
| *Victim:* | No. I'm embarrassed to get medical care. |
| *Nurse:* | What do you find embarrassing? |
| *Victim:* | Oh, I think they'll just laugh at me and not believe me because it was my ex-husband. You hear such awful stories of how victims are treated in ER's, you know. |
| *Nurse:* | Yes, there are a lot of awful situations reported, and it is upsetting. However, there are a couple of excellent hospitals in the area that are sensitive to victims. They see a lot of unusual situations and have a reputation for being understanding. Would you like their names? |
| *Victim:* | Alright. |
| *Nurse:* | (After identifying hospitals) Do you have someone that could go with you? |
| *Victim:* | Yes, I have a friend that will go with me. Thank you for the information. You've been very helpful. You're sure I won't have to report the rape if I just go for medical care? |
| *Nurse:* | Yes. They might encourage you to report the crime, but they won't insist that you do so. |
| *Victim:* | Okay. I think I'll give it a try, and see to it that I'm not hurt. If I need help, can I call you? |
| *Nurse:* | Yes. I am on call all night, and if you want someone to be with you we can send someone to the hospital. |
| *Victim:* | Thanks. That's all I wanted to know. (End of call) Five minutes later: |
| *Victim:* | This is (name) again. I didn't tell you the whole story the first time I called. |
| *Nurse:* | Go on. |
| *Victim:* | Well . . . my friend's a "he." I've lived with him for a year and a half. Will it matter if he goes with me? |
| *Nurse:* | You seem concerned that the nurses will be judgmental. (pause) I don't *expect* that will happen. The nursing staff usually encourage friends or family to be involved at a time like this. What seems to be your concern? |
| *Victim:* | Well, after the rape I went to his apartment and told him about it, and we made love. Will that matter? |
| *Nurse:* | In what respect do you mean? (Nurse privately wonders if he took advantage of the victim.) |
| *Victim:* | Will they think I am terrible? Will they think I am strange? You hear such awful stories of how victims are treated in ER's. I'd rather deal with this by myself than be treated badly. |
| *Nurse:* | The hospitals I referred you to are very good, and I doubt |

that you would receive poor care there. Would you feel better if an advocate met you there for an exam?

*Victim:* I don't think that'll be necessary . . . but, do you think I should get medical care?

*Nurse:* That's really up to you. Do you want to know if your body is damaged physically?

*Victim:* I guess so. Can they tell his sperm from my ex-husband's?

*Nurse:* The crime lab can do some tests to determine the blood type of the sperm of the two men. However, I doubt that they will do that test if you decide not to prosecute. You seem more concerned about how you'll be treated and if you'll be ridiculed.

*Victim:* Yes, I guess I am. Would you call the hospital and tell them I am coming?

*Nurse:* Would you feel better if I called the hospital to tell them you are coming and the nature of your concern?

*Victim:* Oh, yes. I would be greatly relieved and feel more able to go through the ordeal. Would you call (name) hospital for me?

*Nurse:* Yes. Is there anything else I can help you with?

*Victim:* No. You've been very helpful. Thank you.

(End of call)

The objectives of telephone crisis counseling are listed below. To what extent did the nurse in the example meet these objectives? Check your response. (Answers can be used for discussion.)

|  | High | Moderate | Low |
|---|---|---|---|
| 1. To be honest and genuinely interested in helping. This will facilitate rapport between counselor and caller. | ___ | ___ | ___ |
| 2. To assess a problem situation. This includes identifying and clarifying the problem. | ___ | ___ | ___ |
| 3. To be aware of and respect the caller's responsibility to herself and the decisions she makes. To stress the caller's strengths. | ___ | ___ | ___ |
| 4. To be accepting, objective, and non-judgmental. To encourage expression of feelings. | ___ | ___ | ___ |
| 5. To assist the caller in putting things into perspective by helping her to focus on her needs to become aware of her alternatives and resources (including her own emotional strengths). | ___ | ___ | ___ |

|                                                                                                                          | High | Moderate | Low |
|--------------------------------------------------------------------------------------------------------------------------|------|----------|-----|
| 6. To listen carefully to what the caller has to say, allowing her to tell the story her own way and to ventilate her feelings. | ____ | ____     | ____ |
| 7. To reassure the caller and offer her emotional support along with assistance and guidance. | ____ | ____     | ____ |
| 8. To provide pertinent information to the caller regarding her problem. | ____ | ____     | ____ |
| 9. To refer the caller to the appropriate service that can best meet her needs. | ____ | ____     | ____ |
| 10. To reinforce the plan by offering self to caller if she wants to call again. | ____ | ____     | ____ |

What information did the nurse *not* obtain that you think would have been relevant information?

What would you have done if you were the nurse taking this call?

---

## EXERCISE 3. Responding with empathy

*Directions:* In this exercise you are to formulate a response that reflects both the victim's feelings and the content of her statement. It is helpful to attend to the content first and end the response with a reflection of the feeling state. The entire response should have an invitational quality. Listen *only* for the obvious. The goal is to let the victim know that you have perceived what has been said and what she is feeling. Read each situation carefully and identify both surface and underlying feelings. Fill in the blanks to the statements below with reflecting and enhancing responses as quickly as possible so as to retain a conversational style.

In the beginning this exercise may seem very mechanical. However, with practice it will become natural and your responses will flow spontaneously. Forcing attention to surface and underlying feelings will gradually increase your skill in responding to others empathically. (Refer to Table 7-6 for suggestions.)

---

### Situations: Victim to nurse

1. "I can't stand being at parties. I want to scream and run away. I can't bear being around men right now, yet I can't stand being alone either."

   *Reflecting:* You feel (surface) _____ because (content) _____.

   *Enhancing:* You feel (underlying) _____ because (content) _____.

2. "The physician said I shouldn't take it so seriously, that men have a corresponding thing called war. But it's not the same; they have a choice and their bodies are not invaded. They can't become pregnant from war, and they're not under surprise attack. How can he be so narrow-minded?"

*Reflecting:*    You feel (surface) _____ because (content) _____.

*Enhancing:*    You feel (underlying) _____ because (content) _____.

3. "That was my first experience with sex. I didn't know what rape meant until my landlady said, 'She's been raped.' She tried to assure me that married love isn't like that, but I can't stomach the notion of having sex with men."

*Reflecting:*    You feel (surface) _____ because (content) _____.

*Enhancing:*    You feel (underlying) _____ because (content) _____.

4. "I'm afraid to tell my mom what happened. If I hadn't been absent from school, the whole incident never would have happened. Oh, how awful! What can I do?"

*Reflecting:*    You feel (surface) _____ because (content) _____.

*Enhancing:*    You feel (underlying) _____ because (content) _____.

5. "I'm so pessimistic about pressing charges. The pretrial hearing really blew my hopes apart. I can't believe how derogatory that funky prosecuting attorney was. He's sure got a lot of nerve! I felt like throwing my pop can at the bastard when he started suggesting I seduced the guy!"

*Reflecting:*    You feel (surface) _____ because (content) _____.

*Enhancing:*    You feel (underlying) _____ because (content) _____.

6. "I had never had a pelvic exam before, and I just couldn't relax. The doctor didn't tell me what he was doing, and the nurse was so busy she didn't take time to talk with me. I think they thought I was just some specimen on the other end of their tool. I felt so alone and scared. I thought medical people knew how to take care of rape victims."

*Reflecting:*    You feel (surface) _____ because (content) _____.

*Enhancing:*    You feel (underlying) _____ because (content) _____.

7. "I just got out of the hospital. I was in there for 3 days after I was raped. I can't eat and I keep on crying. There's no one for me to talk to. School's out of session and my friends have

gone home. My family would never understand. They warned me not to ever live alone. How do I get control of myself? Do you think this will ever go away?"

*Reflecting:* You feel (surface) ＿＿＿＿＿ because (content) ＿＿＿＿＿＿＿＿＿＿.

*Enhancing:* You feel (underlying) ＿＿＿＿ because (content) ＿＿＿＿＿＿＿＿＿＿.

8. "I told the police not to let the neighbors know they were coming. I'm so embarrassed. The detectives came in an unmarked car, and just as we were leaving the local police drove up with their siren screaming! I was so pissed off, but what the hell could I do about it at that point?"

    *Reflecting:* You feel (surface) ＿＿＿＿＿ because (content) ＿＿＿＿＿＿＿＿＿＿.

    *Enhancing:* You feel (underlying) ＿＿＿＿ because (content) ＿＿＿＿＿＿＿＿＿＿.

9. "I think I'm pregnant from a rape 2 months ago. I thought this whole ordeal was behind me, and now I have this to cope with! How do I find out about abortions? I don't know what to do."

    *Reflecting:* You feel (surface) ＿＿＿＿＿ because (content) ＿＿＿＿＿＿＿＿＿＿.

    *Enhancing:* You feel (underlying) ＿＿＿＿ because (content) ＿＿＿＿＿＿＿＿＿＿.

10. "I won't stay in that apartment until the locks are changed and the windows secured. I just don't feel safe there. Do you think that's ridiculous, a grown woman like me afraid to stay in my own apartment? What do I need to do to get the locks changed? Do you think I'll settle down after that?"

    *Reflecting:* You feel (surface) ＿＿＿＿＿ because (content) ＿＿＿＿＿＿＿＿＿＿.

    *Enhancing:* You feel (underlying) ＿＿＿＿ because (content) ＿＿＿＿＿＿＿＿＿＿.

## EXERCISE 4. Role-play

The following role-play exercises based on actual rape case situations are designed to facilitate the nurse's learning of counseling principles and techniques. Each exercise requires two people to enact the roles of victim and nurse. The remaining students will act as observers/recorders to the demonstration role-plays.

Several teams can be assigned for each exercise. While one team is demonstrating, the other team is out of the room. Team members can spend time coordinating their roles and deciding on types of nursing interventions. The role-plays should be time-limited (5 to 6 minutes).

Students in the audience are to take out a sheet of paper and divide it into two columns: left-hand column for victim's ideas and feelings; right-hand column for nurse's reflected statements. After the exercises are completed, examine the nurse's methods of relating to the victim.

## Exercise A: Teenage traveler

Marion is an 18-year old who has been politically active for women's rights. She is in her first year of college, and this is her first experience in living away from home. Marion is dressed in jeans and a denim blouse.

The victim reports that she decided to "see Europe during summer vacation." Being a student, she did not have much money and could barely afford airfare. A young man in her class convinced her to travel with him since he was also "going her way." While they were in Europe, he raped her in a cheap hotel, beat her, and left her for dead.

The victim is blaming herself for the rape. Her parents had cautioned her before she left for the trip, but she reassured them she could handle the situation. She does not feel that she can tell her parents since she used such "poor judgment." She comes into the health clinic where you are working. The victim is concerned that she might be pregnant and *then* what would she do? The victim cannot get beyond her feelings of self-blame and guilt. How will she ever explain the situation if her folks find out?

## Exercise B: Startled housewife

Joan is a 32-year-old, middle-class, suburban mother of three children. She has chosen a traditional woman's role and is devoted to her duties as wife and homemaker. She believes many myths about rape, particularly that it happens only to "bad" girls who invite it and not to women who stay at home.

Joan reports that she was raped by a man she let into the house to read the water meter. The man said he had been trying for 3 months to read the meter. It was the middle of the afternoon, and the children were napping. So as not to disrupt them, Joan said she would go down to the basement to show the man where the meter was. He pulled a knife and threatened to kill her if she did not cooperate. Joan did not want to wake the children or take a chance on their being harmed, so she complied. She was frightened for her life.

The victim now feels dumb for letting the man in and is blaming herself, wondering what she did to invite the rape. She is in a state of shock, unable to accept the fact that this happened to her in her own home. She cannot decide whether to notify her husband at work. He has a very heavy work schedule that is stressing him, and she does not know whether to burden him with this. He has told her many times not to let anybody in the house, so she is feeling guilty. She does not know how her husband would react, particularly since he is under so much pressure at work and cannot tolerate much more.

### Exercise C: Militant feminist

Barbara is 40 years old, highly self-reliant, and very active in the feminist movement. She believes that as long as men are socialized to be aggressive and women to be submissive, rape will remain a social ill. She has long been concerned about sexual harassment and discrimination against women in work settings. Barbara recently took a self-defense course and was confident she could protect herself. She is dressed in shorts and a halter top.

The victim is escorted to the ED by the police for evaluation and treatment. She is *very* angry as she tells you that she was just raped— in fact, she is furious! You escort her to the examining room while she continues to swear and yell, "The g—d—son-of-a-bitch! I'd like to take his cock and shove it down his throat!" You are startled to hear such language and anger from a woman. Once settled on the examining table, Barbara tells you about how she was on her way out to walk her dogs when a man pulled her into his apartment, raped her and scarred her with a knife, then shoved her out the door saying he'd come after her if she reported to the police. She ignored the threat and called the police who came to the scene of the crime, but they didn't want to arrest the man because of his prominent community "connections." They questioned her about the "company she keeps" and the way she dressed. As she recounts this, the victim looks about ready to explode. She screams and shouts at the nurse who is interviewing her. She *refuses* to talk with anyone, particularly men!

Barbara wants to go out and kill the guy! She knows the conviction rate for rapists is low, and she doesn't trust the bureaucratic legal system. If she can't go after the man, how can she ever settle her rage! Is it *normal* to be so angry? What does she have to do to prosecute? What are the steps? Will he be convicted? Why don't the police arrest him, even if he is powerful? Does justice apply only to the poor? Why *can't* she be examined by a nurse or female physician—she doesn't need to be raped twice! Why *can't* she talk with a female police officer who will respect her?

### Role-play discussion questions

1. What did you think of the nurse's approach?
2. What did the nurse do that elicited a specific response?
3. What do you think was particularly helpful? Or not helpful?

4. Was she emphatic? Nonjudmental? Supportive? Exploring? Explain.
5. Was the nurse sympathetic? Was that helpful? Explain.
6. What clues were there to stalls in the interview process?
7. What did the nurse do to overcome these?
8. What did the nurse feel during the role-play (for example, scared, inadequate)?
9. Did the victim feel that she was understood, listened to? What did you observe or infer to know this?
10. Can you identify with the victim? With the nurse? Explain.

## REFERENCES

1. Aguilera, D.C., and Messick, J.M.: Crisis intervention: theory and methodology, ed. 4, St. Louis, 1981, the C.V. Mosby Co.
2. Burgess, A.W., and Holmstrom, L.L.: Rape: victims of crisis, Bowie, Md., 1974, Robert J. Brady Co.
3. Burgess, A.W., and Holmstrom, L.L.: Rape trauma syndrome, Am. J. Psychiatry **131**:981, 1974.
4. Caplan, G.: Principles of preventive psychiatry, New York, 1964, Basic Books.
5. Frank, E., and others: Past psychiatric symptoms and the response to sexual assault, Compr. Psychiatry, **22**(5):479, 1981.
6. Gazda, G.M., and others: Human relations development: a manual for educators, Boston, 1977, Allyn & Bacon, Inc.
7. Hoff, L.A.: People in crisis: understanding and helping, Reading, Mass., 1978, Addison-Wesley Publishing Co.

## ADDITIONAL REFERENCES

Halpern, S.: Follow-up phone call to rape victims. In Halpern, S., editor: Rape—helping the victim: a treatment manual, Oradell, N.J., 1979, Medical Economics Book Division.
Harrisburg Area Rape Crisis Center: First-night flow chart: victim decisions following a sexual assault. In Harrisburg Area Rape Crisis Center: Training manual, Harrisburg, Pa., 1977.
Interagency Task Force on Rape-Related Services: A handbook for victims, Pittsburgh, Pa., 1979.
Lewis, J.: To be a therapist, New York, 1978, Brunner/Mazel Publishers.

## ANNOTATED SUGGESTED READINGS

Aguilera, D.C., and Messick, J.M.: Crisis intervention: theory and methodology, ed. 4, St. Louis, 1981, The C.V. Mosby Co.
    The first section of this book discusses the phases of development of a crisis and the balancing factors in a stress process. The authors also present an application of crisis theory to the situational crisis of a rape victim.

Banter, S.E.: Crisis theory. In Stuart, G., and Sundeen, S., editors: Principles and practice of psychiatric nursing, St. Louis, 1979, The C.V. Mosby Co.

This chapter is recommended reading for the nurse who has not had a lecture or course of instruction in crisis theory and methodology. It offers an overview of crisis theory and intervention from historical roots to contemporary times and is developed within a nursing process framework.

Burgess, A.W., and Holmstrom, L.L.: Coping behavior of the rape victim, Am. J. Psychol. **133:**413, 1976.

This article is basic to crisis intervention because it describes coping behavior of rape victims under the threat of attack, during the attack itself, and in the period that immediately follows. The authors conclude with a discussion of counseling implications for the nursing care of victims of rape.

Burgess, A.W., and Holmstrom, L.L.: Crisis and counseling requests of rape victims, Nurs. Res. **23:**196, 1974.

The article reports the authors' empirical findings in relation to 146 adult and pediatric rape victims and their crisis and counseling requests. The findings were obtained through follow-up telephone calls and interviews at the hospital where victims received initial treatment. The article presents the study problem and the purpose and method of investigation. Discussion of the findings includes a table describing a sample initial interview guide to use with rape victims; the table identifies the categories of requests and illustrates these with victim and counselor responses.

Burgess, A.W., and Holmstrom, L.L.: Rape: victims of crisis, Bowie, Md., 1974, Robert J. Brady Co.

The authors discuss the importance of the initial counseling interview. They present counselor activities for assessing a rape victim's psychologic distress and determining how to help victims within their social network. Phases of interviewing that are discussed include introductory, working, and concluding phases.

Caplan, G.: Principles of preventive psychiatry, New York, 1964, Basic Books, Inc.

The author presents definitions of crisis and describes both situational and maturational crises. Using a public health model, the author also discusses various levels of prevention.

Clark, T.: Primary health care: counseling victims of rape, Am. J. Nurs. **12:**1964, 1976.

This article discusses counselor experiences and victim needs at the Yale–New Haven Hospital. Specific techniques and services are described from the victim's entrance into the emergency department to counseling phases. Follow-up calls and continued support to rape victims are discussed.

Gazda, G., and others: Human relations development: a manual for educators, Boston, 1977, Allyn & Bacon, Inc.

The manual includes active learning exercises for each of the core qualities essential to effective counseling. Responses for establishing a positive counseling relationship are recommended. Ineffective communication styles in counseling are also presented.

Halpern, S.: Follow-up phone call to rape victims. In Halpern, S., editor:

Rape—helping the victim: a treatment manual, Oradell, N.J. 1978, Medical Economics Book Division.

The author presents an excellent discussion of follow-up contact with rape victims. An outline of essential content includes various victim concerns—emotional, social, and legal.

Hirschowitz, R.: Crisis theory: a formulation, Psychiatric Annals **3**:33, 1973.

This article is a basic reference often used in combination with the work of Aguilera and Messick and that of Caplan to teach students crisis intervention theory and methodology. The content is relevant to nursing care of rape victims, particularly the crisis sequence as it applies to them.

Hoff, L.A.: People in crisis: understanding and helping, Reading, Mass., 1978, Addison-Wesley Publishing Co.

The author illustrates the application of crisis intervention and creative listening through a telephone counseling session with a victim of rape. In one column the verbatim interaction between counselor and victim is presented; in the other column the case example is described in terms of the characteristics of crisis and the intervention techniques.

Hornsby, J., and Payne, F.: A model for communication skills development for family practice residents, J. Fam. Pract. **8**:71, 1979.

The paper presents a communication model that includes definition of the core qualities in effective helping relationships: empathy, warmth, and respect. Although the model is used in a department of family practice for training residents, it is one of the clearest explanations and applications of the creative listening model.

Ivey, A., and Gluckstern, N.: Basic attending skills: an introduction to microcounseling and helping, Amherst, Mass., 1974, Microtraining Associates, Inc.

The text and accompanying videotape are used to train and expand counselor skills in effective helping relationships with clients. The authors offer content and exercises in (1) attending behavior, (2) minimal encouragement (nonverbal communications), (3) paraphrasing, (4) reflecting feelings, and (5) summarizing and integrating counseling skills. The text and videotape are available in some university audiovisual media or learning resource centers.

Johnson, D.: Reaching out, Englewood Cliffs, N.J., 1972, Prentice-Hall, Inc.

The author presents ways in which a person can offer nonthreatening feedback. The book is a good resource for learning and using observational skills—during patient interviews, role-play situations, and exercises—to develop effective communication skills.

Kliman, A.: Crisis: psychological first aid for recovery and growth, New York, 1978, Holt, Rinehart & Winston.

This book, written in an easily readable style, gives the nurse a broad framework for recognizing vulnerability and emotional reactions of persons experiencing a crisis. The author presents her own clinical work and emphasizes the preventive nature of crisis intervention. Situational crisis adjustment measures are emphasized.

Langsley, D., and others: Family crisis therapy: results and implications, Family Process **7**:145, 1968.

The article presents crisis in relation to one's immediate setting, recent stresses, and current events rather than to past history. Crisis therapy is suggested as an alternative to hospitalization. The authors note that an active crisis intervention approach can keep most clients out of the hospital.

Langsley, D., and Kaplan, D.: The treatment of families in crisis, New York, 1978, Grune & Stratton.

The authors report a study of 500 family cases; one half were admitted for in-patient treatment, and one-half were prescribed out-patient crisis intervention. Findings show that those patients who were prescribed crisis intervention did better in these areas: social adjustment ratings, number of days absent from work, family interaction tests, remission figures, symptomatic behavior tests, and antiviolence ratings. The study speaks strongly in favor of not hospitalizing individuals when it can be avoided, but keeping persons functional in their family, social, and work units.

Lewis, J.: To be a therapist, New York, 1978, Brunner/Mazel Publishers.

This book presents one of the most complete discussions of the core qualities requisite to effective relationships in therapy. The author presents and discusses research findings related to the concepts of empathy, warmth, respect, and genuineness. Also discussed are the ways in which the author trained therapists to develop skills in the core qualities that character effective helping relationships. The exercises are adaptable to the education of nurses as counselors with rape victims.

Parad, H., editor: Crisis intervention: selected readings, New York, 1965, Family Service Association.

The book is an excellent resource that offers readings on crisis theory and methodology. The contributing authors address theoretic explorations, maturational and situational crises, and clinical applications of crisis theory.

Paul, L.: Treatment techniques in a walk-in clinic, Hosp. Community Psychiatry **12:**49, 1966.

The author describes a walk-in clinic for problems-in-living that do not require hospitalization and are amenable to crisis intervention. Described are techniques used to achieve social restoration through a quick reversal of decompensation and ways of getting persons to grieve and express their thoughts or feelings.

Pittsburgh Action Against Rape: Training manual, Pittsburgh, Pa., 1979.

This manual is used to train lay and professional volunteers in providing care to rape victims. Its strengths include a comprehensive presentation of information and counseling approaches related to a victim's medical, legal, and psychologic needs. The manual emphasizes use of a creative listening model in counseling rape victims.

Women's Crisis Center: Empathy training manual, Ann Arbor, Mich., 1977, Women's Crisis Center of Ann Arbor, Mimeographed.

The manual presents the concept of empathic understanding and discusses "levels of owning feelings" that persons experience during a growth process in counseling. It shows how the nurse can help a woman own her own feelings by listening, understanding, and communicating understanding. This manual can be used to educate nurses to listen effectively to the feelings of rape victims.

# CHAPTER 8

# Rape victim advocacy

What is currently going on is the natural consequences of the
experience of one's own life. It need bear little or no relationship
to either the *awareness* or the *intent* of the individual. Old pains
are propagated and made stronger by current interaction about
them. *There is hope, then, that anything can change.*

Satir, V.: *Peoplemaking,* Palo Alto, Calif., 1972, Science & Behavior Books, Inc., p.
xi. Reprinted by permission of the author and publisher.

## CHAPTER OUTLINE

## LEARNING OBJECTIVES

After reading this chapter the student will be able to:

1 Define advocacy as applied to rape victims

2 Identify six nursing principles of health advocacy

3 Describe the police investigatory procedure

4 Explain the role of the police at the hospital

5 List and describe at least six guidelines for providing legal advocacy to rape victims during a police investigation

6 Describe the mediation role of the nurse advocate

7 Explain how nurses participate as expert witnesses in court proceedings

8 Describe the role of volunteer advocates in the medical system and the legal system

Rape is a violent assault on the person of a human being. To endure and survive a rape experience is physiologically and psychologically traumatic. Therefore rape frequently precipitates a crisis state for its victims (see Chapters 4 and 7). During periods of crisis it is comforting for victims to have the assistance of an advocate in resolving the rape experience. The concept of advocacy, defined as concern for and actions in behalf of another, is discussed here in relation to meeting the rape victim's needs. A distinction is made between principles of nursing advocacy and the role and functions of volunteer advocates in rape victim care.

## ADVOCACY DEFINED

Traditionally, advocacy has meant an act of concern for and actions in behalf of another at both the individual's and the system's organizational level.[5] Webster defines an advocate as one who "pleads the cause of another."

Advocacy has existed in history "as long as there have been powerless groups in need of a champion."[11] During moments of distress people tend to seek out a champion to back their cause and to help them meet their goals. As long ago as 1948 Herbert Hoover acknowledged the concept of advocacy when he stated:

> It is a curious fact that when we get sick, we want an uncommon doctor; if we have a construction job, we want an uncommon engineer; when we get into war, we dreadfully want an uncommon admiral and an uncommon general.[10]

Sometimes the meaning of advocacy is misunderstood by nurses who are altruistic and eager to help others. All too often such nurses, or others involved in victim care, think of themselves as the victim's advocate and set out to fight for what they (the nurses) think is best for the victim, not what the victim believes is best.[14] Advocacy is *not* doing for, convincing, or coercing the victim to do what the nurse thinks is in the victim's best interest or what the nurse would like to see done—for example, informing others about the rape, collecting evidence through a rape examination, or prosecuting an assailant. As Curtin has stated:

> So often by trying to do what we think is right by our value system, we trespass upon the authenticity of the person. Although in many cases our transgressions are not so great, in some cases they are profound . . . the real question is whether or not the *individual rather than the professional* should make such value decisions. If we decide that a person cannot, how do we reach this conclusion? Can we not, should we not, ought we not to assist the patient in decision making AND YET RESPECT THE PATIENT'S DECISION once it is made?[6]

## PRINCIPLES OF HEALTH ADVOCACY

Advocacy is not new to nursing. It is receiving revived recognition because of societal and professional forces such as "patient's rights" and "accountability to the consumer." Early leaders in nursing who acted as patient advocates include Florence Nightingale, Lillian Wald, and Lavidia Dock.

Regardless of the setting, nurses working with rape victims need to consider principles of nursing advocacy in providing health care to rape victims. A listing and discussion of these principles follows.[14]

1. *Emphasize the individual's assets.* Studies have shown that individuals make more progress toward health when the areas in which they are most able are strengthened or emphasized. Best results are obtained by focusing on the extent to which a person is meeting the goals that they have set for themselves. For example, the nurse may emphasize to a rape victim that she is capable of making sound judgments about who to tell about the rape.

2. *Encourage individuals to explore what is healthy about themselves.* Professional nurses know what comprises a state of health. They help clients to assume responsibility for achieving health. For example, many rape victims express concern over a physiologic or psychologic reaction to the rape experience and have difficulty in determining whether their responses are "healthy" ones. Nurses help victims explore healthy and unhealthy responses.

3. *Emphasize the victim's responsibility for health.* Ultimately each person is responsible for his or her own health care, but all too often people abdicate this responsibility to health care providers. It is important for the rape victim to resume responsibility for her health care in the process of recovery. Active responsibility for one's health implies (1) the use of self as an agent, as the doer; (2) awareness and interpretation; and (3) accountability.[7] Nursing interventions are directed toward helping rape victims interpret information so that they can act in ways that support remaining or becoming healthy.

4. *Help victims gain emotional distance.* Aware that each person is accountable for his or her own health, nurses recognize that in times of stress or trauma a person's ability to think and act clearly is hampered. It is not surprising, then, that rape victims feel vulnerable to abuse, helpless, and highly sensitive to the power that various systems and professionals have in relieving, inadvertently

threatening, or perpetuating suffering. By talking over concerns with an objective, nonjudgmental nurse, a rape victim is able to gain some emotional distance from an issue and determine what to do about presenting concerns.

5. *Provide information needed for health decisions.* Rape victims must have information about alternative treatments, therapies, and follow-up care to determine which options are most in accordance with their life-style, values, and plans. Nurses help rape victims reason through each of the options, enabling victims to decide which alternative is consistent with their own beliefs.

6. *Support health decisions that a victim makes in keeping with the victim's priorities in life.* As stated earlier, the nurse advocate does not impose any advice or decision onto a rape victim. Rather, the nurse supports what the victim believes are the best health decisions at the time.

The following clinical example demonstrates application of the principles of nursing advocacy within a health care setting. The victim is a 17-year-old, black, single woman who was raped by a stranger 3 hours earlier. The nurse interacts with the victim as they prepare for the rape examination.

## CLINICAL EXAMPLE

| Interaction | Principle of nursing advocacy |
|---|---|
| *Victim:* I can't quit thinking about the rape . . . the horrible things he said to me. | |
| *Nurse:* Being raped is a terrible experience. It's normal to be upset about it. After all, it just happened a few hours ago. | Allows expression of victim concerns. Provides information that victim is behaving in a normal manner following a stressful, traumatic experience. Encourages further expression of victim concerns. |
| *Victim:* I feel like I'm out of control . . . like I can't think straight. | |
| *Nurse:* Well, it seems to me that you have made an effort to get control of yourself. You came here to the clinic to get some help. | Nurse reinforces that obtaining medical care is an asset (good judgment) and a healthy behavior directed toward regaining control over one's life. |
| *Victim:* Yeah, at least I have some sense left. I feel really bad about not telling my mom about the rape. | |
| *Nurse:* What stopped you from telling her? | Helps victim to explore her concerns and gain some emotional distance. |

| Interaction | Principle of nursing advocacy |
|---|---|
| *Victim:* I know she'd feel bad. | |
| *Nurse:* Do you plan on telling her? | Helps victim determine which options are available and to decide course of action. |
| *Victim:* Yeah, I do . . . I can't keep secrets from my mom. | |
| *Nurse:* Well, if you or your mom wants help to talk about being upset, there is always someone here for you. | Supports decision and provides further information about alternative treatment for victim and family members. |
| *Victim:* Thanks. Say, I'm right in the middle of my menstrual cycle. Is there anything the doctor can do to make sure I don't get pregnant? | |
| *Nurse:* There are a couple of things you could do. (1) There is a medication called the "morning after" pill (DES) that you could take to prevent pregnancy. However, it has been known to cause cervical cancer in the daughters of women who took it when they were pregnant, and it also causes severe side effects like nausea and vomiting. So not all physicians recommend it. (2) You could ask for a menstrual extraction. That is a suctioning of the uterus that removes the contents. (3) You could wait and see what happens. It's rather rare that women get pregnant as a result of being raped. | Provides information needed for health decision so that victim can select from alternatives. |
| *Victim:* I'm going away to school in 2 weeks. I don't think I could stand waiting to find out if I am pregnant. I want the doctor to give me a prescription for that "morning after" pill. | |
| *Nurse:* Fine, you can discuss your decision with the doctor. | Supports health decision. |

As demonstrated in the example, the rape victim is quite capable of assuming responsibility and determining her own health decisions. The nurse advocate helps the victim work through her concerns, provides necessary information to make sound health care and life decisions, and supports the victim's decisions in a nonjudgmental manner.

## LEGAL ADVOCACY

The nurse's role and responsibilities in relation to the legal process are multidimensional. One aspect of the nurse's role relates to the police investigation; another aspect involves coordinating the victim's care and being sensitive to all concerned parties. Both roles interface as the nurse provides the victim with the best possible care.

Nurses find that rape victims have many questions about the police and the judicial system that they may want to explore while receiving emergency medical care: Do I have to report to the police? Will the police think I am lying? Do I have to tell my parents? If they pick up the man, do I have to say anything to him? What questions will the police ask me? If I prosecute the man, what are the steps I have to go through? What are the chances of his being convicted? Will all the ugly details from the police report be in the newspaper?

Obtaining information has been documented as an important need for victims in the first phase of resolving the rape crisis.[3] Therefore nurses need to know about the legal investigation and the role of the police officer at the hospital in order to explain these matters to the victim.

### Police investigatory procedures

Although police investigatory procedures vary among counties and states, certain aspects of the police investigation have been standardized by the Professional Standards Division of the International Association of Chiefs of Police.

When a rape victim notifies the police of an assault, a set of processes is set in motion to meet her needs, investigate the assault, and bring the assailant to trial. Fig. 8-1 depicts the flow of a rape case from a police perspective and is helpful with the discussion below.

Police officers responding to a sexual assault have a twofold responsibility. They must (1) assist, protect, and provide services to the victim in a professional, sensitive way that recognizes the physical and emotional trauma the victim has suffered; and (2) properly investigate the case, gather and preserve evidence necessary for possible future prosecution of the crime.[8]

When a dispatcher receives a call from a victim, it is the dispatcher's responsibility to ascertain that she is in a safe place. If the victim is in a safe location, the dispatcher then instructs her to remain there until a squad from the police force arrives. Over the phone the dispatcher instructs the victim not to clean up, douche or bathe, or change her clothes because she will destroy valuable evidence. This is difficult for many women because they feel dirty. At this time the services of a rape crisis center (if available) can also be offered.

When the initial investigating officers arrive on the scene, they collect most of the evidence to be used by the prosecution. Usually two officers make this preliminary investigation. The purpose of this interview should be discussed with the victim. In most cases one officer works solely with the victim, interviewing her about the assault, while the other officer gathers and preserves evidence at the scene of the crime. However, in some counties the officers' duties are not split, and both act as a team in completing the investigation.

The initial interview can be extremely stressful for the victim, particularly if she is

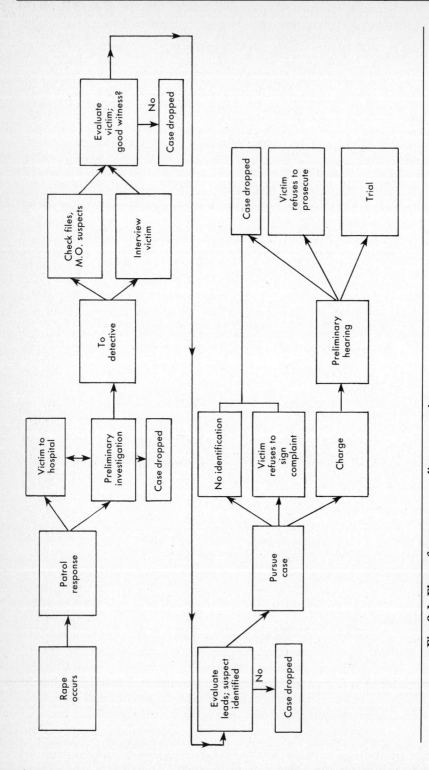

**Fig. 8-1. Flow of rape cases: police perspective.**
Reprinted with permission from Harrisburg Area Rape Crisis Center Training Manual, Harrisburg, Pa., 1977.

doubted, made to feel stupid, or blamed for the rape. For these reasons the Harrisburg Area Rape Crisis Center has developed the following guidelines for police officers to follow when taking the victim's initial statement.

1. Intimate details of the crime are not necessary since a detective will obtain them later.
2. Language such as the "alleged assault" or the "alleged victim" should never be used since it sounds like the officer [or medical personnel] doesn't believe the victim and a defense attorney will bring this out.
3. Writing the victim's statement in the officer's own words is advised [don't use quotes] so if the victim later cannot recall word for word what she said it will not appear as though she is lying.
4. A joint report should never be made—each officer should write his/her own report.[8]

During the initial investigation basic facts about the victim, the rape offense itself, the suspect, and any witnesses to the assault are obtained. The facts may be obtained at the scene of the assault, en route to the hospital in the police squad car, or before or after the sexual assault examination. Data that the officers inquire about include:

1. *Victim*—name, age, home and work address, phone numbers, marital status, number of children, source of income, dates of any prior sexual assaults, and details concerning any prior relationship with the suspect.
2. *Offense*—briefly what happened, exactly when it occurred, just how it occurred, what happened prior to its occurrence and what happened after it occurred, as well as any reason for its occurrence, if one can be ascertained, and exact time and location of the assault.
3. *Suspect*—name and address if known, or full and complete description and any identifying marks. Did the victim know or see the assailant before? How, at what time, where and why did the victim meet up with the suspect on the dates in question? Did the victim ever date the suspect before or have any conversation with him? Obtain highlights of all conversations the victim had with the suspect on the date in question.
4. *Witnesses*—obtain names, addresses and phone numbers of all parties who saw the victim before the incident, who saw or heard any part of the incident and before the police arrived. Statements from those individuals will have to be taken and may provide corroborative evidence at the trial.[8]

It is advisable for one officer to interview the victim and answer any questions that other officers at the scene of the crime may have rather than to have many officers asking questions. The police officer will advise the victim to seek a sexual assault examination for several reasons:

1. To ascertain and document the extent of trauma incurred as a result of the rape and treat injuries as indicated
2. To care for psychosocial needs
3. To collect evidence of the assault in a manner that is legally admissible for prosecution[8]

### Role of police at the hospital

Over the last decade a great deal of work has been done in educating and training police to be sensitive to the victim's emotional needs. Police officers attend to six areas of concern in meeting these needs. First, they respond with warmth and compassion based on their recognition that the victim just endured a violent assault. Second, they attempt to see that the victim is given priority in receiving care in the emergency room. Third, when possible the police delay extensive interviewing of the victim until her pain and physical needs have been taken care of. Fourth, they respect her privacy by (a) securing a private waiting room, (b) interviewing the victim in a private room free from distraction, (c) escorting her in a manner that does not suggest she is a criminal, and (d) excuse themselves from the examining room while evidence is being collected (their presence is not legally required). Fifth, officers allow the victim to ventilate her feelings and discuss any aspect of the assault she so desires. Sixth, they are supportive and tactful with significant others.[8]

The police officer is responsible for receiving the medical evidence that has been collected. The officer is expected to receive the evidence from the nurse or the doctor in the emergency room and *sign* a receipt for any materials turned over to him. A chain of evidence is thereby established. Because there has been a great problem connected with the chain of evidence (that is, evidence has been lost or destroyed) attempts have been made to develop a fail-safe method of evidence collection.[19]

Receipt for release of evidence usually includes the following[8,15]:
1. Victim's name
2. Date and time
3. Victim's hospital number
4. Name of the person collecting the evidence
5. Name of any other person involved in the chain of evidence (e.g., lab)
6. Name of the officer receiving evidence

The officer usually receives the following evidence:
1. Clothing in separate paper bags
2. Debris collected (foreign materials adhering to the body)
3. Foreign hairs:
   a. Pubic hair combings
   b. Head hair combings
4. Standards:
   a. Pubic hair
   b. Head hair
5. Smears and swabs:
   a. Vaginal
   b. Rectal
   c. Oral
   d. Other swabs—if indicated
   e. Control swab
6. Whole blood sample (2 tubes)
7. Saliva sample
8. Fingernail scrapings: right and left hand in separate envelopes
9. Photographic film—if photos are taken in the ED
10. Urinalysis (not required by all crime labs)

When the medical examination has been completed, the officer has a responsibility to ensure the victim's safety and welfare en route to a safe destination of her choice. If a formal statement about the assault has not been taken, at this time the officer may ask the victim to be available the following day for such an interview. Some victims find it reassuring if the officer patrols the area of their residence (if they were assaulted there and are returning home). If the victim does not want to return home, arrangements can be made for alternate housing. Frequently a rape crisis center or local women's group can assist with finding temporary housing.

It is particularly important that the proper police and medical procedures be implemented in the investigation of a sexual assault because it is extremely difficult to obtain a rape conviction—even when the evidence presents a "strong case." Therefore the efforts of the patrolman in a rape case are more important than they are in most other felony cases. Furthermore, police officers have the additional responsibility of intervening in the victim's emotional crisis as well as conducting the investigation of the assault itself.[8] The preparation of police officers to respond to their official responsibilities as well as to victim needs is gaining importance in education programs at police academies. In some sectors of the country, particularly rural areas, much work in this area remains to be done.

The manner in which a police officer investigates a rape case often determines whether or not the victim will cooperate in reporting the data. An attitude of respect and concern for the victim, patience in allowing her to tell her story at her own pace, and sensitivity to her feelings about disclosing the sexual transaction enable the officer to secure the victim's trust and cooperation in the investigation.

The following example demonstrates a well-conducted police interview. In this case an 18-year-old rape victim was brought to the emergency room by strangers who had found her on a highway.

CLINICAL EXAMPLE

Q. [Detective] Ms. Powers, I'm Detective _____ . I work with the Sex and Youth Squad investigating cases of rape. I know this is a tough time for you, but I need to ask you some questions about what happened. Tell me what you remember about what happened from the beginning.

A. [Victim] My car broke down out on the freeway. I was by myself, don't know how to service a car, and don't have any road service like AAA. So I put up the hood of the car to get some help.

Q. It's upsetting enough when your car breaks down and more so when you feel stranded and helpless!

A. Yes. Eventually a trucker stopped to help me, but he couldn't get the car operating. So he offered me a lift to the nearest gas station or phone booth, and I accepted. I didn't suspect anything. Instead of taking me where I could get help he . . . (sobbing) . . . drove off a side exit to a small ravine by a grove of trees. He told me to shut up or he'd kill me and proceeded to rape me. He was real strong.

Q. Where was this exit located?

A. It was exit number 40, about 2 miles from here.

Q. Did you get a good look at this character?

A. Yes, he was about 6 foot. He had dark-brown curly hair and a scar on his chin. He was wearing blue jeans, a tan shirt, and boots.

Q. Did he force intercourse on you?

A. Yes. My arms are bruised from being held down.

Q. Did you try to call for help?

A. Yes. I was screaming with fright, but no one could hear me in that grove of trees.

Q. Did he threaten you in any other way?

A. Yes. He said if I reported him he would come after me and kill me.

Q. How did you get to the hospital?

A. When he was done with me, he shoved me out of the truck and took off. I ran out to the highway and some strangers brought me here. It was awful . . . I had no pants on.

Q. I'm sure it was awful for you and that you were glad to get away.

A. Yeah (crying).

Q. (Pause allowing victim to ventilate) Did you get any other evidence or description of the man?

A. I think I got his license number on the truck, . . . but I was pretty upset. You'll have to track it down. I hope it's right.

Q. Do you want to prosecute this man?

A. You bet! I don't want him free to hurt any other unsuspecting, innocent woman.

In the above interview the detective verified that the incident met the criteria for rape: intercourse, by force, and against the victim's will. He obtained a description of the assailant to put out an alert for his arrest. The detective also made arrangements for the victim to come to the courthouse and file a complaint. When the interview was completed, he called the nurse in to make sure that the bruises the victim reported were recorded on the medical record and made arrangements for photographs of the bruises to be taken for evidence in court. The assailant was arrested later that night.

An interview about a rape experience can be emotionally trying for both the police officer and the victim. A poor interview may leave the victim feeling angry, embarrassed, and disillusioned. By giving the victim warm, empathic, positive support and by dispensing factual information to the victim concerning the police officer's role in the investigation, the nurse acts as an advocate to make the victim's experience with the police a positive one. The Harrisburg Area Rape Crisis Center has developed the following 10 guidelines for providing legal advocacy to victims during a police investigation.

1. *Notifying the police.* If the police have not already been called, the *victim* should determine if they are to be notified or not. It is the victim's decision whether or not to report the assault. Some counties require by law that all cases of rape be reported. Therefore, nurses need to be aware of the legal ruling for their region of employment. In counties that insist all rapes be reported, some hospitals record something less than rape—e.g., traumatic intercourse—if the victim does not want to report the assault. This enables the hospital to provide the victim care that is needed without forcing her to act against her will (a central conflict of the rape experience itself).

2. *Signing consent forms.* Inform the victim that signing consent forms for the medical examination and release of evidence to police agencies does not mean that she is obligated to prosecute. However, in some regions the police officer can file the complaint and take the case to trial. Nurses need to clarify this matter as it applies to their setting.

3. *Offering assistance.* If the police officer brings the victim into the emergency room, the nurse first introduces herself/himself and offers any assistance that can be given. By giving aid to the victim the nurse is assisting the officer. The nurse needs to indicate any way in which the officer can be of assistance to the health team.

4. *Provisions of clothing.* If the victim's clothing is confiscated, see that alternate clothing is provided for her. It is the police officer's responsibility to take photographs of the victim in her attire *before* she undresses and clothing is confiscated.

5. *Restricting exam room.* The officer should never be present in the examining room when the victim is in any state of undress. Inform the physician of the legal requirements if the physician mistakenly believes that the officer's presence is necessary to conduct a (legally) proper examination.

6. *Interviewing the victim.* Although the formal statement-taking does not take place at the hospital, the police will ask the victim basic factual information (discussed earlier) to start the investigation procedure if this has not been done already. Remain with the victim throughout the questioning if an advocate from the rape crisis center is not available and explain to the victim why these questions are necessary.

7. *Observer role.* Do not ask any questions for the police officer. Leave all interviewing to the police personnel. Emphasize to the victim that if she does not know the answer to a question she should indicate that to the police officer.

8. *Omitted evidence.* If the police officer forgets to ask the victim some pertinent question that is important to establishing a strong judicial case, ask to speak to the police officer privately and tactfully mention that it might be important to ask the forgotten question.

9. *Confidentiality.* Do not discuss the details of the case, the crime, or personal notions about the victim's credibility with anyone. The victim has a basic right to both verbal and written confidentiality of information *and* the support of nonjudgmental nurses.

10. *Offensive behavior.* If the police officers appear insensitive in their questioning, the nurse can assertively and tactfully point out what the victim might be feeling at this time. If the nurse believes the behavior of a particular officer is consistently offensive, by the manner in which questions are asked or if improper questions are asked (for example, "Did you have an orgasm?"), discuss the complaint with the officer. If the offensive behavior continues, nurses can report it to their supervisor and other channels of authority such as the local rape crisis center, and the officer's supervisor in a written, signed statement. Nurses ask for some remedy to offensive situations—for example supervision of the officer, inservice education, removal from assignment to rape victim cases, and so forth. [This is discussed further in the next section.]*

*From Harrisburg Area Rape Crisis Center: Training Manual (P.O. Box 38, Harrisburg, PA 17108), 1977. Reprinted with permission.

## MEDIATOR ROLE

Providing nursing care to rape victims in the emergency room is a skill that is learned primarily through experience. Hospitals have begun to develop procedures to ensure that proper care is extended to victims. However, there remains a variety of experiences that nurses are sometimes not prepared for, have not anticipated, and have not given forethought to and which can add needless stress to victims at the most inopportune times. The following discussion presents a number of elements in the advocacy responsibilities of a nurse in a mediating role.[17]

The nurse needs to be well informed regarding the laws in her county in relation to rape and sexual conduct, abortion, the legal age of a minor, treating minors with or without parental consent, and freedom of the informant or the patient's "bill of rights." What is hospital policy is *not* necessarily what is legal. The nurse must be familiar with hospital procedure, guidelines for evidence collection, the similarities and differences in hospital/police/legal/crime lab rules for evidence collection, and the interface between the hospital and professionals in the community. The following example highlights the potential for confusion and conflict.

### CLINICAL EXAMPLE

Jenny is a 16-year-old rape victim who comes into the women's clinic. She states that she is pregnant as a result of a rape and is seeking an abortion. She has not informed her parents about the assault. Jenny also wants the police called because she has decided to prosecute the case. She states that the offender is a classmate at her high school.

In this situation the nurse has to determine how best to assist the victim with her request for help. While assisting the victim, the nurse also has to consider the following questions:

1. What are clinic policies and legal guidelines for performing an abortion on a 16-year-old? Are the parents to be informed, or do they have to give consent to treatment? Does a 16-year-old have the right to privacy? Is Jenny a minor?
2. What is clinic or hospital policy on handling a rape case when the victim reports the rape several weeks after it occurred? Should the nurse notify the police before the examination? Or should she give Jenny time to think about alternative courses of action related to prosecution? Can any evidence be collected at this point in time?

After talking with Jenny in a private room, the nurse asks a volunteer to stay with Jenny while she checks clinical and legal policies relevant to this case. Before leaving the room, the nurse informs Jenny of her intentions and says that she will return shortly.

As demonstrated in this example, the nurse has many considerations and needs more information before deciding on the next appropriate intervention. Because she takes responsibility for providing quality care, the nurse seeks further information about the rules and regulations of the health care and legal systems. She may also consider consultation with her supervisor or another health professional because of the complications of the case. Regardless of the complexity, the nurse does not abandon the rape victim; the nurse reassures the victim that help is available and provides support to the victim while she (the nurse) seeks appropriate guidance.

Research findings report that the police and medical staff are usually cooperative and sensitive to victim needs.[9] However, there will be occasions when police officers or medical personnel are insensitive. The nurse needs to be informed of the proper channels for working through such conflictual situations. The victim does not need to overhear or be caught in a heated dispute between the nurse and another caregiver. It is poor judgment to discuss the offensive handling of a victim's case in front of the victim.

A rational appeal that addresses both an officer's urgency and concerns as well as the victim's position goes a long way in achieving the objectives of both parties in the process of delivering and receiving care. A sensitive, empathic nurse will enlist the cooperation of all persons involved faster than one who uses an authoritative approach directed solely at getting the job done.

There are times when other professionals or family members are experiencing stresses unknown to the nurse. For example, personal conflicts that sometimes impinge on one's job performance or behavior may include marital conflicts, financial stress, children who are ill, or significant others who may have been raped. Therefore the nurse needs to be prepared for unusual or exceptional behavior on the part of professionals or the victim's family.

Understanding that personal stresses exist does not excuse offensive behavior. However, the wise nurse will be aware that factors other than responding to the rape itself may be operating in a person's behavior. The problematic behavior can be best handled through the nurse's creative listening skills—for example:

> I can certainly understand your sense of urgency, Officer Jones. But Sally is really stressed right now. Can we wait until (apply the regulations of your particular region) to complete the interview?

The nurse needs to be not only assertive in potentially conflictual situations, but *empathic* when assertive for effective health team or community relationships to be established and maintained.[12]

The nurse is one person who will, in all likelihood, have extensive contact with the victim. Nurses are perceived by the public as caring persons and, therefore, are often able to readily establish rapport with victims. Thus the nurse is often more able to get information about the assault in interviewing the victim than any other party and can make that clear to all persons collecting such data. If the physician cannot immediately examine the victim, the time spent waiting can be used by either the nurse or the police to gather information about the assault. If police officers interview the victim waiting for medical care, she should be dressed and interviewed in a private room with the nurse or an advocate present. The nurse also explains to the victim or the police officers the current status of the care process. For example:

> *To the victim:* The doctor is a bit delayed and cannot examine you for about 20 minutes. The police will want to get the answers to some of their questions from you at some time, before or after the exam. Would you feel okay answering some of their questions before the doctor comes?
> *To the police:* I have some information from the chart about the victim. This is her address, phone number. . . . What she told me about the assault was. . . . She's upset right now but very responsive to me, and I think I can be of assistance to both of you during the interview.

The police are advised to obtain only a brief intake about the assault and are not to conduct a detailed detective investigation. The extent to which police officers follow that principle depends, however, on who may answer the dispatcher's call, their familiarity with rape investigations, prior positive or negative experiences with victims, human curiosity or indiscretion, and many other factors. The police officer faces a variety of problems that the nurse and the general public often have little appreciation of. These include finding and arresting the suspect; getting the victim to court in the face of repeated, tiring postponements; obtaining an accurate account of the assault to avoid surprises and embarrassment during the trial; securing the necessary witnesses amidst formidable excuses; testing the victim's commitment and motivation before continuing with the prosecution, or risking the victim's decision to drop the charges; buttressing public attitudes toward the police as spiteful enemies not to be trusted; handling problems with parents who do not believe their daughters and refuse to let the victim testify; and dealing with problems with the judicial system that protect the defendant's rights and limit the scope of police power in helping the victim.[8,9] One or more of the concerns cited may affect an officer's behavior. However, understanding these factors does not excuse inappropriate investigatory behavior or procedures.

When an exhaustive investigation develops in the emergency department, it is the nurse's responsibility to remind the officer that a detailed investigation will be obtained later or the following day. The proper setting, timing, and environment for such an investigation should be provided for while following the rules and regulations of the nurse's county. It is these rules and regulations that the informed nurse can enforce as they are within the nurse's realm of responsibility for victim care in the emergency department. During highly stressful times, when a particular professional's concerns are most pressing, the nurse's creative listening skills are most needed *and* effective. For example:

> *To the police:* I know you are really anxious to get a description of the assailant so you can send out an alert and have him picked up. You've got a good reputation for really helping these young women. But . . . Jane is not quite ready to talk with you. She knows you want to help and has asked for just a few more minutes to pull herself together.

The nurse assumes a mediating role by seeing that a victim's care "runs smoothly" while "keeping the peace" among all the forces that come to bear in that task. For example, it would not be unusual for the physician or resident to have a number of people in the emergency department and elsewhere in the hospital needing attention; the clerk may insist upon obtaining the chart and identifying information; the police may be urgent in interviewing the victim to get the facts and apprehend the assailant; and the concerned family or friends may want to know how the victim is feeling or what is going on since the exam is taking so long. As the nurse assesses priorities in the victim's care, she acts to de-escalate pressure operating in any given situation. Regardless of pressures, professional nurse advocates never lose sight of their first priority: quality care to rape victims.

## THE NURSE AS AN EXPERT WITNESS

Very often the nurse is one professional who is first to have intimate contact with rape victims in the emergency department. The nurse is viewed by many people as an expert by virtue of professional education. In rape cases the nurse's skills in patient observation and recording medical assessments are particularly important. In some cases the nurse may be called upon to testify in court proceedings as an expert witness. The nurse is expected to testify in regard to two types of evidence: (1) facts obtained from direct observation of a patient, and (2) conclusions arrived at from facts.[4]

A professional is considered to be qualified as an expert witness when these three criteria are met: (1) the area of knowledge that the expert is testifying to goes beyond the range of knowledge of the average layman; (2) the witness is so skilled or knowledgeable in the field that his/her testimony will facilitate the search for truth; and (3) the area of knowledge must be accrued from clinical practice or extensive reading alone.[13] Guidelines to prepare the nurse for testifying as an expert witness are discussed in this section. Emphasis is placed on how nurses can be unwittingly trapped by defense attorneys who try to discredit or disqualify nurses as expert witnesses. Areas considered include (1) preparation, (2) credibility, (3) testifying, (4) cross examination, and (5) the medical record.

### Preparation

The nurse discusses the presentation with the district attorney (DA) in advance of the scheduled hearing for testimony. The district attorney should be aware of the nurse's knowledge of the case, professional education, and experience—all of which give credibility to testimony.

### Credibility

The prosecuting attorney (DA) will ask the nurse to present professional data to the court prior to testimony to establish professional credibility.

> CLINICAL EXAMPLE
>
> *D.A.:* Ms. Doe, state your name for the record, please.
> *Nurse:* Jane Doe.
> *D.A.:* Would you spell it, please?
> *Nurse:* J-A-N-E D-O-E.
> *D.A.:* Ms. Doe, would you please tell the court about your professional background and education.
> *Nurse:* Yes, I went to (_____ School of Nursing) and obtained my B.S.N. in 1973. Part of my educational training was related to making observations of patients and assessments of their emotional and physical condition, and the reporting of those findings on the chart. Shortly after graduation I began working at the County Hospital in the emergency department. Our director of nursing asked the local rape crisis center to conduct an in-service education program on the care of victims of rape. I attended those sessions and have since been working as a volunteer at the local rape crisis center. I also developed a procedural manual for our ED on the nursing care of rape victims and published several articles on victim care in nursing journals.
> *D.A.:* And you have seen approximately how many victims of rape in that time?
> *Nurse:* Approximately 12 women.

As demonstrated in the above clinical example, nurses are prepared to give name, address, occupation, and information commonly included on resumes, such as education; clinical experience in years and according to nature of the work; certification; any special training or education in the care of rape victims or in evidence collection that qualifies the nurse as an expert—for example, formal education, in-service education, county task forces, rape crisis centers, crime lab experts, procedures and policies written. The nurse states his or her clinical specialty area and its relationship to the subject matter, membership in any professional organizations, and publications that would suggest respect and recognition from professional organizations as well as the general public.

The nurse's credibility as a witness may be challenged primarily through the following lines of questioning.

1. Questions that would show that on previous occasions the nurse has made statements that are inconsistent with present testimony.
2. Questioning that would elicit specifically contradictory testimony, showing that some statements of fact made by the nurse as a witness are, in fact, otherwise.
3. Questions that would show that the nurse is biased because of influences, such as kinship with one party or hostility to another, or motives of pecuniary interest, either legitimate or corrupt.
4. Questioning that would show a defect of capacity in the nurse as a witness to observe, remember, or recount the matters of testimony.
5. Questions that would attack the character of the nurse as a witness.[16]

## Testifying

Nurses can expect to give testimony as to what was said or observed, not opinions or conclusions. Because this objective reporting may include the signs and symptoms of emotional trauma, nurses must be prepared to explain how their education had prepared them to make observations and assessments of a person's emotional trauma. If an opinion is inadvertently given, nurses must demonstrate the basis for such a conclusion by relating it to factual information.

CLINICAL EXAMPLE

D.A.: On the night of June 24, 1979, were you on duty when Ms. Powers entered (name) Hospital for treatment following her rape?

Nurse: Yes, sir, I was on duty.

D.A.: Would you please tell the court what observations you made at that time.

Nurse: Ms. Powers was tearful as she entered the emergency department. However, she quickly pulled herself together. She related the incidents of the rape as she just reported to the courtroom. She stated that the man entered her room about 11:30 that night, had a knife which he put to her throat, and forced sexual relations on her. She was concerned about getting pregnant and asked for medication to prevent that. She was a bit confused about whether or not to report to the police, but I told her it was hospital policy and that I would have to notify them.

D.A.: And what is your opinion about Ms. Powers not reporting to the police?

> *Nurse:* It's a common response of many rape victims that is also reported in the research literature. It is a time of great confusion and crisis for these women. It's not at all unusual.
>
> *D.A.:* I see. And what did you notice about her physical condition?
>
> *Nurse:* I noticed that she had some rope burns on both of her wrists and recorded this on the sexual assault form. In our hospital the nurses have been trained to do most of the interviewing and evidence-gathering. This is more comfortable for the woman. The physician completes the pelvic examination.
>
> *D.A.:* Thank you, Ms. Doe. No further questions. (Looks to defense attorney) Your witness for cross-examination.

In this case the nurse offered a conclusion: that her observation of trauma to the wrists was a rope burn. Although the court does not allow "opinion" testimony as evidence (that is, the nurse must not give an opinion based on "fact"), as a professional the nurse *can* draw, from observation or experience, an inference that constitutes "expert opinion." However, the defense attorney will attempt to invalidate opinion testimony.

## Cross-examination

The nurse can expect to be cross-examined in a manner similar to the questioning of the victim of rape. The defense attorney will attempt to discredit the nurse's testimony and qualifications.

CLINICAL EXAMPLE

> *Def. Atty.:* Ms. Doe, have you had advanced training in the matter of making psychologic and physical assessments?
>
> *Nurse:* I've had training from my baccalaureate nursing education.
>
> *Def. Atty.:* I see. Then you are not a specialist in either psychologic or physical assessments.
>
> *Nurse:* I am skilled as a beginning practitioner.
>
> *Def. Atty.:* I see, a *beginning* practitioner (emphasis). And to be a specialist what kind of training would you need?
>
> *Nurse:* I would need to enroll in a master's program in nursing.
>
> *Def. Atty.:* And that would require how much additional education and preparation?
>
> *Nurse:* Anywhere from 1½ to 2 years, depending upon the program.
>
> *Def. Atty.:* So you are making these *conclusions* as a novice in the field?
>
> *D.A.:* Objection, your honor. The witness is a prepared clinician as recognized by her professional organization.
>
> *Def. Atty.:* I beg the point, your honor. I am talking about this young lady's qualifications as an *expert* witness on the matter.
>
> *Judge:* Objection overruled.
>
> *Def. Atty.:* You say you have seen only about a *dozen* victims?
>
> *Nurse:* Yes, sir.
>
> *Def. Atty.:* Are you *really* suggesting that a handful of cases makes you an expert?
>
> *Nurse:* I am trained in victim care.
>
> *Def. Atty.:* You say that Ms. Powers had rope burns.
>
> *Nurse:* Yes, sir, around both wrists.

> *Def. Atty.:*  Have you ever *seen* rope burns?
>
> *Nurse:*      No, sir. But I've seen burns from restraints used with patients. (inference)
>
> *Def. Atty.:*  So you have *no* experience from which to say that this was a rope burn per se. You have not *seen* rope burns to diagnose the condition.
>
> *Nurse:*      No, sir.

As demonstrated in the clinical example, the nurse answers questions in a matter-of-fact manner, taking each one separately and allowing sufficient time for responses. It is helpful to be aware of any "irrational beliefs" that the adversary process may stimulate. Sometimes it may be useful to role-play the adversary process with the DA to be prepared for cross-examination strategies by the defense attorney. Nurses do not respond to the cross-examination as a personal issue; instead they think of it as a debate or drama to create a desired effect on the jury.

## The medical record

There will be times when the medical record is used as evidence in the courtroom whether or not the professional is present to give testimony. A precise and accurate account of the assault is the strongest supportive evidence to corroborate the victim's testimony. Even though some states have eliminated corrobative evidence as a requirement to prove rape, many juries are reluctant to convict a defendant without it. For example, circumstances deemed corroborative, in the opinion of the United States Court of Appeals of the District of Columbia, include the following:

1. Medical evidence and testimony
2. Evidence of breaking and entering the prosecutrix' apartment
3. Condition of clothing
4. Bruises and scratches
5. Emotional condition of the prosecutrix
6. Opportunity of the accused
7. Conduct of the accused at the time of arrest
8. Presence of blood or semen on the clothing of the prosecutrix and the accused
9. Promptness of complaints to the police
10. Lack of motive to falsify[1]

The medical record should include a precise account of the signs and symptoms of physical and emotional trauma that the victim has endured (see Chapters 6 and 7). *Signs of physical trauma* include all objective data from a complete physical examination and assessment of the victim. Of particular importance are bruises, lacerations, tooth marks, or swelling on the head, neck, and extremities as well as the genital area. *Symptoms of physical trauma* include the victim's verbatim statement describing the nature of the assault, demands made of her, and the types of sexual acts carried out. Questions must be carefully worded by the nurse since victims will simplify or conceal factual data because of their embarrassment, ignorance of terminology (such as fellatio and cunnilingus), fear, and confusion. *Signs of emotional trauma* include a precise description of the victim's behavior during interviews and the physical examination, specifically her emotional style (controlled or expressive) and behavioral evidence of anxiety. *Symptoms of emotional trauma* include the victim's statements about the assailant's threats to harm her, use of weapons, or any method of force employed to subdue her. The defense attorney will attempt to invalidate the credibility of evidence documented in the medical record on inferences drawn from the facts as recorded.[4]

When testifying the nurse may refer to the medical record or the sexual assault form to refresh his or her memory of the case. However, the nurse should discuss referral to the record with the DA in advance of testifying. If the medical record is present in court, the defense attorney may subpoena it as evidence, and the DA may not want the medical record used if it would damage the victim's case. The defense attorney has the right to examine any records a witness refers to; therefore caution needs to be taken in that regard. As one prosecuting attorney has said:

> Look here at this record. The nurse recorded that the victim knew this guy from several previous occasions, and she is telling me that she never met the guy before the night of the party where he raped her. *Because that is written in the record I cannot use it in court;* it would weaken her case if not lose it. All that evidence is down the drain! This is what we mean about reporting facts! It's *so* frustrating to have our hands tied.

Nurse professionals do not like to testify in court any more than the victim does for some of the same reasons: it is unpleasant to be confronted, doubted, and implicated through tricks of questioning and language used in cross-examination. In addition, nurse professionals do not relish disagreeing with colleagues in public or taking time from their professional practice for what seems to be a ridiculous marathon having a slim chance of successful outcome (conviction).[4] Furthermore, professionals are not generally educated in the strategies of testifying within the adversary process and thus often feel unprepared or intimidated in coping with the judicial system. However, gains are being made in assisting victims as more professionals and experts in the field of rape are testifying in court cases. Burgess and Laszlo have summed up the importance of the professional as a witness: "The professional who avoids testifying may be failing an individual just at the moment when he is most needed."[4]

## VOLUNTEER ADVOCACY

A volunteer advocate is someone who works in behalf of another person—usually through an agency. Nurses and student nurses work as volunteer advocates in rape crisis centers. This nursing role developed as a result of the poor quality of care that rape victims have received in health care settings and the disrespect they have endured from judicial systems. Thus, historically, the presence of advocates in emergency departments and courtrooms has been a negative comment on the quality of professional health care. Recently, however, advocates and professionals have begun to work collaboratively, capitalizing on the skills and expertise the other has to offer. This section discusses volunteer advocacy in (1) the medical system and (2) the legal system.

### The medical system

A volunteer advocate from a rape crisis center can be very helpful to the rape victim since the advocate is well acquainted with the medical procedures and can explain them to the victim. The advocate is also familiar with the medical system and how it functions. An advocate helps demystify the health system for the victim by:

1. Explaining simply and clearly what is being done and why
2. Making sure the victim is completely informed about her rights, any medication she is given, or any tests
3. Being assertive with medical personnel to be certain that the victim is being treated with respect and dignity[15]

Given the state of crisis victims experience post-rape, it is not surprising that they often do not understand what is being done to them or why. Because they have just been relegated to a powerless position through rape, it is understandable that victims feel uncomfortable about asserting themselves—even to ask for explanations that they need and have a right to know.

---

### RIGHTS OF THE RAPE VICTIM*

1. To transportation to a hospital when incapacitated.
2. To emergency room care with privacy and confidentiality.
3. To be carefully listened to and treated as a human being, with respect, courtesy, and dignity.
4. To have an advocate of choice accompany her through the treatment process.
5. To be given as much credibility as a victim of any other crime.
6. To have her name kept from the news media.
7. To be considered a victim of rape regardless of the assailant's relationship to the victim, such as the victim's spouse.
8. To *not* be exposed to prejudice against race, age, class, life-style, or occupation.
9. To *not* be asked questions about prior sexual experience.
10. To be treated in a manner that does not usurp her control, but enables her to determine her own needs and how to meet them.
11. To be asked only those questions that are relevant to a court case or to medical treatment.
12. To receive prompt medical and mental health services, whether or not the rape is reported to the police, and at no cost.
13. To be protected from future assault.

*Adapted from Pittsburgh Action Against Rape: Training manual, 1979 (211 Oakland Avenue, Pittsburgh, PA 15219); Foley, T.S.: Counseling the victim of rape. In Stuart, G., and Sundeen, S., editors: Principles and practice of psychiatric nursing, St. Louis, 1983, The C.V. Mosby Co. Reprinted with permission.

In the hospital the advocate gives undivided attention to the victim. The advocate may remain with the victim throughout the entire hospital procedure—providing information, explaining legal rights and alternatives, and assisting the emergency department personnel in meeting the needs of the victim. Having been trained to listen empathically to victim concerns, the advocate also acts as a "watch dog" on the medical system.

### Rights of the rape victim

Sometimes victims do now know what their rights are within medico-legal systems. They may be afraid to ask the professional what their rights are or if the professional has a right to be doing what he or she is doing or about to do. Because, historically, rape victims have been doubly victimized by medico-legal systems and

14. To accurate collection and preservation of evidence for court in an objective record that includes the signs and symptoms of physical and emotional trauma.
15. To receive clear explanations of procedures and medication in language she can understand.
16. To know what treatment is recommended, for what reasons, and who will administer the treatment.
17. To know any possible risks, side effects, or alternatives to proposed treatment, including all drugs prescribed.
18. To ask for another physician, nurse practitioner, or nurse.
19. To consent to or refuse any treatment even when her life is in serious danger.
20. To refuse to be part of any research or experiment.
21. To reasonable complaint and to leave a care facility against the physician's advice.
22. To receive an explanation of and understand any papers she agrees to sign.
23. To be informed of continuing health care needs after discharge from the emergency room, hospital, physician's office, or care facility.
24. To receive a clear explanation of the bill and review of charges, and to be informed of available compensation.
25. To have legal representation and be advised of her legal rights, including the possibility of filing a civil suit.

because they are more vulnerable to abuse post-rape, rape crisis centers have developed a list of rape victim rights as shown on pp. 298-299. This statement of rights was originally developed to protect victims and to ensure that they receive the care that they deserve. Victim rights can be discussed prior to any treatment procedure or throughout an examination process. In some situations, for example, when a victim has to wait for treatment, the victim may be interested in reading a brochure containing a written list of victims' rights and discussing them with an advocate.

Working collaboratively with volunteer advocates from rape crisis centers, nurses can offer better quality care to victims. In some cases health care personnel may not be aware of their belief in myths about rape. They may communicate a hostile attitude toward the victim, thereby lowering the victim's self-esteem. When such conflictual interpersonal relationships develop, the advocate acts as a buffer and works to improve sensitivity toward the victim. At times, tension and conflict arise as advocates work to improve the quality of services to rape victims. This often happens when there is a lack of role clarity in the responsibilities and functions of advocates and professionals.

## The legal system

Victims do not want or need a lot of legal information immediately after a rape assault. They will not remember detailed information. However, the volunteer advocate briefly discusses two subjects, the police interview and the judicial system.

### The police interview

Frequently victims call the rape crisis center *before* they contact the police. Sometimes they contact advocates *after* they call the police. Very often rape victims are frightened, do not know what to expect, and want someone with them when the police arrive or interview them. Victims also have many questions about the police and the judicial system. They may want to explore the following issues while receiving emergency medical care. Do I have to report to the police? Will the police think I am lying? Do I have to tell my parents? If they pick up the man, do I have to say anything to him? What questions will the police ask me? If I prosecute the man, what are the steps I have to go through? What are the chances of his being convicted? Will all the ugly details from the police report be in the newspaper?

Being interviewed by the police immediately after a sexual assault is a frightening experience for some victims. The advocate helps to explain the police investigative procedures, the officer's duties, and the reasons behind some of the puzzling questions asked of the victim. As noted earlier, obtaining information has been documented in the literature as an important need for victims in the first phase of resolving the rape crisis.

Victims report that it is the *attitude* of the person interviewing them or providing care that matters (less than whether that person is a man or a woman).[9] When an officer's attitude is kind and understanding, and when the officer has interpersonal skills that enable him to be sensitive to the victim's unique response style, a police investigative procedure usually proceeds with minimal difficulty. Many women, however, find it comforting to have a female advocate present with them for the police interview. Sometimes victims do not understand the terminology used by the investigating officer (terms such as *fellatio* or *sodomy*) or they are embarrassed to answer what they consider to be very personal questions.

The following example shows how advocates can ease rough spots in the investigative process and explain the importance of giving details to the interviewer.

CLINICAL EXAMPLE

*Victim:*    Do I have to tell you exactly what he did (looking at advocate)?

*Advocate:*  Yes, he (the officer) has to report everything that happened. It will become part of the evidence for the trial.

*Victim:*    Well, I just don't like saying those words out loud, especially in front of a man I don't know.

*Officer:*   I've heard a lot of stories, honey. I know it's rough on you, but these guys are a lot alike. He wasn't makin' love to you, that'd be different. He was hurting you and that is what you need to describe to me, how he forced you to do this thing.

*Victim:*    (blushing) Okay, I'll give it a try. I just haven't had to do this before.

As demonstrated in this example, the volunteer advocate helps explain the police procedure, thus reassuring the victim that the officer's questions are necessary for trial evidence. The victim is embarrassed to answer, but she proceeds to give the information, knowing it is important for her case.

Sometimes adolescents or young adults get into situations they do not want to reveal. Adolescent assault victims may not want their parents or their legal authorities to know about the rape because they fear they will get into trouble. Young adults may do things they would not do if they knew they were going to "get caught" (such as alcohol or drug abuse) or if they realized it would matter "in the long run." It is important that advocates help these victims put such actions into perspective.

Sometimes a rape victim does not know if she wants to prosecute an assailant. A victim may not want to make such a decision immediately after the assault, when she is feeling stressed. In indecisive situations advocates usually recommend that the victim have the evidence collected, report the assault (the case "looks bad" in court if the victim has not filed a prompt complaint), and decide later about whether to prosecute. Prompt medical care and reporting of a rape ensure preservation of the evidence without forcing the victim to make a decision about prosecuting when she is not ready. Sometimes a victim does not even want to have evidence collected or to report to the police. Therefore advocates must be knowledgeable about the legal requirements for the area where they are working. Nurse advocates can help the victim in making a decision by weighing all the pros and cons of any given action.

CLINICAL EXAMPLE

A police detective called the rape crisis center to request that the volunteer advocate who had been with a victim when she sought medical care recontact the rape victim and convince her, as well as her mother, to prosecute the assailant. The detective explained that the assailant had a 25-year history of rape and robbery, multiple prison sentences, was a known murderer, and had been identified by the victim. The detective stated to the advocate:

*Detective:*  I had the plain-clothes policemen call her up on the phone. I had them tell her she had better tell her mom about the rape because *I* was going to talk to her mom, and it would be *better* for her mom to hear it from her first. When I meet with the girl and her mother, I will tell them that by not prosecuting this man they are just being selfish. They are thinking only of themselves and the embarrassment that this would bring to them and not the other victims this guy will get next.

The advocate told the detective that she would contact the victim to *help the victim* regain a sense of control and would support her in working through possible options. The victim related her position to the nurse:

Victim:   I don't want to tell my mom. She doesn't care about me . . . oh, she would in the end, but I don't want to give her any trouble. She's had a lot of trouble with my sister, and I don't want her to think I'm like that. I don't want her to think I'm a delinquent or a prostitute. I'm her baby . . . you know how that is. We don't really relate to each other, we just kind of live in the same house. I've always handled things on my own. I'll handle this on my own also . . . I'll be just fine, don't worry about me. I don't want to upset my mom. She's had lots of problems and I don't want her to know about this.

Rape victim, age 14
Blitz rape

In the above clinical example, the detective *decided for the victim* the action that should be taken (disclose the rape). The detective also pressured the victim into prosecuting the assailant. In contrast, the advocate took a position that was supportive of the victim and explained to the detective:

Advocate:   Your request—for me to convince the victim and her mother to prosecute the assailant—is not an appropriate action in my advocacy position. At this time the victim does not want to disclose the rape to her mother, and I will support her while she works through her decision.

As demonstrated in this clinical example, it is important that advocacy groups and legal authorities cooperate in helping the victim meet her goals. Sometimes these groups are at odds because they have different purposes. For example, it is the work of the police to apprehend and initiate prosecution to an assailant, but it is the responsibility of advocacy groups to support the victim's decisions. *The victim's decision must have first priority* because it helps her regain control over her life and thereby resolve the rape experience.

### The judicial system

It is the responsibility of the investigating detective to explain the legal process to the victim. The advocate, however, has first-hand knowledge about the judicial system and can help the victim understand what is expected of her. Often the victm has established rapport with an advocate by the time her case gets to the preliminary trial stages, and so she relies on the advocate to help her through this process also. The victim looks to the advocate to prepare her for what to expect, to be truthful about what is likely to happen, to inform her about the kinds of questions she will be asked, and to help in handling her feelings in response to matters such as seeing the assailant again and possible trial postponements. The advocate provides emotional support at a time when the victim's anxiety and fear remain high, informs the victim about how to

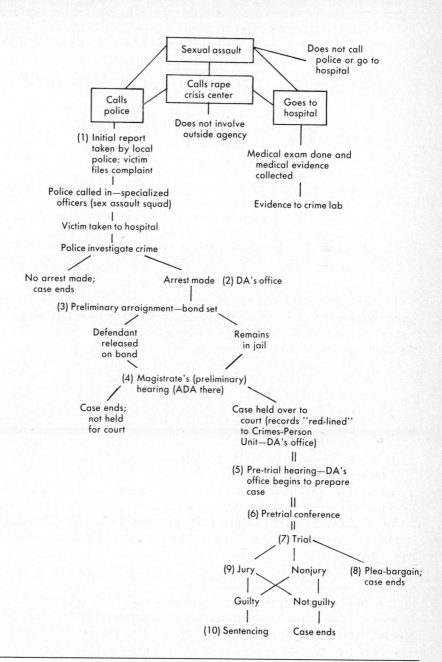

**Fig. 8-2. Flow chart of victim steps in the legal-judicial process.**

Modified and reprinted with permission from Pittsburgh Action Against Rape Training Manual, Pittsburgh, Pa., 1979.

best work with the police and the district attorney, and usually accompanies the victim to all the pretrial hearings and legal proceedings.

Fig. 8-2 shows a flow chart of the steps a victim goes through in the legal-judicial process. (Note that the steps may vary slightly among states and counties.) The process that a victim goes through in the proceedings of a rape case has been written about by many rape crisis centers. The following step-by-step discussion is one account of these criminal procedures that has been synthesized from manuals prepared by the Harrisburg Area Rape Crisis Center, Pittsburgh Action Against Rape, and the Interagency Task Force on Rape-Related Services.*

### Filing of complaint by victim (Step 1)

The normal procedure is for the victim to contact the police, who take the victim's complaint and investigate. If a suspect is arrested, the victim must identify the accused rapist and a complaint showing probable cause for arrest of the accused must be filed before a magistrate. If the victim is a juvenile, her parents or guardian would be responsible for filing the complaint.

A victim may file a complaint privately with the district justice, who then contacts the district attorney's office. The district attorney's office then determines if there is basis for the complaint and if so asks the police to become involved.

### District attorney's office (Step 2)

When a suspect is arrested, the district attorney's (DA's) office becomes involved since it will be the DA's responsibility to prosecute the case if it comes to trial. A private attorney may *advise* the DA or represent the victim in a civil suit. The DA, however, must represent the victim in all criminal courts of law.

Even though the victim has told her story to the police, if her case is considered for trial, she will have to tell the story *again* to the prosecuting assistant district attorney (ADA), and in many cases the ADA will be a man. The victim is encouraged to speak openly to the ADA and give him full details of the incident. An advocate may accompany the victim to the interview, but it is the ADA who will handle the prosecution of the victim's case and full cooperation is essential for thorough case preparation.

Sometimes there will be a change in district attorneys during the preparation of a victim's case. Such a change usually occurs because of scheduling conflicts with the original district attorney and is not an unusual event. If a victim does not like the way her district attorney is handling her case, she may request another attorney (the victim is usually not aware of this possibility).

In most instances the same prosecuting attorney will handle the case from beginning to end. The attorney from the district attorney's office will speak to the police, the advocate, and the medical personnel to help determine whether there is sufficient evidence to charge the accused with the crime of rape. The prosecutor will also decide

---

*Sources: Harrisburg Area Rape Crisis Center: Training manual (P.O. Box 38, Harrisburg, PA 17108), 1977; Pittsburgh Action Against Rape: Training manual (211 Oakland Avenue, Pittsburgh, PA 15219), 1979; Interagency Task Force on Rape-Related Services, Allegheny County, and the Urban League of Pittsburgh, Inc.: A handbook for victims (304 Ross Street, Pittsburgh, PA 15219), 1979.

whether, based on the facts and evidence, any charges in addition to rape should be filed. If the prosecuting attorney decides that charges should not be filed, he or she will usually explain fully the reasons for the decision not to file (if not, the prosecuting attorney can be asked to do so).

### Preliminary arraignment (Step 3)

The accused must be brought before a magistrate, without unnecessary delay, where he is informed of the charges against him and of his right to counsel. The accused does not plead at this time, but bail is set. The victim is not present at the preliminary arraignment, only the accused.

### Preliminary hearing (Step 4)

The preliminary hearing is not a trial. It is exactly what its name implies—a preliminary step that must be taken before the case can actually go to trial. There is never a jury at this stage of the proceedings. The judge at the preliminary hearing is called a magistrate. The hearing takes place 3 to 10 days after the preliminary arraignment before a magistrate in the district where the rape occurred.

An assistant district attorney will represent the commonwealth. The victim is the prosecuting witness. *Under the law, a rape is considered a crime against the state and not against the victim.* For this reason it is not necessary for the victim to have a lawyer. The offender and his defense attorney will be there also. The offender may or may not have a public defender, depending on his financial status.

The preliminary hearing is held in an open courtroom, and anyone may attend. Persons who attend preliminary hearings include the advocate, the victim's family or friends, and the offender's family and friends, and "court bums." The victim will be asked to tell about the rape assault in detail, and she will be questioned by the ADA and by the defense counsel. If, for example, the charge is rape, the victim must speak about penetration, force, and make an identification of the offender. The ADA will ask her questions to be sure that all the information is given. It is important for the victim to have a chance to talk with the ADA before the hearing. Advocates from rape crisis centers can help to arrange this. The police officer and any other witness will also testify.

*Issues in preliminary hearings and rape trials.* The prosecution of a rape case at the preliminary hearing stage, and later at the trial stage, whether by jury or nonjury, usually centers upon one or two major issues. These are commonly referred to as the issue of *identification* and the issue of *consent*. It is a Catch-22 situation: if the victim is not discredited on one account, then an attempt is made to discredit her on the other one.

The issue of *identification* usually arises when the victim and the assailant have never met before. If a woman is dragged off the street by her assailant or attacked as she lies sleeping in her own bed, it is likely that she has never before met the assailant. In cases of this type the major issue is one of identification. Is the person arrested by the police the same person who assaulted the victim? Or how does the victim know that the suspect is the assailant if she was asleep and the room was dark?

The issue of *consent*, on the other hand, is present in those rape cases in which the victim and her assailant had some contact with each other prior to the assault. If the assailant is a neighbor, a friend, or a casual acquaintance, of course there is no problem with identification. However, if the assailant met the victim at a bar, drove her home from a party, or took her out on a date, it is not unusual for the accused to contend that the victim consented to sexual relations. It then becomes the prosecution's problem to prove that the victim was forced to have sexual relations against her will.

*Preliminary hearing verdicts.* It is the prosecution's burden to convince the magistrate that there is probable cause that a public offense has been committed and that the accused is responsible for committing that offense. (Preliminary hearings are usually much shorter than the actual trial because the prosecution is not required to prove as much as at the trial.) If the magistrate is convinced that a crime has been committed—that there is prima facie evidence—and that the accused is the perpetrator, the defendant will be held for court. If the magistrate decides that the prosecution has not met its burden of proof, the charges will be dismissed at the preliminary hearing.

*Bond.* If the charges against a defendant are held for court, the magistrate must set a bond. The defendant has a right under the laws of the United States to have a bond set. The purpose of a bond is to make sure the defendant appears in court every time his presence is requested. In setting the bond the magistrate or judge should consider the seriousness of the crime, the injuries to the victim, and the past criminal history of the defendant—in addition to the length of time he has lived in the community, whether he is employed, and the likelihood of his appearing in court when called. The preliminary hearing is also the last opportunity prior to trial for either party to request raising or lowering the bail.

### Pretrial hearing (Step 5)

Approximately 1 month after the preliminary hearing there will be a pretrial hearing. The pretrial hearing is an organizational step that allows the prosecution to collect evidence, gather police and hospital reports, and interview witnesses for a final time before the DA's office makes a formal presentment of the charges. The victim, the arresting officer, and any witnesses will attend the pre-trial hearing. The offender and his defense attorney will not be there. The victim will be called into a private office to be interviewed by an ADA, who will determine whether or not there is a strong enough case to take it to trial. The victim will *again* have to relate, to another person, the details of the rape incident. The procedure is routine and takes about 15 minutes.

If, after reviewing the evidence and speaking with the victim and witnesses, the prosecuter decides that the state should prosecute the defendant, charges are formally filed in what is called an "information." The "information" contains the final statement of the charges placed against the defendant by the district attorney's office and for which the defendant will stand trial. After the preliminary hearing the DA's office begins preparing its case for trial.

When an indictment is filed, the accused comes before a judge in the court having jursidiction, is informed of the charges against him, is given an opportunity to plead, and *trial date* is set. At the pretrial-hearing screening stage, the DA's office again has the option of dropping the charges but *only* after consultation with the victim and the police. In many cases this important step is not carried out because plea bargaining between the defense and the prosecuting attorney goes on. *Plea bargaining* (see Step

8) is a process whereby the defense attorney barters with the prosecuting attorney for a lesser charge against the rapist. For example, the defense attorney may tell the prosecuting attorney that he or she will settle for a lesser charge than rape (such as simple assault) in exchange for pleading guilty to the charge. The two attorneys may talk about the extent to which the victim has a "good case"—that is, can she win the case. If so, that gives the prosecuting attorney more power in the debate over dropping charges. Since the victim is, in many instances, not consulted about the options (the discussion is held behind closed doors or in court corridors), her rights are violated. The victim is presented with a no-choice situation: "Accept this lesser charge (simple assault) because there is no way you will be able to prove rape." If any of the charges are dropped, the prosecuting attorney is expected to provide the victim with a full explanation of his or her actions. It would be unusual for the DA to determine that there is not a case.

### Pretrial conference (Step 6)

Approximately 1 month after the pretrial hearing the victim will be informed of a trial date. The ADA, who will be the prosecuting attorney, will make an appointment with the victim to discuss what will happen in court. Occasionally an offender will file pretrial motions to either suppress certain evidence or statements or to challenge on identification procedures. The victim usually does not attend hearings on pretrial motions unless asked to testify about identification procedures.

### Trial (Step 7)

In Pennsylvania a person must have a trial within 180 days of the filing of the criminal complaint. (This ruling varies among states.) However, the 180-day rule can be waived by the defendant. *Continuances frequently occur;* that is, often the trial is postponed if the defense or prosecution is not ready to begin. *The victim needs to be prepared for the possibility of continuances.* When trial delays happen, all concerned parties go home and wait for further notification of a trial date. *Waiting* is a tactic frequently used to discourage the victim so she will drop the charges. Usually postponements are about 2 weeks, but they may last several months.

The trial takes place in the county courthouse. The victim first reports to the *witness room* and signs in for the prosecution. She will wait there until her case is called over the loudspeaker. For example, "All concerned with the *State vs John Rapist* report to Judge so-and-so in room such-and such."

The witness room is crowded and noisy. The arresting officer and the other police involved will be there and so will the offender—if he is out on bond. (Some criminal justice systems are making provisions for separate waiting areas for victims and offenders.) *Everyone just waits.* It is possible to wait all day and not be assigned to a courtroom, in which case all concerned parties will report the next day, go through the same process, and wait again. The victim will wait until a jury is chosen. In many cases the victim will wait at least one whole morning and get into the courtroom after lunch.

### Plea bargaining (Step 8)

In some cases the assistant district attorney may enter into what is called *plea bargaining.* This situation arises when the prosecution agrees to recommend a particularly "weak case" or when the victim does not want to testify. In addition to rape, there are other sex-related crimes that may appear on the criminal complaint. A defendant initially arrested for rape may ultimately be charged by the police with a lesser offense or may successfully plea bargain with the ADA to have the charge reduced to a lesser offense (usually referred to as "drop charges"). To *drop charges* means that if the defendant is not found guilty of the primary charge of rape, he can be found guilty of a lesser charge such as indecent assault or simple assault (see Chapter 1 for definitions.) If the defendant is found guilty of rape, then lesser charges *may* be dropped. Lesser charges may also be included in the jury's conviction and in the ultimate sentencing of the offender. Common "drop charges" are (1) indecent assault, (2) corruption of the morals of a minor and statutory rape (if the vicitm is a minor), (3) aggravated assault, (4) simple assault, and (5) involuntary deviate sexual intercourse. The assistant district attorney *should not* enter into any type of agreement or plea bargain without first discussing the nature of the plea bargain with both the victim and the police. Such a discussion will give all interested parties an opportunity to voice their opinions and have input into the outcome of the case.

If the defendant *pleads guilty,* it may not be necessary for the victim to testify at the trial because the defendent will admit his guilt. The assistant district attorney or the investigating officer may summarize the facts of the case for the judge.

If the defendant *pleads not guilty,* the victim is required to testify at the trial. The victim will need to retell every detail she has already told the police, the doctors, and the attorneys who have questioned her. The police, the medical personnel, and any pertinent witnesses will also testify at the trial. The defendant may or may not testify in his own defense, depending on what best helps his case. Physical evidence such as torn clothing, photographs, and evidence collected at the hospital will also be used.

At the time of the trial the defendant has the option to choose either a trial by jury or a trial by a judge. Most defendants elect a trial by jury because of the tendency of jurors to be biased against the victim. If the defendant decides on a jury trial, the victim must wait until a jury is chosen.

### Components of a jury trial (Step 9)

Before a criminal jury trial can begin, a jury, consisting of 12 members and 2 alternates, must be selected. Alternate jurors sit through the entire trial, but they do not participate in verdict deliberations unless they are called upon to replace a juror when an unforeseen event (illness, death, crisis situation) prevents a juror from remaining throughout the entire trial. In most counties potential jurors are selected from voter registration rolls. In order to be eligible for jury duty one need only be 18 years of age or older. No rape myth-awareness test is given to rule out jurors biased against victims.

The jury itself is selected from a larger group known as the *jury panel.* The process of narrowing the jury panel down to the 14 jury members occurs in two ways—through *dismissal by cause* and by *preemptory challenges* from both prosecuting and defense attorneys. *Dismissal by cause* involves general questions to the jury panel from the judge and/or attorneys regarding issues that could affect their ability to hear the case with fairness and impartiality. Examples include questions concerning the existing relationship between panel members and the defendant or the victim, or prior involvement of a panel member in a crime similar to that being tried (either as victim or perpetrator). If a panel member indicates that circumstances do exist that could prevent him or her from having an unbiased view of the evidence, that person can be dismissed "with cause." Each attorney is then allowed to *dismiss* individuals *without cause through preemptory challenges*. The attorneys are allowed 20 challenges for trials involving a capital offense (for example, murder), 7 for all other felonies (including rape), and 5 for misdemeanors.

*Defendent pleas.* The trial is open to the public. In either type of trial, jury or nonjury, *it is the burden of the prosecution to prove the guilt of the defendant beyond a reasonable doubt*. The prosecuting attorney has a heavy burden since the accused rapist is always cloaked with the presumption of innocence.

*Opening address of counsel.* Following the selection of 12 jurors, and in most cases 2 alternate jurors, a criminal trial begins with opening addresses (statements, remarks) directed to the jury from the prosecution and defense attorneys. Court procedure dictates that the prosecuting attorney (DA) deliver his presentation first. He is followed by the defense attorney, who is an attorney in private practice or, if the defendant is unable to afford private counsel, a staff attorney from the public defender's office. (Such services are provided by the state at no cost to the defendant.)

Opening statements provide both attorneys with an opportunity to present to the jury an overview of their case before presenting it in a piecemeal fashion through the testimony of witnesses. In addition to the opening address summary, both attorneys usually point out the important role of jurors in the criminal justice system. Emphasis is placed on the need for "impartiality" and "the presumption of innocence until proven guilty" philosophy upon which the court system is based. The attorneys will request that the jury listen attentively to all the evidence and withhold judgment until all the evidence on both sides has been presented.

In addition, the defense attorney will discuss the prosecutor's responsibility to present evidence of the defendant's guilt "beyond a reasonable doubt." This will take on particular significance in a trial concerning sexual assault because there may be a lack of evidence that can be viewed as positive proof that such an assault took place (see Chapter 2 on sexual dysfunctioning during rape). Therefore the DA will emphasize the "his word against her word" nature of the testimony. Very often the defense attorney will end his opening remarks with a prediction to the jury that the prosecutor will be unable to offer the kind of evidence that establishes the guilt of the defendant "beyond a reasonable doubt."

*Presentation of the state's case.* Following the opening address of counsel, which summarizes each side's version of the case, the prosecuting attorney begins the presentation of the state's case. The prosecutor calls witnesses for the state to take the stand and elicits testimony through a series of questions and answers called *direct examination*. Each witness is subject to further questioning by the defense attorney in what is called *cross-examination*. If cross-examination seems to raise questions or doubts regarding the original testimony, the prosecuting attorney may clarify through *redirect examination* of that witness. The defense attorney can *re-cross-examine* if he or she so chooses. The cross-examination process continues until both sides are satisfied and the witness is dismissed. This is one of the most difficult and trying experiences for both the victim and the witnesses (see Chapter 9).

Prosecution witnesses usually include the arresting and/or investigating police officer(s), experts such as the examining physician and the nurse, and the victim. Often additional witnesses provide corroborative evidence; a common example would be the first person who saw the victim after the attack, offering testimony regarding the victim's mental and physical condition at the time of the incident.

*Presentation of the defendant's case and rebuttals.* Upon completion of the prosecution's case, the defense would present its case with each witness involved in the same process of direct and cross-examination. Although the defendant is given a choice of whether or not to testify, he usually elects to testify in order to avoid the impression of admitting guilt. Additional defense witnesses are usually friends, relatives, prominent community officials, employers, and acquaintances of the defendant called for the purpose of establishing an alibi or the good character of that defendant.

A *rebuttal* to the defense can be launched by the prosecuting attorney if serious doubts and contradictions have arisen. Testimony during a rebuttal must be concerned directly with the evidence raised by the defense; it cannot involve any information that should have been provided in the initial presentation. Any witness called for a rebuttal is subject to cross-examination by the defense attorney. Likewise, the defense attorney has the option to counter a rebuttal with a *surrebuttal*. This process can continue ad infinitum until all issues are resolved. Most court cases do not involve rebuttals and surrebuttals.

*Closing statements.* Following the defense presentation (or rebuttals if they occur), both attorneys summarize, challenge, debate, and clarify all the evidence in closing statements to the jury. This is followed by the judge's *charge to the jury* in which he interprets in layman's terms the various laws that apply to the case. The judge can also highlight certain testimony in terms of its applicability to the law. Finally he charges the jury to objectively consider all the evidence and return with a unanimous verdict of guilt or innocence.

*Jury deliberation.* The jury retires to a separate area to deliberate. This process can take hours or minutes. They return to the courtroom only after a unanimous verdict has been reached or if they consider a unanimous verdict to be impossible. If the latter occurs, they are considered a "hung jury," and a new trial is ordered. A verdict of innocence ends all judicial proceedings. A verdict of guilt is subject to appeal by the defense in a higher court (district, state, and federal). The victim can either wait for the decision or go home (requesting that she be called about the decision). If it is a nonjury trial, the judge can (but may not) decide the verdict there and then.

*Appeal.* The defendant has the right to *appeal* the verdict (if guilty) to a higher court. The appeal must be filed by the defense *within 7 days* of the trial. The victim and other witnesses are not involved in cases under appeal. If there is no appeal, a sentencing will be set and sentence imposed by the judge.

### Sentencing (Step 10)

Sentencing of the defendant can occur immediately after the return of a guilty verdict. More often, however, a *presentence investigation* of the defendant's background is ordered by the judge, and sentencing is deferred until the results of this investigation are available. The sentence is then imposed at a *sentencing hearing,* which usually occurs several months after the trial. The victim can be present at a sentencing hearing although her presence is not required. In addition to appealing the verdict, a defendant is granted the right to *appeal the sentence*. This appeal must be filed *within 30 days* of the sentencing date. During the period in which appeals are being heard and the presentence investigations are being conducted, a defendant may or may not be incarcerated. Incarceration is determined by the judge, who decides whether bail should be revoked, continued, raised, or lowered following the return of a guilty verdict.

## SUMMARY

Philosophically, advocacy is based on the commonality among individuals as human beings. Its underlying assumption is that if persons are given the right kind of support they will be capable of determining what is in their best interest and will assume responsibility to act in their own behalf. Nurses facilitate a rape victim's efforts to work through presenting concerns, arrive at decisions for action, and meet desired goals. The extent to which a rape victim is willing to assume responsibility for her health and life choices, and the extent to which professionals aid or impede that process, influences the way in which the victim lives her life.[14] Nurses implement principles of nursing advocacy in providing care to rape victims, whether that be in hospital emergency departments or in community settings such as rape crisis centers.

A rape victim has survived an experience in which she was made to feel helpless and vulnerable. Therefore the victim often wants a champion who will help her regain a sense of self and strength. The rape victim wants someone who will back her cause while she interacts with doctors, nurses, police officers, attorneys, defendants, witnesses, judges, and bureaucratic systems. Therefore many victims request and appreciate the assistance of a volunteer advocate throughout the rape examination and beyond hospital treatment. Because these victims are fighting a war against violence perpetrated against them, they may seek an "uncommon" leader to plead their cause, to help them regain control over themselves and their lives.

### Learning activities

Nurse consultants use specialized skills to provide consultees with recommendations that will improve their understanding or handling of a work difficulty involving either clients or administration. Through the consultation process they also help consultees learn skills that will help them master similar problems in the future. The following two exercises provide an opportunity for nurses to identify the problem in actual case situations and recommend action for managing the cases.

#### EXERCISE 1. Client-centered consultation

*Case situation:*    *Terrified victim: accessory to sex—inability to consent*

*Profile:*    Marge is a 15-year-old white female attending the local high school. She have been living with her girlfriend's family because her parents disapprove of her

*Stressor:*      relationship with a married man. Marge has refused to have anything to do with her parents.

Marge tells you that this was her first sexual experience. She had been on friendly, casual terms with a man and agreed to go for a ride to his summer cabin. Once there, he forced sexual relations on her and threatened that if she told anyone he would kill her, saying he knew who she was and where to get hold of her. Furthermore, he claimed, no one would believe her anyway because she had gone to the cabin with him. Marge was terrified and just kept quiet until she got home, when her girlfriend's parents brought her to the hospital. she had never had a physical exam before, didn't know what it was about, and was scared to death that it would be like the rape experience. She didn't want to be at the hospital because "people only come here to die, and there are strange doctors around."

*Stress state:*      Marge was crying and wailing at times. She had cried so hard that it was difficult to understand her speech sometimes. She would not let you get near her with any equipment to prepare her for the exam. Marge paced about the room and kept an eye on all the staff, particularly the males. She refused to let anyone touch her. Periodically she would wail, "Oh, my God, what am I gonna do? What if I'm pregnant? My folks said he was no good for me. I don't think I can tell them, but I'm going stir crazy without them.

## Discussion questions

1. What can the nurse recommend to the health care providers?
2. What legal issues would be involved if Marge decides to press charges?
3. What is the nurse's role and responsibility in the following situations?
   a. The police arrive at the emergency department.
   b. The nurse is asked to testify at a court hearing.

## EXERCISE 2. Policy discrimination

Select a local hospital and determine hospital policy in each of the following cases. Then consider what is *legal* in the hospital's community. Compare your findings.

## Case 1:

Susan is an 18-year-old college student who has come to a clinic for menstrual regulation 8 weeks after being raped. She is contending that she is pregnant as a result of the rape. The district attorney sends the nurse a court order requiring that all the products of conception be sent to the crime lab for analysis. (Yet hospital policy states that all products of conception are to be retained.) The crime lab must complete blood typing, chromosomal and other studies on the evidence. The police are asking a lot of questions about what Susan said and did. What would the nurse do in this situation? Does the victim need a psychiatric consultation before being permitted to pursue the abortion? Would the nurse forward the products of conception the crime lab as requested?

## Case 2:

The police are asking to see the medical record in relation to the rape of Janice. However, Janice does not want the police to see the record. Would the nurse let the police see the medical report or not? Do the police need a subpoena to see the medical record against the victim's will?

## Case 3:

Mary is severely traumatized and in need of hospitalization after being raped. It is hospital policy to obtain consent before hospitalizing any teenager. However, Mary is 17 years of age and self-sufficient. She thinks that in a day or two she will be able to tell her parents but not right now. What would the nurse do?

## EXERCISE 3. Role clarity*

*Purpose:* It is important for the nurse to be very clear about role relationships and responsibilities when working with other professionals. The objectives of the following exercise are to (1) clarify your own role; (2) clarify expectations others have of your role; (3) promote renegotiation of role responsibilities; (4) teach a process of role adjustment that can become a group norm.

*Directions*

*Step 1:* Break into groups of three to five with your classmates (or colleagues). Each member of the group is to select one professional

---

*Adapted and reprinted with permission from Harrisburg Area Rape Crisis Center: Focus: volunteer training, 1977 (P.O. Box 38, Harrisburg, PA 17108), pp. 27-28; and Uustal, D.: Values and ethics: considerations in nursing practice, 1978 (4724 E. Shenee, Paradise Valley, Phoenix, Ariz. 85032), p. 78.

or nonprofessional from these listed below, and each group member is to select a different professional/person. It is recommended that those persons most frequently worked with be selected for the exercise.

a. volunteers to community action group
b. medical advocate from rape crisis center
c. physician
d. nurse
e. police officer
f. detective
g. social worker
h. counselor
i. resident or intern
j. nursing supervisor
k. head nurse
l. therapist
m. chaplain or clergy
n. layman, concerned neighbor
o. lawyer
p. jury
q. judge
r. district justice
s. magistrate
t. state trooper
u. parent

*Step 2:* In silence write your response to each of the aspects listed below. For each of the categories—role expectations, conception, acceptance, and behavior—answer *two* of the available questions. You need not agree personally with what you think others perceive about that person and his/her role. Your awareness and difference of opinion will assist the group in determining variables that affect the interaction in different groups.

a. *Profile:* Describe this person/professional as you typically view him/her—i.e., age, race, sex, clothing, equipment, behavior, and demeanor.

b. *Role expectations:* What others think that person is responsible for and how he/she should do it.
   1. List 3 responsibilities this person/professional has to you as a nurse; a female/male; a citizen.
   2. List 3 responsibilities you have toward this same person/professional in the same areas.
   3. Are there any limitations inherent in these responsibilities—e.g., dominance-submission, power-helplessness, or change agent-follower?
   4. How do nonassertive, assertive, and aggressive behaviors relate to sex roles?
   5. Which behaviors are common to the person/professional you are discussing?
   6. How does trust with that colleague person/professional affect your willingness to give feedback and your receptivity to give feedback?

c. *Role conception:* What others think that person's job is. How he/she has been taught to do it.
   1. List 3 responsibilities this person/professional has to a victim of rape.

   2. List 3 responsibilities this person/professional has to one other health team member (pick a person from the list on the opposite page).

   3. List 3 assumptions made by society-at-large concerning this person/professional's role, class, power, status, control over others, and flexibility to change.

   4. Which behaviors (assertive, nonassertive, aggressive) are common among nurses? Why?

   5. What rights do you believe people should have in their relationship with the professional you are discussing? Explain. And with nurses? Explain.

d. *Role acceptance:* What this person is *willing* to do (usually) as it relates to victims of rape.

   1. List 3 indicators that that person/professional accepts his/her role.

   2. List 3 indicators that that person/professional rejects his/her role.

   3. What are your thoughts and feelings about the appropriate times to give feedback and be self-disclosing with the colleague/person/professional you are discussing?

   4. When do you want that colleague/person/professional to give feedback to you and be self-disclosing?

e. *Role behavior:* What that person/professional *actually* does (usually) in relation to victims of rape.

   1. List 3 behaviors indicating that that person has implemented that role.

   2. List one sanction should that person *not* implement the expected role.

   3. Would you like to change the way you behave now with that colleague/person/professional?

   4. What changes in your behavior would be productive and useful to develop better relationships with that colleague/person/professional?

*Step 3:* Once you have written your responses, share your answers with your group members in a round-robin fashion, noting:

a. What are the *confirmed* and *misperceived* expectations?

b. What are their areas of concern in relating to that person/professional? For example:

| | |
|---|---|
| 1. authority | 8. territoriality |
| 2. power | 9. monitoring or being monitored |
| 3. decision-making | 10. accountability |
| 4. planned change | 11. reverberation/repercussion |
| 5. manipulation | 12. competence |
| 6. resistance | 13. self-esteem/self-image |
| 7. limit setting | 14. conflict management |

## EXERCISE 4. Role-plays for assertiveness in professional interactions

### Purpose:

At times it is necessary for nurses to ensure that a victim receives good care in a manner that is sensitive to the victim's needs. The following sketches depict actual case situations that require assertive nursing interventions. Select those most useful in meeting your learning needs and role-play them as directed below.

### Directions:

1. Break into groups of three.
2. One person is to enact the role of the nurse.
3. A second person is to enact the role of the other party—for example, a physician, police officer, or supervisor.
4. A third person is to act as observer-recorder and identify (a) which interventions the nurse used, (b) which interventions were most effective, and (c) which interventions were least effective.
5. When the role-play is completed, the group is to discuss the situation.
6. For subsequent role-plays the group members are to rotate role enactments until each member has an opportunity to enact the nurse's role.

### Sketches

1. The physician tells the nurse, who is about to enter the examining room, that "this is a real nutty one, really messed up." The physician says he is not sure she even knows what rape is since she is "just a mental case." The physician wants to get rid of the case quickly since it is a "waste of time to be up in the middle of the night with this nuisance."
2. The physician is unduly rough with the victim during the physical examination and insensitive to the victim's discomfort. The physician yells at the victim for "not cooperating" with the procedure and does not explain what he is doing or why.
3. A resident "on call" completes the rape examination. The resident physician has not had previous experience with the medical protocol of rape victim care. The nurse notices that the physician inserted a wet swab in a dry test tube, only took one swab (instead of the two required) of the pertinent areas, and did not do a routine oral or anal exam because the patient denied these types of assault. The nurse is aware that evidence is not being properly collected.
4. Prior to giving the medico-legal evidence to the police, the nurse completes a checklist to see that everything is accurate. The nurse notes that the physician entered personal opinions and nonmedi-

cal conclusions about the victim in writing a general description of the examination results and the victim's report of the rape. The nurse is aware that this may damage the victim's character in court.

5. The police bring a rape victim into the emergency department. A nursing colleague assists the nurse assigned to the case by helping with the victim's care in the examining room. After the victim is settled, the nursing colleague states that she will help by notifying the victim's family (without the victim's consent having been obtained), call for an advocate from the rape crisis center, and tell the police officer to come interview the victim while the staff wait for the physician.

6. The nurse in the emergency department is trying to establish rapport with a rape victim when the physician arrives and orders the volunteer advocate out of the room. The nurse has not had a chance to explain to the victim that she has a right to have an advocate present during the examination. The nurse is very busy, low-staffed, and would appreciate the advocate's assistance.

7. The rape examination is completed and the police are preparing to interview the victim. The victim does not have an advocate with her, so the nurse says that she will stay but is told by the police that this is unnecessary. The nurse observes the victim's discomfort in being alone with three male investigating officers. The officers begin to ask the victim questions about sexual acts during the rape (cunnilingus and fellatio), but the victim appears not to comprehend the questions. Her facial expression is one of confusion. The victim starts to cry when the officers ask why she did not resist the assailant.

8. It is 1:30 in the morning and the rape examination has just been completed. The police officer begins to interview the victim about the rape. The interview turns out to be a long-winded account of the officer's life story "on the beat" with "cases like this." The officer spends more time asking the victim about her relationship with the accused assailant, a local officer on the force, than inquiring about the rape.

## REFERENCES

1. *Allison vs United States,* 209 F 2d 445, 1969.
2. Belden, L.: Why women do not report sexual assault, Aegis: magazine on ending violence against women, Winter-Spring: 5, 1980.
3. Burgess, A.W., and Holmstrom, L.L.: Rape: crisis and recovery, Bowie, Md., 1979, Robert J. Brady Co.
4. Burgess, A.W., and Laszlo, A.T.: Courtroom use of hospital records in sexual assault cases, Am. J. Nurs. **1**:64, 1977.
5. Chapman, J., and Chapman, H.: Behaviors and health care: a humanistic helping process, St. Louis, 1975, The C.V. Mosby Co., p. 60.
6. Curtin, L.: The nurse as advocate: a philosophical foundation for nursing, Adv. Nurs. Sci. **1**:1, 1979.

7. Gustafson, J., and Laney, J.: On being responsible, New York, 1968, Harper & Row.
8. Harrisburg Area Rape Crisis Center: Training manual, Harrisburg, Pa., 1977.
9. Holmstrom, L.L., and Burgess, A.W., editors: The victim of rape: institutional reactions, New York, 1978, John Wiley & Sons.
10. Hoover, H.: On the uncommon man. In address upon the American road: 1948-1950, Stanford, Calif., 1951, Stanford University Press.
11. Kahn, A., Kamerman, S., and McGowan, B.: Child advocacy report on a national baseline study, New York, 1972, Columbia University School of Social Work.
12. Lange, A.J., and Jakubowski, P.: Responsible assertive behavior: cognitive/behavioral procedures for trainers, Champaign, Ill., 1976, Research Press.
13. McCormick, C.: The law of evidence, St. Paul, Minn., 1969, West Publishing Co.
14. Nowakowski, L.: A new look at client advocacy. In Hall, J.E., and Weaver, B.R., editors: Distributive nursing practice: a systems approach to community nursing, Philadelphia, 1977, J.B. Lippincott.
15. Pittsburgh Action Against Rape: Training manual, Pittsburgh, Pa., 1979.
16. Slovenko, R.: Psychiatry and the law, Boston, 1973, Little, Brown & Co.
17. Stern-Kiernan, M.: Personal communication, Aug. 1980, Pittsburgh Action Against Rape, Pittsburgh, Pa.
18. Sutherland, S., and Scherl, D.: Crisis intervention with victims of rape, Social Work 17:34, 1972.
19. Terzian, J.A., and Martin, B.G.: Rape cases: is your test handling failsafe? In Halpern, S., editor: Rape—helping the victim: a treatment manual, Oradell, N.J., 1978, Medical Economics Co. Book Division.

## ADDITIONAL REFERENCES

Christy, T.: New privileges . . . new challenges . . . new responsibilities, Nurs. '73 11:8, 1973.
Dock, L., and Stewart, I.: A short history of nursing, New York, 1925, G.P. Putman's Sons.
Gambrell, L., and Wilson, R.: Focusing on the strengths of children, Belmont, Calif., 1973, Lear Siegler/Fearon.
International Association of Chiefs of Police: Interviewing the rape victim, Training Key No. 210. In Center for Women's Policy Studies: Rape and its victims: a report for citizens, health facilities, and criminal justice agencies, Washington, D.C., 1974, Law Enforcement Assistance Administration, U.S. Department of Justice.

## ANNOTATED SUGGESTED READINGS

Bard, M., and Ellison, K.: Crisis intervention and investigation of forcible rape. In Center for Women's Policy Studies: Rape and its victims: a report for citizens, health facilities, and criminal justice agencies, Washington, D.C., 1975, U.S. Department of Justice.
    The authors emphasize the manner in which both law enforcement and

human service functions are combined in an officer's response to a victim of forcible rape. They describe ways in which the police can use psychologic knowledge to benefit the victim, apprehend assailants, and close cases satisfactorily. The authors give a brief background on crisis theory and the aspects of crisis; characteristics of successful intervention; viewing rape as a crime against the person versus a sexual act; implications for the investigator; and guidelines for the investigation process.

Burgess, A.W., and Laszlo, A.T.: The professional as a court witness, J.E.N. **2:**25, 1976.

This article gives examples of the professional as a witness in cases of sexual assault and the linguistic strategies used by the defense counsel and the prosecutor. The authors describe the history of the adversary system; the rules of evidence establishing qualifications of an expert witness; the nature of direct observation; hypothetical situation and opinion rule testimony, including the restrictions of each; and main lines of attack on credibility of the witness.

Center for Women's Policy Studies: Rape and its victims: a report for citizens, health facilities, and criminal justice agencies, Washington, D.C., 1975, U.S. Department of Justice.

The material presented here is based on national surveys and reflects innovation in approaches to cases of rape. It suggests guidelines for improving procedures and reflects the highly interdependent nature of all agencies involved. It also identifies programs, policies, procedures, and techniques that have been particularly effective in response to victim needs and investigative processes.

Drapkin, I., and Viano, E., editors: Victimology: a reader, Lexington Mass., 1974, Lexington Books.

The book presents reading selections that provide the reader with major achievements in the field of victimology. Five major areas of interest are presented: (1) development of victimology as a specialized concern within criminology; (2) relationship between offender and victim; (3) victim and society; (4) justice system issues; and (5) victim compensation and treatment.

Halpern, S.: Police role. In Halpern, S., editor: Rape—helping the victim: a treatment manual, Oradell, N.J., 1978, Medical Economics Book Division.

This brief chapter offers a succinct, point-by-point account of the police role in interviewing victims of rape. It addresses psychologic considerations such as the officer's attitude, case priority, the setting, and rapport. The chapter also discusses ways to interview children and elements to consider in relation to psychosexual development.

Holmstrom, L.L., and Burgess, A.W., editors: The victim of rape: institutional reactions, New York, 1978, John Wiley & Sons.

The authors describe the complicated process set in motion when the rape victim reports an assault and the resulting experiences, which are often more than the victim bargained for. "Entering the Criminal Justice System" describes (1) reporting the rape—who does this and how victims feel about others making the decision for them; (2) the police encounter—the interview, the officer's evaluation of the case and concerns, the victim's reaction to the police encounter; (3) the decision to press charges—the authority of the state, the victim's feelings about pressing charges; and (4) police referral to the hospital.

International Association of Police Chiefs: Interviewing the rape victim. In Halpern, S., editor: Rape—helping the victim: a treatment manual, Oradell, N.J., 1978, Medical Economics Book Division.

The article describes a tactful and compassionate communication that should exist between the police officer and a victim who has suffered a psychologic and physical assault. It describes the legal elements of rape; the psychologic reactions of victims during and after the assault—self-concept, responses to being interviewed; the interview—the officer's attitude, physical comfort, the setting, opening remarks, ventilation period, investigative questioning, and ending the interview.

Keefe, M.L., and O'Reilly, J.T.: Changing perspectives in sex crimes investigations. In walker, M.J., and Brodsky, S.L., editors: Sexual assault: the victim and the rapist, Lexington, Mass., 1976, Lexington Books.

The authors describe the effort by New York City to establish a model for police investigation of rape that is both effective and sensitive to victim needs. The article describes a training program designed to develop constructive attitudes and helping skills; the program included content on crisis intervention techniques and psychologic intervention techniques. The police trainees were given specific guidelines for crisis intervention with rape victims that applied to investigating sexual assaults.

Klemmack, S., and Klemmack, D.: The social definition of rape. In Walker, M.J., and Brodsky, S.L., editors: Sexual assault: the victim and the rapist, Lexington, Mass., 1976, Lexington Books.

The authors note that the normative standards defining rape are inconsistent internally as well as in relation to the legal code. The probability of a situation being defined as rape is noted to be inversely related to the victim-offender/stranger-acquaintance status.

Quinney, R.: Who is victim? In Drapkin, I., and Viano, E., editors: Victimology: a reader, Lexington, Mass., 1974, Lexington Books.

The author's concern in this paper is how victims are characterized. Conceptions of victims and victimization are optional and discretionary. All crimes have a victim; if a victim cannot be imagined, a criminal law is neither created nor enforced. The "victim" is described as a social construction.

Sanders W.B.: Rape and woman's identity, Beverly Hills, Calif., 1980, Sage Publications.

The author analyzes rape by examining the drama of detective work with rape victims. He discusses the socially assigned roles that victims and police officers adopt, the manner of their interaction, the ways in which they present themselves, and the results of such self-portrayals.

Sredl, D.R., Klenke, C., and Rojkind, M.: Offering the rape victim REAL HELP, Nurs. '79 7:38, 1979.

The authors describe one treatment program for victims of rape. The program includes clinical help, protection against pregnancy and venereal disease, psychologic support, and legal backing to victims. Of particular usefulness is a table ("Rape: The Legal Process") that describes the process from gathering evidence to arresting a suspect and going to trial.

## CHAPTER 9

# Counseling victims through the court process

Psychological problems can be mastered by sharpening discriminations, correcting misconceptions, and learning more adaptive attitudes.

Beck, A.: In *Cognitive therapy of depression,* 1979.[1]

## CHAPTER OUTLINE

## LEARNING OBJECTIVES

After completing this chapter the student will be able to:

1 Describe two components of the cognitive behavior therapy model that can be used in counseling rape victims

2 List and define five steps in the cognitive behavioral exercise of a daily record of dysfunctional thoughts

3 Cite five reasons that victims choose not to prosecute their assailants

4 Describe the importance of preparing the victim for the court process, emphasizing information related to attorneys, cross-examination, and coaching

  5  Identify five victim concerns that occur throughout the court process

  6  Describe five nursing intervention strategies that help rape victims handle their concerns throughout the court process

  7  Explain anticipatory guidance as a strategy used in preparing a victim for the verdict

Rape victims have a variety of problems for which they seek longer-term counseling including: (1) prolonged anxiety reactions, (2) continued fears, and (3) depression. Nurses who counsel rape victims use different models and approaches to care. Many of these counseling models are learned in nursing school; others are used within a work setting or health care system.

There are no "cookbook rules" in counseling rape victims; a variety of approaches have been descriptively cited as beneficial to rape victims. This chapter describes several approaches to longer-term counseling of rape victims and one model of care that has not been previously discussed in this text: the cognitive-behavioral model. We have found this model to be effective in helping rape victims achieve desired changes in their lives. Special attention is given to concerns of rape victims who decide to prosecute their assailants. It is hoped that the reader will develop an appreciation of the importance of professional nursing interventions that help rape victims beyond the immediate aftermath of the rape and with "the next ordeal,"[5] testifying at the trial and its outcome.

## LONGER-TERM COUNSELING

Predominant models used by nurses in providing services to rape victims include (1) the medical model, (2) the psychosocial model, and (3) the behavioral model. Table 9-1 presents the basic principles, goals, and nursing interventions of these three models of care. The table is intended to serve as a guideline for differentiating the models; it is not all-inclusive.

### Medical model

The medical model emphasizes the physical treatment and medical care of rape victims. (The medical model of care is discussed in detail in Chapter 6). Within this model, nurses ensure adequate medical care for rape victims and provide services that are goal directed to give rape victims relief from physical pain, trauma, and disease as a result of the rape. In longer-term counseling, nurses implementing a medical model watch for somatic disturbances and gynecologic problems and direct patients toward appropriate medical treatment.

### Psychosocial model

Psychosocial models of care are based on the assumption that early developmental events leave a person vulnerable to stress resulting from the interaction of psychosocial variables. The counseling relationship focuses on helping rape victims meet identified needs and cope with social networks. For example, the nurse develops an empathic

**Table 9-1. Models of care**

| Model | Principles | Goals | Nursing interventions |
|---|---|---|---|
| Medical | Focus is primarily on the illness. | Relief from physical pain<br>Somatic treatment | Attempt to ensure adequate medical care for victims.<br>Watch for somatic disturbances and gynecologic problems. |
| Psychosocial | Life events, stress, and personality structure influence responses.<br>One's social network provides model for appropriate and inappropriate behaviors. | Interactional events can influence emotional responses and life adjustment.<br>Maintain or establish adequate supportive systems(s). | Help a victim reorder her life and gain control: crisis intervention.<br>Facilitate a victim's active involvement with extended family, social network, and relationships with others.<br>Initiate referral/contact with appropriate support systems that provide victim with reassurance of worth. |
| Behavioral | Emphasis on environmental influences and situational changes over time. | Focus on how to arrange circumstances to decrease anxiety. | Decrease painful effects of experience through desensitization process or negative practice.<br>Attempt to increase victims self-confidence and self-esteem. Nurses are a social reinforcer. |

relationship with the rape victim and guides the victim in (1) reordering perceptions of the event and (2) learning adaptive coping mechanisms, such as use of appropriate social support systems (see Chapters 4, 5, 6, and 7).

### Behavioral model

Behavioral care models are based on theories related to the learning process, the sciences of physiology and psychology, and the assumption that all behavior is learned. Behavioral models focus on the behavior of the individual in terms of social adaptiveness and the magnitude and frequency of behaviors. Focus of treatment within the behavioral model becomes observable behavior, and longer-term counseling is aimed at change towards desirable behaviors.

Professional nurses who apply the behavioral model consider "the real problem" as the observable behavior, rather than any deep unconscious conflicts. Behavior is viewed as continuing because it induces positive feedback (for example, relief from anxiety) or avoids negative feedback (for example, family or societal disapproval). Major theorists in the behavioral field include Pavlov, Watson, Skinner, Wolpe, Bandura, and Selgman.

Steps in the behavioral model treatment process include (1) identification of the behavior to be modified, (2) determination of the circumstances around which the behavior occurs, (3) determination of reinforcers that foster persistence of the behavior, (4) selection of treatment conditions or therapies, and (5) scheduling behavior retraining. With rape victims behavioral treatment strategies are applied to behaviors that result from the rape—specifically the phobic symptoms (anxieties and fears). Frequently, post-assault, a victim's anxieties and fears generalize and interfere with personal and social functioning. Since anxiety is believed to be the mediating mechanism of symptomatic difficulties, the therapeutic goal of behavioral treatment is to decrease the victim's fears and anxieties while increasing the victim's self-esteem and self-confidence.

### Cognitive behavior therapy

Cognitive behavior therapy, one model used in counseling rape victims, has been proven to be effective in alleviating symptoms that rape victims report.[6] This therapy incorporates treatment approaches characterizing behavioral care models. The following discussion presents the components of cognitive behavior therapy used in counseling rape victims.

Cognitive behavior therapy is an active, semistructured, time-limited, and goal-directed approach used to treat a variety of problems such as anxiety, phobias, and depression. The therapy model was designed for empirical research and treatment of emotional problems. However, certain features of the model have been adapted to counseling rape victims to help alleviate their distress. The counseling is based on the theoretic rationale that a person's "affect and behavior are largely determined by the way in which he structures the world."[1] That is, *the way a person feels and behaves is determined by the way he or she thinks*.

Two components of cognitive behavior therapy are (1) cognitive restructuring strategies and (2) behavioral techniques. Through a mutual collaborative relationship with the victim the nurse explains "we are partners in a project."[7] The ultimate goal of cognitive restructuring strategies and behavioral techniques is for the victim to "view herself as competent, powerful and able to direct her life."[7,8]

**Table 9-2. Types of error in thinking**

| Cognitive error | Assumption | Example |
|---|---|---|
| Overgeneralization | If something is true in one case, it is true in all similar cases. | "My boyfriend left me; I can't keep a good relationship with anyone!" |
| Arbitrary inferences | Conclusions are drawn without supporting evidence. | "I feel someone is trying to break into my apartment." |
| Selective abstraction | The only events that matter are failures, deprivation, etc. | "I got up late, missed my bus, and probably failed my exams." |
| Excessive responsibility | I am responsible for all bad things, failures, etc. | "I ruined my children's lives by not being a good mother." |
| Catastrophizing | Always think of the worst. | "My life is miserable. I'm hopeless! I'll never recover." |
| Dichotomous thinking | Everything is either one extreme or the other (good or bad). | "I can't do anything right; I'm a total failure!" |

Adapted from Beck, A., Rush, A., Shaw, B., and Emery, G.: Cognitive therapy of depression, New York, 1979, The Guilford Press, p. 261.

### Cognitive restructuring techniques

Cognitive restructuring is defined as a process by which a person becomes aware of thought patterns that lead to ineffectual behaviors and then changes these patterns to ones that lead to effectual behaviors.[14] By using cognitive restructuring techniques, nurses teach rape victims to master problem situations in which they feel helpless or vulnerable. The therapeutic techniques challenge a victim's negative life assumptions or life-style. The major focus of intervention in this model is disputing faulty attitudes, assumptions, and processing of information.[1]

Table 9-2 outlines six types of errors in thinking that, if present, are brought to a rape victim's attention during counseling. As outlined in the table, thinking errors are derived from some type of assumption. Examples of statements made by victims are included in the table to help illustrate the cognitive errors. In cognitive restructuring, rape victims are encouraged to challenge their basic assumptions actively. Once assumptions are challenged, victims can then act against the assumptions.

### Behavioral techniques

The second component of cognitive behavior therapy is the use of behavioral techniques to elicit thought processes associated with specific behaviors and to change certain behavior patterns. One of the best-known behavioral intervention strategies is *desensitization.* Systematic desensitization is a procedure specifically designed to relieve symptoms of anxiety and behavior associated with anxiety. Two methods of systematic desensitization are used in treatment: (1) in vivo desensitization and (2) systematic desensitization. *In vivo desensitization* is a process of gradually facing in real life a stimulus that is feared. For example, with rape victims, in vivo desensitization takes the form of the victim approaching the site where she was raped or returning to the vicinity of the rape. The process of in vivo desensitization is designed to give victims a sense of mastery over themselves and their lives. It instills a sense of competence and self-confidence so that the rape no longer holds power over them by dictating their behavior—where they will go or what they will avoid. Another form of desensitization, *systematic desensitization,* consists of a gradual exposure to stimuli that are feared. The specific stimulus varies according to the victim. However, it can encompass behaviors such as going out on a date or to a party, specific sexual activities, and seeing the rapist again. The effectiveness of systematic desensitization as a treatment intervention to the responses of rape victims post-rape is currently being investigated.[6]

Other behavioral strategies include (1) weekly activity schedules, (2) mastery and pleasure schedules, (3) graded task assignments, and (4) a daily record of dysfunctional thoughts. The *weekly activity schedule* is a diary in which a victim keeps a record of her hourly activities during the week. The diary allows the nurse to see at a glance where the victim is having difficulty or functioning well. On the *mastery and pleasure schedule,* the victim rates on a scale from 0 to 5 the degree of mastery (M) and pleasure (P) associated with each activity. With this schedule the nurse helps the victim see where repeated thoughts (such as "I don't get *anything* done") are not accurate and that certain activities bring pleasure or slight relief from unpleasant feelings. *Graded task assignments* consist of the nurse helping the victim achieve a goal by setting and achieving smaller goals in a graduated, sequential order so that the overall goal is ultimately reached. By shaping behavior over a period of time, the victim is able to achieve goals that otherwise seem impossible for her. When the victim can see that she is able to master and derive pleasure from graduated tasks, she is less inclined to entertain negative thoughts such as "I'll never get over this rape." The preceding behavioral strategies are discussed in more detail by Beck[1] for nurses interested in adapting these strategies to counseling rape victims. The fourth strategy, the *daily record of dysfunctional thoughts* is a cognitive technique that helps rape victims perceive the relationship between negative conditions, unpleasant affects/emotions, and non-productive behaviors as well as develop a realistic perception of the rape event and its sequel. The nurse gives the victim a sample of the daily record of dysfunctional thoughts form and teaches her how to use it and complete the exercise. Once the form is completed (see, for example, Table 9-3), the nurse retains copies of those the victim has completed to evaluate underlying false assumptions and progress in treatment.

Doing a daily record involves five steps: (1) situation, (2) emotion, (3) automatic thoughts, (4) rational response, and (5) outcome. The following clinical example demonstrates how the daily record is used to help identify target behavioral symptoms and cognitions that are nonproductive for the rape victim.

### CLINICAL EXAMPLE

Marcy is a 20-year-old black female who was raped by a friend of her brother. She is determined to press charges against the man but is seeking counseling because of panic attacks that occur each time she leaves her home. After receiving some instruction from the nurse, Marcy is asked to complete the daily record for the next situation that precedes an unpleasant emotion.

The next morning Marcy is determined to improve her situation. She remains relatively calm as she leaves her home, but she soon becomes fearful at the bus stop. She has difficulty breathing and suddenly feels vulnerable and helpless. Marcy returns home and calls the nurse who reassures Marcy that she is safe. The nurse then encourages Marcy to complete the daily record and bring it to their session that afternoon.

Table 9-3 shows the completed form that Marcy and the nurse used in their counseling session. As illustrated in the table, the victim records a *situation* that precedes an unpleasant emotion. In this example the victim is waiting for the bus and thinks about seeing her assailant in the courtroom. As the victim envisions the courtroom scene, she experiences the *emotions* of fear, vulnerability, and helplessness. She is asked to rate her emotions using a numerical scale of 0 (intensity—a trace) to 100 (the most intense possible). She then reports her *automatic flow of thoughts:* that the rapist will divulge her past sexual history during the court testimony and ruin her reputation. The victim is then asked to rate her belief in the automatic thoughts on a percentage scale of 0% (not at all) to 100% (completely). During the counseling session the nurse helps the victim to: (1) determine a *rational response* to the automatic thoughts previously listed and (2) rate her belief in the rational response using a numerical scale of 1 (a trace) to 100 (the most intense possible). In this example the victim is informed that the jury will determine the verdict based on facts of the case and not on her past sexual history, which is not admissible evidence in the trial. The *outcome* section of the daily record is then completed by asking the victim to now (1) re-rate belief in the automatic thoughts on a percentage scale of 0% (not at all) to 100% (completely) and then (2) specify and re-rate subsequent emotions on a numerical scale of 0 (a trace) to 100 (the most intense possible). As indicated in this example, the victim feels less fearful and helpless. Confidence in her lawyer also allows Marcy to feel less vulnerable.

Table 9-3. Daily record of dysfunctional thoughts

| Date | SITUATION<br>Describe:<br>1. Actual event leading to unpleasant emotion, or<br>2. Stream of thoughts, daydream, or recollection, leading to unpleasant emotion. | EMOTION(S)<br>1. Specify sad/anxious/angry. etc.<br>2. Rate degree of emotion, 1-100. | AUTOMATIC THOUGHT(S)<br>1. Write automatic thought(s) that preceded emotion(s).<br>2. Rate belief in automatic thought(s), 0-100%. | RATIONAL RESPONSE<br>1. Write rational response to automatic thought(s).<br>2. Rate belief in rational response, 0-100%. | OUTCOME<br>1. Re-rate belief in automatic thought(s), 0-100%.<br>2. Specify and rate subsequent emotions, 0-100. |
|------|------|------|------|------|------|
| 3/1/82 | Waiting for the bus and thinking about seeing the rapist in the courtroom. | 1. Fear<br>2. 80<br>1. Helpless<br>2. 80<br>1. Vulnerable<br>2. 60 | 1. (The rapist) will divulge my past sexual history.<br>2. 80%<br>1. (The rapist) will ruin my reputation.<br>2. 80%<br>1. I have no one to protect me.<br>2. 80% | 1. The jury will determine the verdict based on the facts of the case.<br>2. 60%<br>1. My past sexual history is not admissable in the trial as evidence.<br>2. 80%<br>1. My lawyer will defend me.<br>2. 60% | *Automatic Thoughts*<br>1. 10%<br>2. 25%<br>3. 10%<br>*Emotions*<br>Fear = 30<br>Helpless = 30<br>Vulnerable = 20 |

EXPLANATION: When you experience an unpleasant emotion, note the situation that seemed to stimulate the emotion. (If the emotion occurred while you were thinking, daydreaming, etc., please note this.) Then note the automatic thought associated with the emotion. Record the degree to which you believe this thought: 0% = not at all; 100% = completely. In rating degree of emotion: 1 = a trace; 100 = the most intense possible.

Table format reprinted with permission of Beck, A., Rush, A., Shaw, B., and Emery, G.: Cognitive therapy of depression, New York, 1979, The Guilford Press, p. 403. Copyright © 1978 by Aaron T. Beck, M.D.

The next section explores the reasons victims decide to press or not to press charges against their assailants. The professional nurse who counsels rape victims does not try to influence the victim's decision. Rather the nurse supports whatever decision is made by the victim about prosecuting the assailant and attempts to help the victim feel comfortable with her decision.

## REASONS VICTIMS CHOOSE NOT TO PROSECUTE

Because of the social climate surrounding the crime, it is understandable that many women do not report rape. Rape myths generally held in our society tend to degrade the victim and excuse the assailant. Nonreporting is also affected by the depersonalized and humiliating care some victims receive in medical, police, and legal systems. Reasons cited by Holmstrom and Burgess[12] for victims pressing or not pressing charges include the following:

| Reasons for pressing charges | Reasons for not pressing charges |
|---|---|
| 1. To protect other women from a similar attack | 1. To avoid the ordeal of court |
| 2. Outrage at the assailant's behavior | 2. Afraid the assailant will take revenge |
| 3. To punish the assailant and have justice done | 3. To avoid sending a person to jail |
| 4. Fear for one's own safety if charges are not pressed | 4. What is the use—he'll get away with it anyway |
| 5. Assailant is sick | 5. Feeling sorry for the assailant |
| 6. Other miscellaneous reasons | 6. Just want to forget the whole thing |
| | 7. Scared of identifying the wrong person |
| | 8. Would look bad on my record |
| | 9. Other miscellaneous reasons |

There are many reasons rape victims decide not to prosecute an assailant. Some reasons are personal—for example, "I just want to forget it and get on with my life" or "I know my family, and I don't want to create any more hardships." Other victims choose not to prosecute assailants because of an awareness of the way victims are blamed for the crime, the extent to which the rapist can rape with impunity (according to current conviction rates), and the ordeal of the court process. Medea and Thompson[16] advise that when a woman is deciding whether or not to prosecute her assailant she needs to consider how women are currently treated in the criminal justice system. Rather than suffer further abuse, many rape victims choose not to prosecute their assailants.

## PREPARING FOR COURT

As stated in the last section, women who press charges have highly individualized reasons for doing so. However, the legal process is similar for all victims. Three areas are selected for special emphasis here: (1) the attorneys, (2) cross-examination, and (3) coaching.

### The attorneys

Preparing the victim for court testimony is usually done by the district attorney's office. However, in expanded roles the nurse may see the victim for counseling during and/or after the court proceedings. Lawyers are professionals trained in the use of language to win a point; this is part of their education and job. Victims and witnesses will encounter linguistic techniques at any time during the criminal justice proceedings, not just in the courtroom. During the trial the predominant mode of interviewing is the question-and-answer method.

The attorneys for victims and offenders use polarized terminology in discussing the same aspect of an assault to imply to the jury a point of view or attitude that supports their respective positions. The prosecuting attorney for the victim, most often called a district attorney (DA), *uses language that suggests violence or portrays an image of force and aggression:* "He held you down with the weight of his body?" or "He restrained you by twisting your arm in back of you and making you lie on it?" The DA *describes physical actions as brutal and threatening:* "He made you douche at gunpoint?" or "He kept a knife at your throat and made you crawl around the apartment floor?"[12]

The prosecuting attorney for the victim will primarily limit questions to facts about the rape in order to prove that the essential elements of the crime exist in order to meet the criteria for a legal conviction. The DA may also inquire about the nature of any prior relationship between the victim and the offender. If possible, the DA *implies emotional distance* in the relationship with the offender: "You had not met this man before the night in question?" or "You had refused to date him?" When suggestions about romance or irrelevant evidence arise, the DA objects to such questions: "I object to the suggestion that he escorted you to the office party!"[10]

In contrast, the defense attorney for the accused offender *uses terms to convey sexuality:* "You were hitchhiking in a halter top?" or "You were sunbathing on the front lawn in your bikini?" He *portrays an image of romance and sexiness:* "You were alone on the porch swing?" Physical acts are described as romantic: "His strength was exciting!" or "It was a lovely evening when he drove you through the park." The defense attorney *implies consent to intercourse* through friendship and emotional closeness with the offender: "When you're out on a date, don't you usually let a man put his arm around you?" or "It's hard to refuse a man you've invited up to your apartment, isn't it?" Finally, the defense attorney *plays upon traditional sex-role stereotypes* that the general populace holds: "If you are a respectable woman, what were you doing in a bar alone?" or "It's against the law for teenagers to be drinking beer, and you did that without your parents' knowledge!"[10]

### Cross-examination

Preparing the victim for court includes providing information about the types of questions to be expected during the trial. During the court process the defendant does not have to take the stand to testify. However, the victim must do so, and she is subjected to a cross-examination style *full of trickery* rather than aimed at eliciting the facts. Three ways questions are frequently phrased include (a) an accusatory form, (b) declarative sentences, and (c) forced-choice questions.

The *accusatory form* of questioning is used to portray an image of the victim as responsible for the assault. The victim is then asked to agree with it: "Isn't it true you dated the defendant on numerous occasions?" or "Isn't it a fact that you pulled your pants down?" or "Oh, so now you're telling me your mom came in on you and that's why you decided to cry rape!" Even though accusatory questions may be stricken from the record by the DA's objections, the impression the accusatory form of questioning leaves in the minds of the jurors cannot be erased.[4,11,12]

*Declarative sentences* can be used by the defense attorney to sneak a suggestive comment or image "in the back door" that would otherwise be excluded by law in the cross-examination process. This strategy allows the defense attorney to portray an image of the victim and the assault that ultimately discredits her testimony and character: "You've been committed for therapy in the past, haven't you!" or "You're actually confused about what happened that night!" Again, the suggestive ideas to discredit the victim have been planted in the minds of the jurors even though they can be stricken from the written account of the trial.[4,11,12]

*Forced-choice questions* require the victim or witness to answer a question that follows a statement with only a "yes" or "no" reply. A forced-choice question presents the facts out of context, does not reflect the interaction between the victim and the offender in relation to the assault, and is generally frustrating to the person testifying. After the victim answers "yes," the defense attorney usually interrupts and asks the next question, thereby keeping mitigating evidence from being considered by the jury: "Isn't it true that you didn't resist his advances in any way whatsoever?" or "Isn't it true you had a chance to jump out of the car at the stoplight, and you didn't?" or "He forced you to stop for something to eat, and you failed to say anything to the waitress?" A victim has the right to explain her answers and can ask the judge to let her do so fully.[4,11,12]

### Coaching

Webster defines *coaching* as "to train intensively by instruction, demonstration, and practice" whereas *to prepare* is defined as "to make ready beforehand for some purpose, use or activity . . . to work out the details . . . to plan in advance." The victim gets caught in the middle of legal jargon, intimidation, and a semantic argument. Defense attorneys often make the victim feel that to seek counseling during the trial process is to do something "evil" or illegal when, in reality, the victim is simply doing what most healthy persons do in anticipation of stressful events.

Victims may be cross-examined about whether they were *coached* for the trial, and therefore it is helpful to prepare victims to consider how they might respond to intimidating or trick questions about being coached. One way victims can be prepared for the trial is by role-playing the cross-examination adversary process around questions on being coached.

*Role-playing* is defined in this text as the acting out of real or imagined situations by two or more persons. Through role-playing the nurse can take the defense attorney's position in cross-examining the victim or reverse roles and play the role of the victim to offer ideas on how the victim could answer questions. Role-playing provides a safe setting in which to try out new or unexpected behaviors and new ideas, to test principles, and an opportunity to use the nurse as a sounding board in the learning process. The "pretend" quality of the enactment makes the experience safe because the person can choose to admit to, deny, or minimize any of its elements. Through this protective strategy the victim gains confidence in herself and can develop coping skills that will be useful during a cross-examination process (as well as in later life situations of a comparable nature). The victim is given a vicarious opportunity to use the nurse as a role model for responding to threatening questions.[13] Role-playing as an intervention approach for preparing victims for the rape trial has only begun to be discussed in the literature, perhaps because of the defense attorney's intimation that such counseling approaches comprise illegal "coaching." The following discussion presents some questions victims should consider in preparing to answer inquiries about whether or not they were coached for the trial.

When introducing the victim to a role-play session on questions about being coached, it is helpful for the nurse to briefly review the victim's general pattern of response in coping and, in particular, the victim's coping style in relation to the trial. An introduction about the nature of role-playing sets the climate for the victim to view the role-play as an exercise in cognitive restructuring and also encourages the victim to view the cross-examination process as a drama or debate rather than a personal attack. For example, the nurse might say:

> I've been reviewing the notes from a number of our sessions in getting ready for today. You seem to have a pattern of responding to questions that suggests you feel vulnerable or helpless. You tend to respond, for example, with "Oh, my God. How terrible the questions are (or will be)," rather than thinking, "This is the 'great debate!' How can I go about fielding the questions?" Today I want to work on some exercises with you to help you feel more confident in fielding questions. What we are going to do is . . . (and the nurse explains the role-play method to the victim).

The following discussion presents questions often asked of victims about whether they have been coached to determine if they were illegally prepared for the trial or are "telling the truth." The discussion contains ideas on ways victims can answer cross-examination questions that nurses can use in role-plays to prepare rape victims for the trial.[4,11]

*Did anyone coach you?* Victims answer this question in a variety of ways. Some victims reply with a straight "no." Others answer with a question, "What do you mean, *coach* me?" and look puzzled. It is the victim's attitude as much as the literal response that the jury will weigh in deciding if the victim was told a "false" story to give as testimony.

*Did anyone talk to you about coming to court?* The question is another version of the first question. Again, it is helpful if the victim questions the defense attorney about what he means by that question because its intent is not clear. The defense attorney might become annoyed when unable to catch the victim off guard and shout, "Just answer the question 'yes' or 'no'." Nurses can inform the victim that it is perfectly suitable to indicate a second time, "I don't understand the question." The victim might even suggest to the defense attorney something benign related to a misunderstanding of the questions, for example: "Do you mean was I told to be here today?" or "Do you mean did the district attorney's office notify me to be present to give testimony?" One victim responded to the role-play on being coached about coming to court as follows:

> *Victim:* That question would really screw me up . . . (pause) I was told about going down to the courthouse (sounding puzzled).
> *Nurse:* He might ask you, "What were you told?"
> *Victim:* Just the procedure to expect . . . . Is the defendant coached? I would think he is told word for word what to say! Why does it matter if I'm helped out?

*What were you told?* It is always best to ask the victim what does *she* remember asking about the trial. From a brief recall of what it is the victim wanted to know, she can easily formulate her own reply to the question. Some victims reply, "To tell the truth" or "Not to falsify anything" or answers of a more absurd and humorous nature such as "That the judge would sit up high on a bench and the jury would be in rows off to the side." Victims also respond by describing what they were told about how the courtroom and waiting areas would appear. At times the defense attorney can look ridiculous by persisting with a "what were you told" question or even by the victim's response to the question in a manner that implies its absurdity. To continue absurd questioning damages the image the defense attorney is trying to convey to the jurors and the purpose he hopes to achieve by questioning the victim (discrediting the admissibility of her testimony in court).

*Were you told what to wear?* Inquiry about attire is usually a fairly straightforward question to answer. For example, victims reply with "No" or "No, I wear what I want to wear." Some victims report wishing someone would tell them what to wear to make the proper impressions. Victims also express anger that it is necessary to conform to a set of social norms for an effect on the minds of jurors rather than being judged on the facts of the case or their self-evaluation of intrinsic worth. One victim discussed attire as follows:

| CLINICAL EXAMPLE | Comment |
|---|---|
| *Victim:* I wish someone would tell me what to wear. I want to wear a dress but my good dress has a slit in it. I don't want to look tempestuous. | Awareness of social norms. |
| *Mother:* You mean like a sexpot? You've got nice clothes, none of them are sexy looking. | |
| *Victim:* (with humor) Gee, Mom, thanks a lot! I just want to look like an average 17-year-old girl, not like I'm out looking for sex. | Humor: sign of healthy family system. |
| *Nurse:* So what do you have to wear to look that way? | Activating the victim's cognitive skills. |
| *Victim:* Blue jeans and a T-shirt, a nice dress, or a pair of pants with a blouse. | |
| *Nurse:* Do you have that clothing? | |
| *Victim:* Yes. | |
| *Mother:* Her closet is bulging so much she has trouble deciding what to wear, that's her trouble! | Humor: sign of healthy family system. |

|  | | **Comment** |
| --- | --- | --- |
| *Victim:* | (with humor) I've so many choices it's no fun. | Joining with mother in use of humor. |
| *Nurse:* | So you *can* come up with something. | |
| *Victim:* | Yeah. The first time I was afraid to wear a dress. I didn't want to show my legs, but then I figure we all got 'em! | Choice of attire reflects victim's sensitivity to social misperceptions of rape as a sexually motivated act. |

*Did you talk with the rape crisis counselor in front of the district attorney?* The question implies that the counselor and the district attorney are in a conspiracy to falsify the victim's testimony in some manner. The question suggests that, if there was a joint conference to prepare the victim for court, the victim's testimony has been tampered with and that the victim is therefore being less than honest or reliable. Some victims answer the question with a question; for example, "Oh, do you mean did she talk with me at the pretrial hearing?" On occasion techniques discussed earlier such as pausing, looking puzzled, and hesitating are also effective.

When victims pause to think about the questions they are asked, it soon becomes obvious that they are not falsifying information and that telling the truth is the simplest approach in handling trick questions. It is, rather, the *unexpected* question that gets the victim off guard. The net effect of an unexpected question is similar to the case of an adolescent who expects to be awkward, therefore acts awkward, which in turn makes him or her feel awkward—and a vicious cycle is established. Similarly, victims who anticipate being tricked or tripped up feel uneasy or frightened and answer questions awkwardly, thereby making a poor impression on the jury. When the nurse role-plays the questions to be asked under cross-examination before the trial, the exercise helps prevent the victim from taking the role she believes others expect of her or trick her into—that is, acting in a manner that suggests *she* is at fault for the rape.

The next section looks at specific victim concerns raised in counseling sessions. Nurse counselors explore anxieties, fears, and insecurities experienced by rape victims during the court process. Nurses establish trust with rape victims since people in distress are inclined to trust professionals, and nurses in particular, as caring persons.

## VICTIM CONCERNS

Frequently victims find prosecuting the assailant to be a threatening situation. In most trials the defendant attempts to be acquitted. However, rape trials differ from other trials in that the victim is commonly attributed fault for the crime by the jurors, believed to have invited assault, and in essence is accused of having brought an unfair claim against the assailant.[12] The victim feels that she is on trial rather than the defendant. It is not surprising, therefore, that many rape victims experience high levels of anxiety and fear when prosecuting assailants.[17]

*Anxiety* occurs when individuals find some value they hold essential to their personality to be threatened or when they anticipate an impending ill of some unidentifiable nature.[15] The emotion of anxiety is usually accompanied by physiologic changes. Because the source of the anxiety is not identifiable, the victim finds it difficult to find a recourse of action that will bring relief. Thus the anxious victim feels helpless, isolated, powerless, and insecure—that is, the feelings experienced during the rape persist. *Fear,* on the other hand, has an identifiable stimulus and is experienced as a strong emotion caused by anticipation or awareness of danger. The danger is external to the person, and, because the danger can be identified, the victim is able to take action to relieve the discomfort.[10] For example, a victim may feel *anxious* while anticipating the trial as an impending disaster (unidentifiable danger) in the form of "not knowing what to expect"; at the same time the victim might be *fearful* of seeing the rapist on the street or in the courtroom (identifiable danger). Rape victims report that anxiety and fear often occur together. When these emotions persist at high levels for long periods of time, the victim's crisis period is prolonged, and she is handicapped in resolving the rape crisis. In such a case the victim finds the rape trial an additional stressor to her current crisis state. (See Chapter 7 for a discussion of crisis theory.) Therefore it is important that nurses intervene to reduce anxiety and fear when counseling victims through the court process. The following discussion describes five concerns, anxieties, and fears that victims attempt to work through in counseling sessions: (1) information, (2) credibility, (3) delays, (4) task performance disruption, and (5) harassment. Use of the cognitive behavioral technique of a daily record of dysfunctional thoughts is demonstrated for several victim concerns.

### Information

One way a person gains self-control and environmental control is by finding out as much as possible about what to expect from an unfamiliar situation. Learning what to expect is particularly important if the person has never before experienced that situation; for example, a victim who is prosecuting a rapist. It is a basic principle of crisis intervention and advocacy that clients be given information for planning and making decisions (see Chapters 7 and 8). Being informed of what to expect is a form of anticipatory guidance. When the victim feels secure in knowing what to expect, her level of anxiety decreases, she is able to get on with the rest of her life, and the trial becomes only one of several current life events. Questions victims commonly ask nurse advocates include the following:

1. What happens next? What are the steps I have to go through?
2. How long before the trial begins?
3. What will he (the assailant) be charged with?
4. Why are certain charges dropped?
5. Can I go out of town (e.g., on vacation), or do I have to stay available?
6. What are the chances for a guilty verdict?
7. How long does the trial last?
8. How much do I have to tell on the stand? (Will my family hear it all?)
9. What will my witnesses be asked?
10. Is my past sexual (or psychiatric) history admissible in court?
11. Why do I keep talking to different detectives?
12. Will you (the advocate) be with me on the day of the trial? (This is a very important question to the victim.)

Victims who are unfamiliar with the judicial system do not understand why they are shuffled between so many different people. The following clinical example demonstrates how the nurse can help the victim by explaining a judicial system process.

| CLINICAL EXAMPLE | Comment |
|---|---|
| *Victim:* Why do I have to keep talking to different police and district attorneys? At the pretrial hearing there was one set, now there's another set. | Counseling request for information. |
| *Nurse:* It's like an assembly line. The set of officers who take the initial report may not be the experts qualified to do the investigation. Then one detective determines if there is sufficient evidence to take the case to trial. Next, an expert attorney in rape trials is assigned to the case, and so forth. | Reflective response. Giving information to help the victim gain control over events. |
| *Victim:* It's like me and (the rapist) just help, and it's the two attorneys who are engaged in battle, not us. | Sense of depersonalization and loss of control. Magnification. |
| *Nurse:* It's unpleasant to be shuffled around, not to be able to fight your own battle . . . to be a spectator some of the time. | Creative listening to the feelings behind the question. |
| *Victim:* Yeah, I don't like it. | Emotional response. |

In the preceding example the nurse explained the investigatory procedures and pretrial information so that the victim could understand what events were occurring. At the same time the nurse reflected the victim's concern over loss of control and helped the victim to continue discussing her feelings.

Giving information about what to expect at the trial includes questions about *how the offender will participate*. Because the victim is truly preparing "to do battle," she wants to know what the "other side" will do. The following example demonstrates how one nurse responded to a question frequently asked by rape victims.

| CLINICAL EXAMPLE | Comment |
|---|---|
| *Victim:* What will they ask the rapist? | Seeking information. |
| *Nurse:* He might not testify. It's not always to his advantage to testify. He'll work out that strategy with his attorney. If he does testify, he will probably tell the same story you do but give a different version of it. For example: | Nurse provides information relating to the polarized testimony of the respective positions. |

| *You will say:* | *He will say:* | |
|---|---|---|
| 1. He forced me. | 1. She agreed to go drinking and have sex. | Consent issue. |
| 2. I was worried about getting home. | 2. She cried rape to prevent parental disapproval. | False accusation. |

In the preceding clinical example the nurse provided the victim with information relating to the court testimony of the assailant. Victims who have not been prepared to hear polarized testimony often experience high levels of anxiety and anger in response to the offender's implications of sexuality and romance. In contrast, victims who are adequately prepared can think rationally: "This is what the offender's lawyer has instructed the offender to say so that he (the offender) will be acquitted."

Another point of information that victims seek an answer to is: "How could anyone defend a rapist?" Often the victim's question masks underlying feelings of outrage ("How *could* the attorney defend him!"). It is difficult for the victim to understand how an attorney can defend a client who admits privately (to the attorney) that he raped the prosecuting victim. This situation stimulates a state of cognitive dissonance for the victim—that is, it does not make sense to the victim to defend a guilty man. The following example demonstrates how a victim tries to resolve the tension experienced from cognitive dissonance by searching for a logical explanation and by ventilating feelings of frustration.

CLINICAL EXAMPLE | Comment
--- | ---
*Victim:* Will the rapist have to tell his lawyer he raped me? | Seeking information.
*Nurse:* His attorney will ask him to describe what happened, just as the DA asked you to do. But you must remember, often men who rape believe that they seduced you or that your description of their behavior is out of proportion. Sometimes the man admits to raping the victim. | Giving information (see Chapter 3).
*Victim:* How can the attorney defend a man who is guilty? | Questioning an illogical action.
*Nurse:* That's a difficult question. It seems illogical to you, doesn't it? | Reflective technique.
*Victim:* Yes. Isn't it harder to prove his innocence if his attorney knows he is guilty? | Trying to make logic out of cognitive dissonance.
*Nurse:* Well, it's his job to defend his client as "not guilty beyond a reasonable doubt." | Giving information.
*Victim:* *He* should have to prove he's innocent beyond a reasonable doubt instead of *me* having to prove I'm not guilty! | When the system's logic fails, the victim's feelings of anger and frustration surface along with a firm conviction in her own belief system.
*Nurse:* It would be nice to feel assured that you could win the case if his (the rapist's) attorney felt unethical about defending him. | Creative listening enhancing response.
*Victim:* Yeah, I just wish I knew that I could win my case. | Fantasizing. Fearful of losing case.

As demonstrated in this clinical example, the nurse helped the victim talk about feelings of anger and frustration related to cognitive dissonance. By offering a logical explanation for the lawyer's behavior, the nurse tried to alleviate the victim's distress. At the same time the nurse allowed for open expression of feelings.

### Credibility

Rape victims want to appear credible in court; that is, they want to offer reasonable grounds for being believed. But most victims realize that there will be some effort to make them appear unreliable. One way of discrediting the victim's credibility is through the style in which the defense attorney cross-examines the victim about her testimony. It is not uncommon for the victim to feel trapped; she tries to answer questions honestly but anticipates that tricks will be played upon her so she will lose the case. The defense attorney may play upon social norms ("You weren't wearing a bra?") or confuse the victim by the way questions are constructed. (See preceding discussion of "Preparing for Court" in this chapter.)

Another way of attacking the victim's credibility is through assessment of her "character" by police, attorneys, significant others, and the victim herself at different points in the prosecution process. According to Webster, *character* is defined as "the attributes or features that make up and distinguish the individual." If others perceive the victim as having an "undesirable character" (or if she perceives herself this way), often the victim will drop the charges or be told by the attorneys that her case is not strong enough to take to court. For example, an "undesirable character" in rape victim cases may be associated with the use of alcohol or drugs, prostitution, lesbianism, or sexually active behavior by adolescents or young adults.[12]

There are times when victims have a sufficiently strong case to prosecute the assailant, but because they have engaged in "undesirable" behavior the defense attorney will raise doubts about their credibility. According to social norms, some behaviors are less desirable than others—for example, prostitution or drug abuse is generally judged as less socially acceptable than the use of alcohol at the time of the assault. Research indicates that even the use of alcohol frequently results in victims encountering "negative responses from associates and medical and legal systems that exist to serve them, which may severely impede the resolution of the rape trauma."[18] In the following example a victim wants to discuss behavior labeled as deviant or undesirable, which might be used to cast doubt on her credibility or defame her character.

CLINICAL EXAMPLE

| | | Comment |
|---|---|---|
| *Victim:* | What bugs me is I told the detective I had some beers, two beers. His (the rapist's) attorney said I had three beers. I recall the first and second beer but not the third beer. | Feeling powerless; externalized focus of control; high level of anxiety and fear. |
| *Nurse:* | Then stick with what you know. You have to report what you remember, he (the rapist) will report what he remembers, and the jury will make their own judgment. The jury will listen to more than facts; they will appraise your attitude as well. | Preparation for cross-examination. |

CLINICAL EXAMPLE                                   **Comment**

*Victim:* How can they tell how I feel?          Seeks clarification and
                                                 reassurance.

*Nurse:* For example, do you sound as if you     Nurse provides specif-
account are certain? Do you change your          ic examples based on
account under questioning? Do you                knowledge of the
seem to know what you are talking                court process.
about?

Now, the defense attorney might try              Anticipatory guidance
to use the issue of three beers to               related to the issue of
make it appear that you were drunk               credibility.
and therefore unaware, unreliable,
and confused.

*Victim:* I could have had a *six-pack* and not  Feeling solid, confi-
gotten drunk that night!                         dent of own position;
                                                 internalized locus of
                                                 control.

*Nurse:* You also need to be ready for some      Preparation for cross-
of the types of questions the attor-             examination continues.
ney will ask you, for the way in
which the questions will be asked.

*Victim:* Like what?

*Nurse:* How would you answer if the attor-      Role-playing to pre-
ney asked you a "yes" or "no" ques-              pare victim for tactics
tion such as, "Don't you know it's               of defense attorney.
against the law to drink?"

*Victim:* I was too scared of (the rapist) to    Prior counseling ses-
refuse the beer, even though I know              sions of role-playing
I'm under the legal age and it's                 in preparation for trial
against the law.                                 evaluated as helpful to
                                                 victim.

*Nurse:* Good. You're catching on. The jury      Positive reinforce-
will judge the attorney for his                  ment. Uses analogy to
behavior just as much as they will               demonstrate ideas;
evaluate your behavior and attitude.             tries to make situation
It's like the theater—it's a stage and           more realistic for vic-
a drama, so play it up to the jury               tim to understand.
who are the audience that judge the
play.

*Victim:* It's true. I *was* scared the minute   Feeling more confi-
after he pulled out of the bar!                  dent of own position.

*Nurse:* Well, then you have nothing to fear.    Challenging assump-
You are not lying even if the defense            tion that "Jury will be-
attorney makes it seem that you are.             lieve defense attorney,
Now, why does it matter if the                   not me"; challenging
attorney makes you seem like a                   need for public ap-
liar?                                            proval. Emotional de-
                                                 tachment frees client
                                                 to evaluate fears about
                                                 credibility.

Table 9-4. Daily record of dysfunctional thoughts

| Date | SITUATION  Describe: 1. Actual event leading to unpleasant emotion, or 2. Stream of thoughts, daydream, or recollection, leading to unpleasant emotion. | EMOTION(S) 1. Specify sad/ anxious/angry, etc. 2. Rate degree of emotion, 1-100. | AUTOMATIC THOUGHT(S) 1. Write automatic thought(s) that preceded emotion(s). 2. Rate belief in automatic thought(s), 0-100%. | RATIONAL RESPONSE 1. Write rational response to automatic thought(s). 2. Rate belief in rational response, 0-100%. | OUTCOME 1. Re-rate belief in automatic thought(s), 0-100%. 2. Specify and rate subsequent emotions, 0-100. |
|---|---|---|---|---|---|
| 3/1/82 | The defense attorney accused me of having 3 vs 2 beers. | 1. Frightened 2. 90 | 1. It looks like I'm lying or don't know what is going on. It's against the law, and I'll get charged for an offense. 2. 80% | 1. All I can do is report what I remember. I could've had 6 beers and still been sober that night! I won't get charged for drinking. They just want to make my judgment look poor. At most I'd be put under my parents' surveillance. 2. 80% | *Automatic thoughts* 20% *Emotions* Frightened = 10 |

EXPLANATION: When you experience an unpleasant emotion, note the situation that seemed to stimulate the emotion. (If the emotion occurred while you were thinking, daydreaming, etc., please note this.) Then note the automatic thought associated with the emotion. Record the degree to which you believe this thought: 0% = not at all; 100% = completely. In rating degree of emotion: 1 = a trace; 100 = the most intense possible.
Table format reprinted with permission of Beck, A., Rush, A., Shaw, B., and Emery, G.: Cognitive therapy of depression, New York, 1979, The Guilford Press, p. 403. Copyright © 1978 by Aaron T. Beck, M.D.

Table 9-4 shows a completed daily record of dysfunctional thoughts for the victim in the above clinical example. By using this technique in the counseling session, the nurse asisted the victim in determining a rational response to concerns about credibility. The outcome was productive: the victim felt less frightened.

## Delays

One of the most stressful situations for the victim is the numerous delays or postponements of the trial. Delays occur for a number of reasons, which should be discussed with the victim: the defense attorney may need more time to prepare the case; the judge or the attorneys may be on vacation (particularly in summer months); records and witnesses need to be subpoenaed; a jury must be selected; and a change in trial lawyers may have occurred.

In legal jargon, delays or postponements are referred to as "cooling the mark."[12] *Cooling the mark* means that the victim's perseverance and degree of motivation to prosecute the assailant are tested; the assailant and defense attorney hope the victim will become discouraged and drop the charges. Indeed, many victims do become discouraged and drop charges. The following example demonstrates how a professional nurse helped one rape victim work through feelings about a court delay.

| CLINICAL EXAMPLE | Comment |
|---|---|
| *Victim:* They postponed the trial! How *could* they! I don't understand how they can postpone it for so long. I'm *furious!* It's okay for maybe a month, but not for 2 months. | Victim's feeling state: enraged. |
| *Nurse:* What were you told about why it was postponed? | Seeking information. |
| *Victim:* They said that the judges were on vacation. Also, he (the rapist) got a new attorney. The other attorney wanted $2000.00 up front and (the rapist) didn't have the money. So he got a new attorney, and that guy needs time to prepare the case. | Realistic reason for postponement. Possibly a tactic of "cooling the mark." |
| If he's not tried in 180 days (county regulation), will he go free? | Victim's personal goal threatened. Request for information. |
| *Nurse:* No. Not if the judge set the trial back. Usually the defendant has to sign permission for the trial to continue. Would you like me to check on that? | Nurse provides information to allay fears that the trial will be dropped; helps victim maintain control over life by providing secondary social network support. |
| *Victim:* Yeah, I'd feel better . . . wouldn't worry about it getting dropped. Why is it so hard to get a jury? They tried Tuesday, Wednesday, Thurs- | Coping style: search for logical reasons to handle frustration. |

**Comment**

day, and Friday of last week. What questions do they ask to make it so difficult?

Request for information.

*Nurse:* Sometimes the attorneys ask the prospective jurors questions like: "Would you be willing to give a prison sentence?" (that is, is the prospective juror willing to consider the full range of sentencing?). Sometimes people get off jury duty with a letter from their employer and have to be replaced. Sometimes either attorney can dismiss a jury member for no cause; each has a certain number of times he's permitted to do that and often exercises that right to eliminate jurors perceived as likely to hurt his case.

Giving information to allay victim's fears and to provide logical reasons for length and confusion of the court process.

*Victim:* I don't like our system; it's confusing. It makes me mad. There isn't anything I can do about it.

Victim feeling angry and helpless.

*Nurse:* Yeah. It can be pretty rotten. It's hard to keep waiting. What if the attorney is just using a delay tactic to get you to drop the charges?

Creative listening. Evaluating the victim's motivation to continue with the prosecution process.

*Victim:* Not me. I'll not drop it!

Victim remains goal directed.

*Nurse:* Sometimes that is one strategy to test the victim. Some women *do* get discouraged and *do* drop the charges.

Presents reality of postponement tactics.

*Victim:* Not me! I've been discouraged, but I'll not drop it!

Victim's motivation assessed as strong; wants to continue prosecution.

The nurse in the above clinical example helped the victim express feelings of frustration and anger over the court delays. The nurse also decided to use the daily record of dysfunctional thoughts to assist this victim through the waiting period. Table 9-5 shows one example of a record completed by this victim. As demonstrated in the record, the victim did not lose her determination to press charges against her assailant. Rational responses help to change the victim's automatic thoughts into productive behaviors. The victim becomes less angry and less discouraged; she is committed to prosecuting her assailant.

### Task performance disruption

Task performance disruption consists of difficulty or inability to resume one's usual role responsibilities such as wife, mother, student, or employee.[2] Such disrup-

**Table 9-5.** Daily record of dysfunctional thoughts

| Date | SITUATION<br>Describe:<br>1. Actual event leading to unpleasant emotion, or<br>2. Stream of thoughts, daydream, or recollection, leading to unpleasant emotion. | EMOTION(S)<br>1. Specify sad/anxious/angry, etc.<br>2. Rate degree of emotion, 1-100. | AUTOMATIC THOUGHT(S)<br>1. Write automatic thought(s) that preceded emotion(s).<br>2. Rate belief in automatic thought(s), 0-100%. | RATIONAL RESPONSE<br>1. Write rational response to automatic thought(s).<br>2. Rate belief in rational response, 0-100%. | OUTCOME<br>1. Re-rate belief in automatic thought(s), 0-100%.<br>2. Specify and rate subsequent emotions, 0-100. |
|---|---|---|---|---|---|
| 7/15/80 | Trial was postponed for 2 months. The judge is on vacation. The offender got a new attorney who needs time to prepare for the trial. | 1. Angry<br>   Discouraged<br>2. 90 | 1. I want to get this whole thing over with and go on vacation. It's unfair. I don't *want* to be treated this way. I feel so insignificant. They expect me to drop the charges as if *I* were guilty.<br>2. 80% | 1. This will give *me* more time to prepare for cross-examination. This ordeal has brought my family closer together, and we may not have otherwise developed bonds so close. The world doesn't live by fairness. I can *tolerate* the delay; there are a lot of things in life one has to wait for. I am not insignificant. I can go on vacation now and put my energy into active sports. I can't control others, but I can control my thoughts/feelings and feel good about that. I *won't* drop the charges.<br>2. 80% | *Automatic thoughts*<br>10%<br>*Emotions*<br>Angry = 20<br>Discouraged = 20<br>Committed to prosecuting |

EXPLANATION: When you experience an unpleasant emotion, note the situation that seemed to stimulate the emotion. (If the emotion occurred while you were thinking, daydreaming, etc., please note this.) Then note the automatic thought associated with the emotion. Record the degree to which you believe this thought: 0% = not at all; 100% = completely. In rating degree of emotion: 1 = a trace; 100 = the most intense possible.

Table format reprinted with permission of Beck, A., Rush, A., Shaw, B., and Emery, G.: Cognitive therapy of depression, New York, 1979, The Guilford Press, p. 403. Copyright © 1978 by Aaron T. Beck, M.D. Further information about this scale may be obtained from Center for Cognitive Therapy, Room 602, 133 S. 36th St., Philadelphia, PA 19104.

tions occur for many victims when the trial is scheduled and then delayed. Again and again the victim has already taken a day off from home, school, or work; hired a babysitter; and/or paid the cost of transportation to the trial.

Repeated absences from regular responsibilities are costly in terms of the loss of earned income, the expenses involved in attending hearings, and the emotional drain of coping with repeated delays.[12] Some states provide victims with partial compensation for being present at trial hearings; however, not all victims are aware of available reimbursements. Ultimately, the victim and her social network must decide how much time they can afford to be absent from their responsibilities. The following clinical example demonstrates how one victim handled the effects of task disruption.

### CLINICAL EXAMPLE

| Interaction | Comment |
|---|---|
| *Victim:* I can't take any more time off school. My grades dropped right after the rape; then there were all the trial postponements. | Victim finds it difficult to resume her usual role of student. |
| *Nurse:* All the delays are certainly frustrating. | Recognizes the emotional cost to the victim; uses empathic listening. |
| *Victim:* I've got a test coming up too. I want to do well so I can go to college. This business is really a bummer; sometimes I don't know why I'm doing it (prosecuting) or if it's worth it. | Victim's perseverance and degree of motivation to prosecute the assailant are tested; victim shows some discouragement and thinks about dropping the charges. |
| *Nurse:* Many victims do drop charges because of all the hassles. Of course, we could work on ways to handle your problems with school. | Testing the victim's motivation. Offers assistance at problem-solving the victim's task disruption. |
| *Victim:* I want to finish what I've started. I just get discouraged . . . Let's work on how to make my school situation better. | Victim makes own decision. |
| *Nurse:* Fine, let's start by identifying your most pressing concern. | Assists victim in identifying specific stressor. |
| *Victim:* My upcoming test—I'm not prepared at all. Do you think it would help to talk with my teacher? | Begins problem-solving process. Comes up with a constructive method of coping. |
| *Nurse:* What would you talk about? | Encourages victim to elaborate further and plan upcoming actions. |

### CLINICAL EXAMPLE

| Interaction | Comment |
|---|---|
| *Victim:* Why I'm missing class. My teacher's a female—she might understand my situation. | Envisions encounter and feels positive about outcome. |

As demonstrated in the above example, task performance disruptions can emotionally distress rape victims. Feelings of discouragement, hopelessness, and frustration occur when victims cannot resume their usual role performances. Nursing interventions with victims who experience task disruption include (1) recognizing the financial and emotional costs to the victim; (2) assisting the victim in identifying specific responsibilities that are being disrupted; (3) helping the victim find healthy coping mechanisms for handling the problem; and (4) supporting the victim in self-care decisions.

## Harassment

Sometimes accused assailants threaten victims in an effort to get them to drop the charges. Harassment can take a variety of forms: incessant and/or obscene phone calls; threats of harm from the assailant's relatives or friends who meet the victim in the ladies' room at the courthouse; driving by the victim's house; or confronting the victim in public. It is important for nurses to explore with victims what is identified as "harassment." The following example demonstrates nursing interventions with a victim who felt harassed.

### CLINICAL EXAMPLE

| Interaction | Comment |
|---|---|
| *Nurse:* How are you feeling? | Opening remark. |
| *Victim:* Sick! Especially since the rapist's brother talked to me! | Identifies stressful situation. |
| *Nurse:* He talked with you? | Surprised. Seeks additional information. |
| *Victim:* Yeah, on the phone Friday. Said he wanted to come to the house to talk with me. Thought I might like a visitor. | Relates fear from perceived harassment. |
| *Nurse:* What did you say? | Encourages further description. |
| *Victim:* I told him I'd call the police if I see him anywhere near my house! I was sure scared! | Relates appropriate handling of situation. |
| *Nurse:* It's very frightening to get a call like that. What was his response? | Reflective response. |
| *Victim:* He just laughed. Then said he lived nearby and might drop by sometime. | Another harassing threat. |
| *Nurse:* Then what did you do? | Encourages verbalization of action taken. |
| *Victim:* I hung up on him. Thank goodness my mom was home. She was real supportive. | Appropriate response to caller. Support available from victim's mother. |

| Interaction | Comment |
|---|---|
| *Nurse:* She helped you feel less frightened? | Implied in victim's statements. |
| *Victim:* Yeah . . . How do you think he found me? | Seeks information. |
| *Nurse:* Well, your name and number are listed in the phone book; and you said (the rapist) dropped you off in front of your house the night of the rape. He may have given your address to his brother. | Offers information that provides logical reason for rapist's brother to have victim's address and phone number. |
| *Victim:* Yeah, I forgot about that. Should I tell my lawyer about this? | Accepts explanation. |
| *Nurse:* Yes. Your attorney has ways to deal with this problem. But it also sounds like you handled a difficult situation quite well. | Provides information about appropriate use of attorney. Positive reinforcement for victim's coping mechanism. |
| *Victim:* Thanks . . . I just hope it doesn't happen again. | Outcome is positive. Victim has realistic perception of event. |

As demonstrated in the clinical example above, rape victims will call nurse counselors when they feel anxious and fearful about harassment. Nurses who have developed supportive relationships with victims can help them determine how to act (or not act) in response to a threatening situation. Sometimes referral to a more appropriate supportive person (in this case, the victim's lawyer) is indicated. Other times the assistance of the police or the district attorney's office may be necessary to ensure a victim's safety.

## THE VERDICT

The final step in the court process is the trial verdict, which presents rape victims with a legal decision regarding the guilt of their assailant. Preparing the victim to cope with the verdict is a major responsibility of the nurse counselor. Through a strategy called anticipatory guidance, nurses help rape victims become aware, *prior to the verdict,* of the thoughts and feelings that a guilty or not-guilty verdict will arouse in them.

*Anticipatory guidance* is defined as a method of leading a person through an anticipated stressful event or period "by exploring, in advance, possible alternatives for action and supporting reasonable problem-solving mechanisms, so that he or she can undergo the stress without being catapulted into a crisis."[9] Caplan has described anticipatory guidance as a form of "emotional innoculation" that prepares a person for a hazardous event prior to its occurrence so that when the event does occur the person is less likely to experience a crisis.[3] Anticipatory guidance can be considered as a practice session for the upcoming stressful event in which a person is guided through all the expected problematic areas and can plan ways to manage them. This type of guidance makes a person more prepared to problem-solve and less vulnerable to the expected stressor. When a person has a vivid anticipation of the problems that lie ahead, poten-

Table 9-6. Daily record of dysfunctional thoughts

| Date | SITUATION Describe: 1. Actual event leading to unpleasant emotion, or 2. Stream of thoughts, daydream, or recollection, leading to unpleasant emotion. | EMOTION(S) 1. Specify sad/ anxious/angry. etc. 2. Rate degree of emotion, 1-100. | AUTOMATIC THOUGHT(S) 1. Write automatic thought(s) that preceded emotion(s). 2. Rate belief in automatic thought(s), 0-100%. | RATIONAL RESPONSE 1. Write rational response to automatic thought(s). 2. Rate belief in rational response, 0-100%. | OUTCOME 1. Re-rate belief in automatic thought(s), 0-100%. 2. Specify and rate subsequent emotions, 0-100. |
|---|---|---|---|---|---|
| | Guilty verdict | 1. Sad Happy. 2. Sad = 10 Happy = 80 | 1. I hope he's put away for life. I shouldn't feel elated; it's wrong to be happy about hurting him. He's sick; he *deserves* what he got. I won a victory; I got revenge. Now what? Everything seems so meaningless. I feel numb after all the commotion/excitement. It's awful to create such turmoil in his family. It's terrible to send someone to prision. 2. 80% | 1. I don't care if he's hurt; he didn't care about me. Feelings are feelings, neither right nor wrong. He'll get help this way. He needs treatment, not just prison/punishment. It's *good* to get on with my life and put this behind me now; I've got every right to feel great! I filed the charge; I'm not responsible for the sentencing or his family responsibilities—he should've thought of them first. 2. 90% | *Automatic thoughts* 5% *Emotions* Sad = 5 Happy = 90 |

EXPLANATION: When you experience an unpleasant emotion, note the situation that seemed to stimulate the emotion. (If the emotion occurred while you were thinking, daydreaming, etc., please note this.) Then note the automatic thought associated with the emotion. Record the degree to which you believe this thought: 0% = not at all; 100% = completely. In rating degree of emotion: 1 = a trace; 100 = the most intense possible.

Table format reprinted with permission of Beck, A., Rush, A., Shaw, B., and Emery, G.: Cognitive therapy of depression, New York, 1979, The Guilford Press, p. 403. Copyright © 1978 by Aaron T. Beck, M.D.

tially growth-producing solutions can be facilitated by the nurse. Grace, Layton, and Camilleri assert:

> Anticipatory counseling in all its forms is an effective tool for nurses to use in working to prevent the maladaptive coping that frequently occurs when people have not been adequately prepared for the crisis situation they face. (p. 319)[9]

The cognitive behavioral strategy of the daily record of dysfunctional thoughts, explained earlier in this chapter, is presented in the discussion that follows as a way for nurses to help victims anticipate trial outcomes.

### A guilty verdict

During the trial some victims focus entirely on the goal of getting a conviction. They temporarily ignore the impact or meaning of that outcome for them. Even though a guilty verdict is the victim's goal of prosecution, nurse counselors must *prepare* victims to cope with a guilty verdict.

Although it is helpful for nurses to be aware of common thought patterns victims report in response to guilty verdicts, it is important that they be attentive to a victim's unique response patterns and identify which thoughts are dysfunctional for a particular victim. Nurse counselors can use a cognitive behavioral approach by asking the victim to report feelings and thoughts on the daily record of dysfunctional thoughts and to complete the cognitive restructuring exercise with the nurse in the counseling session so that the response pattern can be discussed. Together the nurse and the victim can work to identify intense nonproductive feelings or thoughts and find ways to refute them.

In helping a victim prepare for a guilty verdict, the nurse guides the victim in considering a range of feelings and thoughts. Victims may find it hard to consider many possible responses to a guilty verdict; often they cannot imagine feeling anything other than delight at achieving a conviction. Through the use of guided imagery and fantasy, the nurse suggests that the victim list feelings and thoughts that the victim views as totally absurd or "crazy" in response to achieving her goal—for example, sadness and concern for the rapist's family if the rapist is sent to prison.

Table 9-6 depicts one victim's efforts to apply cognitive restructuring strategies in anticipation of a guilty verdict. As demonstrated in the table, a rape victim can have many feelings that emerge, some of which might appear contradictory. For example, the paradoxical response of sadness and happiness following success is not so puzzling. Successes and achievements are often followed by sadness or depression.[1] Such responses have been attributed to the fact that achievement of a goal has placed new responsibilities on the person and that something of the past has been lost.

Rape victims sometimes feel a sense of responsibility for what happens to the rapist. Although the victim was seeking justice through prosecution, the harsh reality of a prison sentence, a life-term or lengthy sentence, or the disruption of the offender's social network may come to the victim's attention more fully following the trial. Other rape victims feel elated over a guilty verdict, as demonstrated in the following case example.

## CLINICAL EXAMPLE

Carolyn is a 20-year-old, white, single female. On her way home from work Carolyn was accosted by a man who had a cast on his arm. He brutally raped and beat Carolyn, making her perform oral sex. Carolyn was badly bruised from the struggle. Throughout the trial she focused on fears that the man would not be convicted. Her fears seemed unfounded to objective observers: Carolyn had the support of the police, the crisis center, many friends, and an "ideal" case in terms of evidence. Carolyn had identified her assailant; she had identified the cast used against her by the writing on it; and a witness knew the assailant had been within one block of the specified location of the assault. A guilty verdict was returned, and the rapist received a sentence of 45 years in prison. Carolyn felt tremendous relief with the guilty verdict; she felt no remorse or guilt. She was joyful and went out celebrating—drinking and partying the way most people celebrate an outstanding success. The anxiety Carolyn felt during the trial dissipated and was replaced by warmth and appreciation toward those who had been supportive of her throughout the trial process.

The clinical example above shows a victim who responded to a guilty verdict with happiness and relief. However, sometimes victims feel guilty about experiencing intense elation over a guilty verdict. Although it pleases them that justice has been met, some victims feel that it does not seem "quite right" to be so happy about a guilty verdict.

Nurses may be inclined to think that "everything will be just fine" after justice has been done. In reality, the victim may find that time and energy are available for reflective thought about the meaning of the whole event in her life, and that many conflicting, ambivalent feelings, assumed to have been settled, have once again arisen. Further, some victims realize that a guilty verdict does not begin to settle other losses endured—for example, a broken marriage or an altered body image. Fear of being harmed by the rapist (if he is released from prison) also worries some victims; this fear tends to be more intense if the rapist has threatened to take revenge or to see that his friends get back at the victim.

### A not-guilty verdict

In many states the probability is high that a rape victim will not obtain a guilty verdict when prosecuting an assailant.[12] Therefore, the nurse must discuss with the victim the possibility of a not-guilty verdict. Again, the nurse can use a cognitive restructuring exercise to help the victim consider, in advance of the fact, what thoughts would be useful in helping to cope with feelings about a not-guilty verdict. Initially the victim identifies what she expects to feel if a not-guilty verdict is returned—for example, outrage or anger, disappointment, disgust, sadness, or numbness.

Victims' thoughts about a not-guilty verdict usually fall into one or more of the following patterns:[12]

1. Desire to protect others ("I don't want him hurting other women. I'd hate to think he might get one of my friends.")
2. Belief that the rapist should be punished ("What he did was wrong. He deserves to go to prison. I hope somebody rapes him.")

**Table 9-7. Daily record of dysfunctional thoughts**

| Date | SITUATION Describe: 1. Actual event leading to unpleasant emotion, or 2. Stream of thoughts, daydream, or recollection, leading to unpleasant emotion. | EMOTION(S) 1. Specify sad/ anxious/angry. etc. 2. Rate degree of emotion, 1-100. | AUTOMATIC THOUGHT(S) 1. Write automatic thought(s) that preceded emotion(s). 2. Rate belief in automatic thought(s), 0-100%. | RATIONAL RESPONSE 1. Write rational response to automatic thought(s). 2. Rate belief in rational response, 0-100%. | OUTCOME 1. Re-rate belief in automatic thought(s), 0-100%. 2. Specify and rate subsequent emotions, 0-100. |
|---|---|---|---|---|---|
| 6/1/80 | Not-guilty verdict | 1. Angry Fearful 2. 70 | 1. I may seek my own revenge and kill him. He may seek revenge. How could they not convict him—believe him and not me? I didn't lie. There isn't any justice in this world. He violated me, my whole person. How can anyone let him back on the streets? This is a rotten, sexist society! I'll get *really* depressed and unable to function. 2. 70% | 1. I don't want to spend my life in jail for murder. He is not allowed to come near me. I can always move to a new state. Somebody will get him convicted because he's done it before and will probably do it again. Our system of injustice is changing slowly for the better. Even so, I've done my duty; it's not my fault if society is stupid. I told the truth; that's all I can do. I can use my energy to help the rape prevention program. 2. 80% | *Automatic thoughts* 25% *Emotions* Angry = 40 Fearful = 20 |

EXPLANATION: When you experience an unpleasant emotion, note the situation that seemed to stimulate the emotion. (If the emotion occurred while you were thinking, daydreaming, etc., please note this.) Then note the automatic thought associated with the emotion. Record the degree to which you believe this thought: 0% = not at all; 100% = completely. In rating degree of emotion: 1 = a trace; 100 = the most intense possible.

Table format reprinted with permission of Beck, A., Rush, A., Shaw, B., and Emery, G.: Cognitive therapy of depression, New York, 1979, The Guilford Press, p. 403. Copyright © 1978 by Aaron T. Beck, M.D.

3. Failure to convince the jury to believe the victim's account ("I feel rotten. How could they believe him and not me?")
4. Fear of the assailant ("Now he'll really take revenge, just like he threatened. I'm not safe anymore.")
5. Denial of the verdict as real ("I'm stunned. I can't believe it. Are you *sure* you're talking about *my* case?")
6. Hope that eventually the rapist will be convicted ("He's done this before so he's bound to go to prison sometime; maybe not this time, but somebody will get him.")

As stated earlier, victim response patterns depend on the individual woman and her unique situation. Table 9-7 demonstrates one victim's thoughts and responses to a not-guilty verdict. As demonstrated in the table, the victim uses cognitive restructuring to become aware of her thought patterns and to change these patterns so that more effectual behaviors and thoughts can emerge. In this case the victim sought counseling after the trial to work through her response to the not-guilty verdict and to make a good adjustment so that the remainder of her life would be positively influenced.

## SUMMARY

There are no "cookbook rules" for counseling rape victims through the court process. Victims have a variety of needs, and nursing interventions are planned according to (1) the nurse's education and clinical judgment, (2) the results of research specifying effective interventions, and (3) the health care or community setting.

A model of care known as cognitive behavior therapy is presented in this chapter because it has been found helpful in counseling rape victims throughout the court process. Cognitive behavior therapy is a semistructured, time-limited approach used to treat a variety of problems and concerns that rape victims bring into a counseling session in relation to the court process. Through cognitive restructuring strategies and behavioral techniques, nurses help rape victims view themselves as competent, powerful, and able to direct their lives. The major focus of intervention in this behavior model is disputing faulty attitudes, assumptions, and processing of information. One exercise that helps rape victims recognize and modify dysfunctional thoughts is called a daily record of dysfunctional thoughts. Its purpose is to help rape victims discriminate emotions and to refute nonproductive automatic thoughts. We suggest formal training for those nurses interested in applying the cognitive behavior therapy model in their interventions with rape victims.

In expanded roles nurses often counsel rape victims during and after court proceedings. Nurses who understand the court process can adequately prepare victims for court. This preparation for courtroom activities reduces the victim's intimidation and fear. Because the judicial process is often lengthy, victims are sometimes discouraged from prosecuting assailants. Also, processes such as the cross-examination by attorneys can be stressful and unpleasant.

Rape victims who decide to prosecute their assailants have various feelings and concerns throughout the court process. Many experience high levels of anxiety and fear during prosecution. Other common emotions are helplessness, powerlessness, and insecurity. One way a victim gains self-control and control over her environment is by learning what to expect in the court process. An important function of the nurse counselor is to explain to the victim the general procedures relating to court testimony, cross-examination, and attorney behaviors. Many victims also have concerns about their credibility, their past sexual history being exposed during the trial, and the involvement of significant others.

Other stressful situations for the victim include trial delays or postponements and task performance disruption. Delays occur for a number of reasons, and the nurse can provide information to the victim about the reasons for court delays. During the court process many victims experience a disruption in their normal life activities. They often express concerns about repeated absences from their responsibilities. Through counseling sessions rape victims work with nurses to decide how to problem-solve task disruption. Sometimes victims are concerned about harassment. It is important for the nurse to explore with the victim what is identified as harassment and to assist the victim in securing her safety.

Because the probability is high that a rape victim will not obtain a guilty verdict, nurses prepare victims to cope with both guilty and not-guilty verdicts. Using anticipatory guidance, they prepare victims for a stressful event before the actual situation occurs. Both anticipatory guidance and cognitive behavior strategies are helpful in preparing rape victims for the stressful experience of a verdict.

In general, both victims and nurses find the court process to be stressful. Counseling victims who prosecute assailants is an expanded role for nurses who recognize the vulnerability of victims and their need for support both during and after a trial process.

## Learning activities

### EXERCISE 1. Clinical situation

The following exercise consists of a clinical situation and nursing interventions that apply content from this chapter. An answer key is provided at the end of the Learning Activities.

Mary Jo is a 17-year-old high school girl who is very popular with her classmates. Recently she was chosen as a school cheerleader, and she holds a class office. On Saturday evening Mary Jo went shopping at the mall and met some of her girlfriends there. On the way out of the parking lot a car full of young boys from her high school pulled up to ask for directions. The girls chatted with the youths, who were older (about 19 years old) because they were complimented by the approach. Suddenly several of the youths jumped into the girls' car and forced them to drive near the high school to a deserted field; they were followed by the car with the remaining youths. There were five young men who raped the three girls. After insults, laughter about their appearance, degrading remarks, physical abuse, and rape by more than one male in the gang, the girls were returned to the shopping mall with threats of more physical harm if they told anyone. As soon as the young men departed, the girls found a shopkeeper and reported the incident. The girls have been brought to the emergency room where you are working to obtain a physical examination and treatment.

*Directions:* The following questions relate to the above situation. Answer each question as directed. (More than one response may be correct.)

1. Mary Jo has been told that when she testifies on the witness stand the defense attorney may ask her a number of leading and apparently innocent questions in an attempt to discredit her testimony. However, she can prepare for these strategies during a conference with the nurse at the community mental health center or local rape crisis center. The nurse will help prepare her for the courtroom experience with which of the following information?
   a. Even though Mary Jo is a popular girl at school, her past sexual history cannot be used in court unless directly related to the defendant.
   b. The defendant can be charged with statutory rape and has no defense about mistaking Mary Jo for older than 15 years of age.
   c. The law no longer requires that the victim show proof that she resisted during the attack, only that intercourse was by threat of force.
   d. The victim should not be alarmed by the judge's cautioning the jury in their consideration of her testimony because the law mandates that he deliver such instructions.

2. As the trial proceeds, Mary Jo reports to the nurse that she is distressed by the courtroom experience, specifically the defense attorney's linguistic strategy. The nurse tries to help her prepare to cope with the defense attorney's delivery style by conveying which of the following information?
   a. It is best to respond to questions that are out of sequence by trying to find a logical pattern or sequence and not admitting to any confusion.
   b. It is acceptable to answer leading questions with short, simple answers and explanations.
   c. Apparently innocent questions that continue in a series are best answered by simple and short statements.
   d. In all probability the lawyer will use a variety of techniques rather than a few favorite ones to catch Mary Jo off guard.

3. The nurse is aware that the courtroom experience has the potential of creating as much of a psychologic crisis as the rape experience did. In responding to Mary Jo's stress state resulting from the courtroom experience, the nurse intervenes in which of the following ways?
   a. Elicits Mary Jo's feelings of fear, anger, and embarrassment stimulated by reliving the rape experience through testifying.

b. Informs her that she need not look at the defendant or the defense attorney; says she can look at the jury or friends in the room when testifying.

c. Validates that Mary Jo is not alone when she feels extremely fearful of retaliation, scared, and nervous because many women feel that way.

d. Suggests that she be realistic about the court process, which is designed to create skepticism and suspicion about her testimony.

## EXERCISE 2. Prejudging the rape victim*

This exercise is intended to develop nurses' awareness of the way defense attorneys, by playing on stereotypes that jurors hold about rape victims, prejudge victims and attribute fault to them. For example, a woman who is hitchhiking is doing so because she wants a ride, not because she wants to be raped. However, her behavior is evaluated negatively by jurors in most cases, and the victim is attributed fault for the crime.

*Directions:* In Column 1 the account of the robbery of Mr. Smith is reported. In Column 2 the nurse is to write a statement describing the similarities in questions asked of the robbery victim and those of a rape victim—identifying any implication, prejudgment of the victim, or expectation conveyed by the type of question.

| COLUMN 1 | COLUMN 2 |
|---|---|
| Cross-examination of robbery victim, Mr. Smith | Implication and prejudgment when applied to a rape victim |
| *Defense Attorney:* Mr. Smith, you were held up at gunpoint on the corner of First and Main? | |
| *Witness:* Yes. | |
| *Defense Attorney:* Did you struggle with the robber? | |
| *Witness:* No. | |
| *Defense Attorney:* Why not? | |
| *Witness:* He was armed. | |
| *Defense Attorney:* Then you made a conscious effort to comply with his demands rather than resist? | |
| *Witness:* Yes. | |
| *Defense Attorney:* Did you scream? Cry out? | |
| *Witness:* No. I was afraid. | |
| *Defense Attorney:* I see. Have you ever been held up before? | |

*Reprinted with modifications by permission of the American Bar Association Journal, April, 1975.

| COLUMN 1 | COLUMN 2 |
| --- | --- |
| Cross-examination of robbery victim, Mr. Smith | Implication and prejudgment when applied to a rape victim |
| *Witness:* No. | |
| *Defense Attorney:* Have you ever *given* money away? | |
| *Witness:* Yes, of course. | |
| *Defense Attorney:* And you did so willingly? | |
| *Witness:* What are you getting at? | |
| *Defense Attorney:* Well, let's put it like this, Mr. Smith. You've given money away in the past. In fact, you have quite a reputation for philanthropy. How can we be sure that you weren't contriving to have your money taken from you by force? | |
| *Witness:* Listen, if I wanted . . . | |
| *Defense Attorney:* Never mind. What time did this holdup take place, Mr. Smith? | |
| *Witness:* About 11:00 PM? | |
| *Defense Attorney:* You were out on the street at 11:00 PM? Doing what? | |
| *Witness:* Walking. | |
| *Defense Attorney:* Just walking? You know that it's dangerous being out on the street that late at night. Weren't you aware that you could have been held up? | |
| *Witness:* I hadn't thought about it. | |
| *Defense Attorney:* What were you wearing at the time, Mr. Smith? | |
| *Witness:* Let's see . . . a suit. Yes, a suit. | |
| *Defense Attorney:* An *expensive* suit? | |
| *Witness:* Well—yes. I'm a successful lawyer, you know. | |
| *Defense Attorney:* In other words, Mr. Smith, you were walking around the streets late at night in a suit that practically advertised the fact that you might be a good target for some easy money, isn't that so? I mean, if we didn't know better, Mr. Smith, we might even think that you were *asking* for this to happen, mightn't we? | |

## EXERCISE 3. Role-play situations disputing negative cognitions

*Purpose:* The purpose of this exercise is to give the nurse *practice* in countering negative cognitions frequently verbalized by victims of rape. It is similar to a drama, offering freedom to be creative and expressive by improvising responses to a situation. Therefore the nurse can feel free to express intense feelings such as anger, rudeness, dissatisfaction, or joy. It is expected that the nurse will feel more confident, competent, and better prepared to intervene in real situations with rape victims after practicing these cognitive restructuring strategies.

*Guidelines:* The following role-plays are for class discussion; they are not intended for a course grade. Therefore the nurse can purposefully do something "wrong" or something that violates the principles for an effective helping relationship in order to highlight, compare, and contrast counseling interventions, and/or stimulate discussion. It can be helpful to think of the role-play as a game, not reality. There are no winners or losers. The nurse is essentially playing against herself/himself to learn effective cognitive restructuring skills that will help victims receive quality care. As the person enacting the role, strive to present situations that reflect a conflict of feelings, response patterns, motives, choice, indecision, and values. Conflictual situations reveal the greatest differences in responses and can prepare nurses for the unexpected situation.

*Directions:* Although the emphasis of this exercise is on cognitive restructuring responses, the nurse is to begin with a creative listening response ("That was a terrible experience."), follow with an assessment of the victim's crisis state ("You think you are to blame because you didn't fight back." = perception of the event), and close with a cognitive restructuring statement ("You did all you could to survive. Do you think it makes sense to risk being murdered?"). The emphasis here is on the learning of the students in disputing negative cognitions.

Each nurse is to receive a set of victim statements (listed on the next page), reflecting varying stress states, to enact in a role-play. These can be written on 3 × 5 cards for ease in implementing the exercise (put about 5 statements on one side of a card). The nurse can then glance at the card for statements that reflect the given stress state for the role-play being enacted. Allow 10 minutes for each role-play, and close with a discussion of the exercise (see the following page).

## Victim statements for cognitive restructuring role-play situations*

*Stress state: Fear/anxiety*

1. He said he'd kill me if I called the police.
2. I will *never* sleep again!
3. Oh, God. I'm sure I'm pregnant!
4. How can I *ever* go out alone again?
5. He'll come back and hurt me again, only worse next time.
6. He might hurt the kids.
7. He's my husband's best friend—my husband will kill him if he finds out!
8. He said he knew where I lived, where to get me.
9. I'll never be normal again.
10. I'm upset and edgy all the time.
11. I can't eat or sleep. I think I'm going crazy!
12. I'm too scared to go to work.
13. I can't concentrate. I can't even make simple decisions anymore.
14. Laughing is better than crying.
15. He keeps driving by the house!
16. His family is harassing me on the phone to drop the charges or they'll get my kids in trouble.
17. I keep hearing his voice and smelling his awful smell!
18. I can't even walk the street.
19. What if I catch VD!

*Stress state: Anger*

1. I don't want to talk about it!
2. Leave me alone!
3. Don't touch me!
4. Get out of here.
5. That ____! I'll kill him if I see him again.
6. How could he do such a thing!
7. Why doesn't *he* pay the cost of my ER care!
8. Why do I have to go through this (exam)!
9. I wish I had a gun!
10. I could kill my girlfriend for introducing him to me.
11. No police! Get them out of here.
12. My supervisor had the nerve to be upset because I didn't come to work.
13. My husband's out looking for the guy now, and he'll give it to him for me if he finds him.
14. I could have torn him apart with my bare hands.

---

*The authors wish to thank Mary Stern-Kiernan, M.S.W., Counselor, Pittsburgh Action Against Rape, for her assistance in developing victim statements for the cognitive restructuring role-play situations.

*Stress state: Belief in the myths/myth conception*

1. I asked for it.
2. I deserved it.
3. I'm dirty.
4. I'm a bad person.
5. I had no bra on.
6. I should not have hitchhiked.
7. He looked honest to me.
8. I led him on.
9. I was drunk.
10. I didn't resist.
11. I was so powerless—I am powerless, I had no control.
12. I should not have been out alone.
13. I should not be living alone.
14. It's not his fault—I started the fight.
15. This wouldn't have happened if I had sex more often with him.
16. I didn't think it was rape; he's my husband.
17. God is punishing me.
18. My folks told me not to go to that party and I wouldn't listen.
19. I'm not a virgin anymore.
20. My folks will know I had sex.
21. I'm so stupid.
22. Nobody will believe me; we've been dating.

*Stress state: Guilt/self-blame*

1. I should never have hitched that ride!
2. Why did I leave the bar with him?
3. How could I have left the door unlocked?
4. He looked like a nice man.
5. All I did was take the short cut through the park—that was a dumb thing to do.
6. I thought I knew him. I'll never forgive myself.
7. I just want to die.
8. I didn't fight back or even scream.
9. I shouldn't have been smoking reefers at the party.
10. I was wearing shorts.

*Stress state: Shame/self-blame*

1. I can't believe I let this happen.
2. I'm so embarrassed.
3. No one will believe me.
4. I can't go home.
5. The other man was just watching the whole time.
6. I'm a religious person.
7. Sex outside marriage isn't okay.

8. I should have had my Freon whistle with me.
9. Please don't let my folks know.
10. I had to take a shower—that was the wrong thing to do.
11. I wish I had called the police.
12. I was drunk (on drugs).
13. I let him into the apartment.
14. I've never been unfaithful to my husband.
15. I can't live with myself anymore. I feel dirty.
16. Why didn't I take karate lessons?
17. I was out jogging alone.

*Stress state: Shock/disbelief*

1. I can't believe this happened to me.
2. No, I'm fine. I don't need any help.
3. I don't think what I do matters.
4. Mute or silent, smiling, restless.
5. Crying, sobbing, hysterical.
6. I feel numb.
7. I just want to forget it.
8. What he did was so dirty and perverted!
9. I don't know what I'm going to do now.
10. This is the worst experience in all my life.
11. I wish he had killed me.
12. This'll probably hit me later.
13. I feel so tired.
14. It doesn't seem real.
15. I'm dumbstruck.

## SUGGESTED DISCUSSION QUESTIONS

1. Which situations were the *most difficult* to role-play?
   a. Explain.
   b. Did you feel helpless? Stuck for an answer?
2. Which situations were the *easiest* to role-play?
   a. Explain.
   b. What made the easiest situations different from the difficult ones? For example, were the situations focusing on anger more difficult than those that involved anxiety or guilt? Were the situations that centered around sexual concerns more difficult than those that focused on self-blame?
3. What intervention strategies seemed to be *most* useful, to work best?
   a. Explain.
   b. Did it help to begin with creative listening and assessment of the victim's status before moving into cognitive restructuring strategies? Explain.

4. Which intervention strategies seemed to be the *least* useful, not to help?
   a. Explain.
   b. What seemed to make the victim's symptoms intensify—make her more defensive, angry, or assert that you were not understanding?
   c. Did it help to return to creative listening at a time when the victim became upset by cognitive restructuring strategies? Explain.
5. Closure:

   It takes time to acquire familiarity and integration of new skills. However, with practice, cognitive restructuring strategies will become an integral part of the nurse's interventions with rape victims. With these skills the nurse can intervene when a rape victim has negative or nonproductive cognitions in relation to resolving the experience.

---

## Answer key to Exercise 1: Knowledge and clinical practice

*Rationale for answer selection*

(1)   *1. a and c
     2. b and d
     3. b and c
     4. a and d

*a. Past sexual history cannot be admitted in court unless directly related to the defendant (see chapter text).
 b. The elements for statutory rape do not exist in the case situation.
*c. The requirement that the victim show proof of resistance during the attack has been dropped from the law in most states.
 d. The law mandates that the credibility of the victim's testimony be judged the same as that of witnesses in any other crime.

*Rationale for answer selection*

(2)   1. a and b
     2. a and d
    *3. b and c
     4. b and d

 a. There is no logical sequence or pattern; this is done to confuse the witness. She should relax, take time to think, and answer each question totally independently of the others. It is acceptable to admit confusion.
*b. This is considered the best response to leading questions.
*c. These questions are similar to leading questions and are best answered in a similar manner.
 d. The defense attorney usually uses a few favorite techniques rather than a wide variety of delivery styles.

---

*Asterisk indicates correct answers.

*Rationale for answer selection*

(3) *1. a,b,c
    2. b,c,d
    3. a,c,d
    4. a,b,c,d

*a. The nurse acts as a support system by acknowledging and listening to feelings, allowing for ventilation, and exploring perception of the event.

*b. This is a behavioral strategy effective with both adults and children; it focuses the victim's attention away from threats to the self.

*c. Provides a sense of universality by confirming that the victim's experience is quite normal, not unique or "crazy."

d. Tends to ignore and cut off the victim's reaction to court; can be viewed as a lecture that is insensitive to her feelings.

---

*Asterisk indicates correct answers.

---

## REFERENCES

1. Beck, A., Rush, A., Shaw, B., and Emery, G.: Cognitive therapy of depression, New York, 1979, The Guilford Press.
2. Burgess, A.W., and Holmstrom, L.L.: Rape: its effect on task performance at varying stages in the life cycle. In Walker, M.J., and Brodsky, S.L., Editors: Sexual assault: the victim and the rapist, Lexington, Mass., 1976, Lexington Books.
3. Caplan, G.: Principles of preventative psychiatry, New York, 1964, Basic Books, Inc.
4. Cox, H.: A courtroom guide for rape and sexual assault victims, Allegheny County Police Department, 1979. Mimeographed.
5. Davenport, J.A.: Role playing helps rape victims prepare for next ordeal, Innovations, 5:35, 1978.
6. Frank, E., and Turner, S.: The rape victim: her response and treatment, Pittsburgh, Pa., 1982, Western Psychiatric Institute and Clinic.
7. Frank, E.: Cognitive-behavioral therapy, Pittsburgh, Pa., 1979, Western Psychiatric Institute and Clinic. Mimeographed.
8. Frank, E.: Personal communication, Pittsburgh, Pa., 1982, Western Psychiatric Institute and Clinic.
9. Grace, H., Layton, J., and Camilleri, D.: Mental health nursing: a socio-psychological approach, Dubuque, Iowa, 1977, Wm. C. Brown Publishers.
10. Graves, H., and Thompson, E.: Anxiety: a mental health vital sign. In Longo, D., and Williams, R., editors: Clinical practice in psychosocial nursing: assessment and intervention, New York, 1978, Appleton-Century-Crofts.
11. Harrisburg Area Rape Crisis Center: Training manual, 1979.
12. Holmstrom, L.L., and Burgess, A.W.: The victim of rape: institutional reactions, New York, 1978, John Wiley & Sons, Inc.
13. Kalkman, M.: Models of psychiatric treatment. In Kalkman, M., and Davis, A.: New dimensions in mental health–psychiatric nursing, New York, 1974, McGraw-Hill Book Co.

14. Lange, A., and Jakubowski, P.: Responsible assertive behavior: cognitive/behavioral procedures for trainers, Champaign, Ill., 1976, Research Press.
15. May, R.: The meaning of anxiety, New York, 1950, Ronald Press.
16. Medea, A., and Thompson, K.: Against rape, New York, 1964, Farrar, Straus & Giroux.
17. Shore, B.: An examination of critical process and outcome factors in rape, report to the public, December 1979, and final summary report submitted to NIMH, January 1980.
18. Stevens, D., and Ousley, N.: Sequelae of chemically-involved sexual assault, Seattle, Wash., 1981, Harborview Medical Center.

## ADDITIONAL REFERENCES

Baril, C., and Couchman, I.: Legal rights, Society **13:**15, 1976.

Brownmiller, S.: Against our will: men, women and rape, New York, 1975, Simon & Schuster.

Bruch, H.: Learning psychotherapy: rationale and ground rules, Cambridge, Mass., 1964, Harvard University Press.

Burgess, A.W., and Holmstrom, L.L.: Rape: crisis and recovery, Bowie, Md., 1919, Robert J. Brady Co.

Burgess, A.W., and Holmstrom, L.L.: Rape: victims of crisis, Bowie, Md., 1974, Robert J. Brady Co.

Burgess, A.W., and Holmstrom, L.L.: Crisis and counseling requests of rape victims, Nurs. Res. **23:**196, 1974.

Burgess, A.W., and Laszlo, A.T.: Courtroom use of hospital records in sexual assault cases, Am. J. Nurs. **1:**64, 1977.

Burgess, A., and Lazare, A.: The social context of mental illness. In Burgess, A., and Lazare, A.: Psychiatric nursing in the hospital and the community, Englewood Cliffs, N.J., 1976, Prentice-Hall, Inc.

Calhoun, L.G., and others: The effects of victim physical attractiveness and sex of respondent on social reactions to victims of rape, Br. J. Soc. Clin. Psychol. **27:**191, 1978.

Calhoun, L.G., Selby, J.W., and Warring, L.J.: Social perception of the victim's role in rape: an exploratory examination of four factors, Hum. Relations, **29:**517, 1976.

Carbary, L.: Treating terrified victims, J. Pract. Nurs. **2:**20, 1974.

Davis, J., and others: The decision process of 6- and 12-person mock juries assigned unanimous and two-thirds majority rule, J. Pers. Soc. Psychol. **32:**1, 1975.

Davison, G., and Goldbried, M.: Clinical behavior therapy, New York, 1976, Holt, Rinehart & Winston.

Ellis, A.: Humanistic psychology, New York, 1973, McGraw-Hill Book Co.

Ellis, A., and Harper, R.: A new guide to rational living, North Hollywood, Calif., 1975, Wilshire Book Co.

Feldman-Summers, S., and Lindner, K.: Perceptions of victims and defendants in criminal assault cases, Criminal Justice Behav. **3:**135, 1976.

Foley, T., and MacDonald, C.: Models of treatment, lecture notes, Pittsburgh, Pa., 1975-1976, University of Pittsburgh School of Nursing.

Frieze, I., and others: Women and sex roles: a social psychological perspective, New York, 1978, W.W. Norton & Co.

Freud, S.: Insterpretation of dreams, New York, 1950, Modern Library.

Gager, N., and Schurr, C.: Sexual assault: confronting rape in America, New York, 1976, Grosset & Dunlap.

Goldstein, A.: Behavior therapy. In Corisini, R., editor: Current psychotherapies, Champaign, Ill., 1973, F.E. Peacock Publishers.

Gottschalk, L.: How to understand and analyze your own dreams, New York, 1975, Jason Aronson.

Hall, C.S.: The meaning of dreams, New York, 1966, McGraw-Hill Book Co.

Hayman, C.: What to do for victims of rape, Med. Times **101**:49, 1973.

Hoffman, S., and Dodd, T.: Effects of various victim characteristics on attribution of responsibility to an accused rapist, paper presented at the twenty-first annual meeting of the Southeastern Psychological Assocation.

Holmstrom, L.L., and Burgess, A.W.: Rape: the husband's and boyfriend's initial reactions, The Family Coordinator **7**:321, 1979.

International Association of Chiefs of Police: Training key no. 210: interviewing the rape victim. In Center for women's policy studies; Rape and its victims: a report for citizens, health facilities, and criminal justice agencies, Washington, D.C., 1974, Law Enforcement Assistance Administration, U.S. Department of Justice.

Jones, C., and Aronson, E.: Attribution of fault to a rape victim as a function of respectability of the victim, J. Pers. Soc. Psychol. **26**:415, 1973.

Klemmack, S., and Klemmack, D.: The social definition of rape. In Walker, M.J., and Brodsky, S.L., editors: Sexual assault: the victim and the rapist, Lexington, Mass., 1976, Lexington Books.

Kliman, A.: Crisis: psychological first aid for recovery and growth, New York, 1978, Holt, Rinehart & Winston.

Lazare, A.: Hidden conceptual models in clinical psychiatry, New Engl. J. Med. **288**:345, 1973.

Leighton, A.: Conceptual perspectives. In Kaplan, B., Wilson, R., and Leighton, A.: Further explorations in social psychiatry, New York, 1976, Basic Books.

Lidz, T.: The person: his and her development throughout the life cycle, New York, 1976, Basic Books.

McLaughlin, W.: Address to Suffolk superior court jury, Juris Doctor, **4**:26, 1974.

Pennsylvania Coalition Against Rape: Personal communication, November, 1979.

Rimm, D., and Masters, J.: Behavior therapy: techniques and empirical findings, New York, 1974, Academic Press.

Rosenbaum, C., and Beebe, J.: Psychiatric treatment: crisis/clinic/consultation, New York, 1975, McGraw-Hill Book Co.

Schachter, J.: Clinical consultation, Pittsburgh, Pa., 1980-1981, Pittsburgh Psychoanalytic Center, Inc.

Segal, S.: Imagery: current cognitive approaches, New York, 1971, Academic Press.

Sheen, P.: The function and nature of imagery, New York, 1972, Academic Press.

Singer, J.: Imagery and daydream methods in psychotherapy and behavior modification, New York, 1974, Academic Press.

Sloane, P.: Psychoanalytic understanding of the dream, New York, 1978, Jason Aronson.

Smith, R.E., and others: Role and justice considerations in the attribution of responsibility to a rape victim, J. Res. Pers. **10:**346, 1976.

Snyder, J., and Wilson, M.: Elements of a psychological assessment, Am. J. Nurs. **2:**253, 1977.

Symonds, M.: The accidental victim of violent crime. In Pasterneack, S.A., editor: Violence and victim, New York, 1975, Spectrum Publications, Inc.

Topalis, M., and Aguilera, D.C.: Psychiatric nursing, ed. 7, St. Louis, 1978, The C.V. Mosby Co.

Welch, K.: Derogation of rape victims, unpublished doctoral dissertation, 1977, The University of Alabama Department of Psychology.

## ANNOTATED SUGGESTED READINGS

American Psychological Association: Principles for therapy and counseling of women, APA Monitor, p. 6, December 1978.

The Division of Counseling Psychology of the American Psychological Association has drafted 13 principles for therapy and counseling with women that appear in this issue. These principles were recommended in the American Nurses' Association Pacesetter, Newsletter of the Council of Specialists in Psychiatric and Mental Health Nursing, **4:**5, 1979. Nurses can obtain copies of the principles for therapy by writing to the cochairman of the Ad Hoc Committee on Women: Laurel Oliver, Army Research Institute, 5100 Eisenhower Avenue, Alexandria, VA 22333.

Beck, A.: Cognitive therapy and the emotional disorders, New York, 1978, International Universities Press.

This book introduces nurses to the basic principles and techniques of Beck's cognitive therapy. The author describes the procedure of tapping one's irrational internal communications and cognitions, which Beck asserts underlie erroneous interpretations of experience and psychologic disturbances such as depression and other neuroses. Beck concludes with a discussion of the place and contribution of cognitive theory in the current treatment of emotional disorders.

Beck, A., and Greenberg, R.: Cognitive therapy with depressed women. In Franks, V., and Vasanti, B., editors: Women in therapy, New York, 1974, Brunner/Mazel Publishers.

The chapter briefly discusses the tendency of women to be depressed; theories about the nature of depression; symptoms of depression, including accompanying cognitive factors; a perspective on and discussion of cognitive therapy, including an illustration of its use; and an integrated discussion of socialization factors that contribute to depression in women. The authors also provide an excellent list of references.

Beck, A., Rush, A., Shaw, B., and Emery, G.: Cognitive therapy of depression, New York, 1979, The Guilford Press.

The book presents step-by-step guidelines for implementing cognitive therapy. It is explicit and offers excellent illustrations of the techniques employed. The authors discuss the basic principles of cognitive therapy; the role of the emotions in determining depression; the therapeutic relationship with the client; the structure of the initial interview and the interview itself; session-by-session treatment illustrating a typical course of therapy; application of behavioral and cognitive techniques; focusing on target symptoms; applications with specific problems such as suicide and depression; the role of depressogenic assumptions; the use of homework assignments; technical problems; and supporting research studies. When combined with supervised clinical practice, this book is an excellent manual for nurses interested in applying cognitive-behavioral therapy with rape victims.

Brodsky, A., and Hare-Mustin, R., editors: Women and psychotherapy: an assessment of research and practice, New York, 1980, The Guilford Press.

This book represents the work of leaders in the field of psychotherapy research. It addresses five major areas: (1) research on gender differences in therapy (therapist attitudes, the process of therapy, therapy outcomes); (2) traditional approaches (psychodynamic, behavioral, use of medication); (3) highly prevalent disorders (depression, anxieties, phobias, marital and family conflict); (4) crisis intervention (for violence against women, reproductive crises, marital transition); and (5) alternative approaches (nontraditional treatments such as feminist therapy, consciousness-raising groups, self-help groups). Written in nontechnical language, the book is useful for professionals who are beginning to confront the special needs of women. It offers a synthesis of research and clinical experience, dispels old myths, and provides a solid foundation for treating problems specific to women.

Bruch, H.: Learning psychotherapy: rationale and ground rules, Cambridge, Mass., 1974, Harvard University Press.

In teaching the beginning nurse practitioner the art and skill of functioning as a psychotherapist, the author communicates the wisdom of a lifetime. The fundamental issues of psychotherapy are addressed in a way that is useful to the experienced clinician as well. Nurses will find the content applicable to the counseling of rape victims and their families, particularly these sections: (1) When Strangers Meet; (2) Personality in the Making; (3) The World Around: Significant Others; (4) The Patient Speaks; (5) On Talking and Listening; and (6) The Therapeutic Experience.

Ellis, A.: Humanistic psychology, New York, 1973, McGraw-Hill Co.

The author presents a full exposition of rational-emotive-therapy (RET). The book contains many essays from other volumes and revisions of speeches delivered to professional groups and university audiences. The author compares and contrasts RET to other theories and approaches in therapy.

Ellis, A.: Rational-emotive-therapy. In Corisini, R., editor: Current psychotherapies, Itasca, Ill., 1973, F.E. Peacock Publishers, Inc.

The chapter presents an overview of rational-emotive-therapy as developed by Ellis, including (1) the 8 basic concepts of the theory, (2) 13 biological proclivities of man, (3) 4 reasons why irrational beliefs are empirically invalid, (4) the mechanism of psychotherapy, and (5) the process of treatment in individual therapy. It is useful to nurses interested in developing skill in identifying negative or nonproductive cognitions that become the focus of treatment interventions in counseling rape victims and their families.

Ellis, A., and Harper, R.: A new guide to rational living, North Hollywood, Calif., 1975, Wilshire Book Co.

This book is written for the lay person and presents a full discussion of rational-emotive-therapy, including an analysis of 12 irrational beliefs identified by Ellis. The authors offer many examples to illustrate their approach in refuting irrational beliefs, including an attitude of hopefulness that is conveyed to the client ("You have control, you can get better or change") and attacks on perfectionistic shoulds, oughts, and musts.

Fishel, A.: What is a feminist therapist? Ms. **6:**79, 1979.

The author succinctly defines and describes the nature of feminist therapy, comparing and contrasting it briefly with other therapeutic approaches in counseling. The focus is on embracing power and a redefinition of power in regard to personal choices and power politics. The article includes a Consumer's Guide to the Right Therapy that underscores the basic premises of feminist therapy. It also offers a consumer's Bill of Rights as delineated in suggested questions for clients to answer after completing an initial evaluation session with a therapist. The article contains an excellent resource list to help readers identify feminist agencies and locate feminist therapists.

Golan, N.: Treatment in crisis situations, New York, 1978, The Free Press.

The author provides nurses with a chart illustrating a step-by-step breakdown of the crisis intervention model present. One column of the chart identifies what may transpire in the interview and includes typical remarks made during crisis intervention with the client. The other column offers guidelines and explanations of why the intervention approach was implemented. We have found this source useful in teaching nurses the process of crisis intervention with rape victims and their families.

Heppner, P., and Heppner, M.: Rape: counseling the traumatized victim, Personnel and Guidance J. **10:**77, 1977.

This article describes phenomena commonly reported in the literature about response to rape—for example, the impact of rape myths on victim response and the response of significant others. The authors discuss the special needs of rape victims, immediate counseling goals, deep psychologic needs, and future possibilities in meeting the needs of rape victims. The article is particularly helpful in illustrating the application of cognitive restructuring techniques with rape victims.

Karasu, T., and Bellack, L.: Specialized techniques in individual psychotherapy, New York, 1980, Brunner/Mazel Publishers.

The book covers a wide range of clinical areas and provides the practitioner with varied approaches and techniques known to be effective with different patient populations seeking psychotherapy. Expert clinicians discuss the theoretic basis for diagnosis, realistic therapeutic goals, and the specialized techniques most useful in reaching those goals. Each chapter includes helpful, specific clinical examples and case studies. Subjects useful to nurses counseling rape victims and their families include (1) brief and emergency psychotherapy; (2) psychotherapy of the depressed patient; (3) psychotherapy of ambulatory patients with severe anxiety; psychotherapy with suicidal patients, with the elderly, and with bilingual patients; (4) racial issues in psychotherapy; (5) family and marital therapy combined with individual psychotherapy; (5) behavioral techniques in conjunction with individual psychotherapy; and (6) brief psychotherapy of stress response syndromes.

Kell, B., and Mueller, W.: Impact and change: a study of counseling relationships, Englewood Cliffs, N.J., 1966, Prentice-Hall, Inc.

The authors present their theory about how change occurs in the process of counseling. This interpersonal theory has been derived from their own clinical practice and that of colleagues and from hours of analyzing tape recordings of counseling interviews. The book is useful to anyone responsible for those who seek counseling to change themselves. Of particular benefit to nurses counseling rape victims and their families is Part 1, which focuses on (1) introduction to the dynamics of change; (2) dimensions of a counseling relationship; (3) the impact of client dynamics and conflicts on the counselor; and (4) the counselor: a human being who helps. This book is helpful to nurses learning the process of psychotherapy or counseling clients.

Lange, A., and Jakubowski, P.: Cognitive restructuring procedures. In Lange, A., and Jakubowski, P.: Responsible assertive behavior: cognitive/behavioral procedures for trainers, Champaign, Ill., 1976, Research Press.

The recommended chapter provides nurses with an overview of cognitive restructuring techniques used as interventions with rape victims and emotionally distressed clients. The authors discuss and illustrate each of Ellis's irrational beliefs/ideas and apply RET to assertiveness training. The last section of the chapter discusses internal dialogues or negative cognitions and ways to cope with these. It includes suggestions for refuting self-statements related to anger, confrontation, arousal, and conflict; for preparing for a stressor, reacting during a stress-producing situation, and coping with being overwhelmed.

Lindemann, E.: Symptomatology and management of acute grief. In Parad, H.J., editor: Crisis intervention: selected readings, New York, 1965, Family Service Association.

The author presents findings on the nature of bereavement from a study of the Coconut Grove Fire. The reading describes acute grief; symptomatology of normal grief; the course of normal grief reactions; morbid grief reactions; prognostic evaluations; psychiatric management, including transforming distorted phenomena into a normal grief reaction with resolution; and anticipatory grief reactions. Since resolving a rape experience involves working through a grief process, it is recommended that nurses who counsel rape victims and their families have a working knowledge of grief and bereavement.

McMullin, R., and Casey, B.: Talk sense to yourself!, Lakewood, Colo., 1975, Counseling Research Press.

This manual is written for the layman and therefore is easily readable. It is intended to supplement professional instruction in cognitive restructuring therapy and can be of help in teaching rape victims or their families cognitive restructuring strategies. The manual addresses (1) thoughts that cause problems; (2) six irrational thoughts; (3) analyzing your thoughts; (4) eliminating an irrational thought; (5) the habit of realistic thinking; (6) self-punishment/self-reward thinking exercises; (7) things you can do on your own; and (8) an appendix listing (a) thoughts that cause problems, (b) sabotages or sure-fire ways to fail, and (c) suggested readings.

Raimy, V.: Misunderstandings of the self, San Francisco, 1975, Jossey-Bass Publishers.

The author asserts that cognitive variables—such as faulty beliefs, convictions, and misconceptions—are responsible for psychologic disturbances. Further, if the misconceptions can be eliminated or modified, improved adjustment results. Because the approach suggested by the author does not depend on any given set of methods or techniques, it can be widely applied. The book discusses changing misconceptions, presenting evidence, cognitive review, the role of affect and insight, and contributions to psychoanalysis. The book is excellent supplementary reading to the writings of Beck.

Raths, L., Harmin, M., and Simon, S.: The clarifying response. In Smith, M.: A practical guide to value clarification, La Jolla, Calif., 1977, University Associates.

The authors present 30 useful clarifying responses to be used in combination with value clarification and self-care decision processes. The purpose of the responses is to raise questions that will prod a person to gently examine his or her life, actions, and ideas in order to clarify understandings, purposes, feelings, attitudes, and beliefs. The clarifying responses are helpful in counseling rape victims when used with cognitive behavior therapy.

Rimm, D., and Masters, J.: Behavior therapy: techniques and empirical findings, New York, 1974, Academic Press.

This book addresses two fundamental questions: (1) How does one design and execute a program of behavior therapy? and (2) Why should a given technique of behavior therapy be selected? The authors provide a detailed account of behavior therapy techniques and describe empirical findings that demonstrate the effectiveness of a given technique, thereby validating their application in appropriate settings. Nurses who use behavioral approaches in counseling rape victims or their families will find the book an excellent resource for readings on behavior therapy.

Snyder, J., and Wilson, M.: Elements of a psychological assessment, Am. J. Nurs. **2:**235, 1977.

The authors describe 10 elements basic to an eclectic approach in the psychologic assessment of clients that the generalist or specialist nurse is expected to be capable of completing. These elements are (1) response to stress: coping and defense mechanisms; (2) interpersonal relationships; (3) motivation and life-style; (4) thought processes and verbal behavior; (5) nonverbal behavior; (6) awareness and handling of feelings; (7) support systems; (8) talents, strengths, and assets; (9) physical health; and (10) the interview and the self of the nurse. The authors discuss each element in detail and suggest questions for conducting an interview.

Weiner, I.: Principles of psychotherapy, New York, 1975, John Wiley & Sons.

This book is primarily a manual of principles for conducting psychotherapy in clinical practice and is addressed to the practitioner. The author provides guidelines for the conduct of interviews from initial evaluation sessions through the working and terminating phases of treatment. These guidelines are amplified with illustrations of what the therapist can say or do in a given situation or under various circumstances. The book is a major resource for nurses learning to be primary psychotherapists with clients and therefore is valuable as a reference for nurses responsible for counseling rape victims.

# CHAPTER 10

# Child sexual abuse

Recognition of child molestation is entirely dependent on the willingness of the individual to admit that the condition may exist.

Sgroi, S.M., in Holley, K.C.: *Sexual misuse of children: tools for understanding.*

## CHAPTER OUTLINE

## LEARNING OBJECTIVES

After completing this chapter the reader will be able to:

1 Define child sexual abuse and incest

2 Describe how the incidence of child sexual abuse is determined and the scope of the problem

3 List ten myths related to child sexual abuse and the facts from reported cases that refute these myths

4 Describe three common stress reaction indicators of child sexual abuse

5 Explain three types of family member response to a disclosure or discovery of child sexual abuse

6 Identify two social systems that work with child victims and their families

7 Describe five goal-directed nursing interventions related to the areas of interviewing the child, medical management of the child, and psychologic management of the child's parents

8 Explain two approaches to the prevention of child sexual abuse

Child sexual abuse is often a taboo subject because the public likes to believe that such abuse does not exist or is not prevalent enough to warrant discussion.[16] Professional nurses recognize that child sexual abuse *does exist;* it represents a growing problem for American society and a challenge for health care providers.

Professional nurses have two major responsibilities: (1) to acquire a knowledge base about child sexual abuse through a critical review of existing research, literature, and statistics on the subject and (2) to use the existing information to deliver quality nursing interventions to child victims and their families. This chapter presents current information related to defining child sexual abuse, the scope of the problem, and common myths about child sexual abuse. Facts that refute the myths are presented so that nurses will know the most current information on the subject.

Not all child victims and families respond to sexual abuse in the same manner. Each victim and family has unique reactions to the problem; their responses are influenced partially by the nature of the abuse. Professional nurses assess each individual case of child sexual abuse to determine the particular circumstances involved and to choose interventions that will facilitate healthy adjustment. Nurses who are sensitive to victim and family needs are a major source of support during a most difficult time.

## DEFINING CHILD SEXUAL ABUSE

As with the study of rape, professional nurses who begin to study child sexual abuse ask one very important question: How are the terms under study being defined? Any professional who takes a serious interest in learning about child sexual abuse must consider two issues: (1) How do researchers, clinicians, or statisticians define a *child* so that information and statistics are accurately and uniformly collected? and (2) How is *sexual abuse* defined so that understanding of the term is consistent, especially when describing and reporting cases of child sexual abuse?

The issue of defining the term *child* is important because professional nurses who review literature, research studies, or collected statistics learn to evaluate the reported conclusions by looking carefully at the population being studied. For example, when adolescents are included in child sexual abuse studies or statistics, the results may look quite different from those that do not include adolescents.

Depending on the research design, professional judgment, or state legislative definitions, the population under study may vary regarding the definition of a child and the terminating year of childhood. For this text, a *child* is defined as "a young person between infancy and 12 years of age (inclusive)." We consider a young person between the ages of 13 and 18 years to be an adolescent. The sexual abuse of adolescents involves different variables, reactions, and dynamics—some of which are addressed under the section on victim responses in this chapter.

Nurses who attempt to understand child sexual abuse can also be confused or misled by terms such as *sexual abuse, sexual relations, sexual misuse, sexual assault,* and *incest.* For example, Breen defines child *sexual assault* as "manual, oral, or genital contact by an offender with the genitalia of the victim without the victim's consent."[2] Berliner considers the developmental level of the child as reflected in the definition of *sexual misuse* as "the exploitation of a child who is not developmentally capable of understanding or resisting the contact or who may be psychologically and socially dependent upon the offender."[1] The terms sexual abuse, sexual misuse, and sexual assault are often used interchangeably. According to Webster's dictionary, *abuse* is defined as "improper use, action or treatment" whereas *assault* is defined as "a violent physical or verbal attack."

For the purpose of this text *child sexual abuse* is defined as *the forcing of any sensory (visual, physical, or verbal) sexual contact onto another person.* The sexual contact involves fondling, genital manipulation, oral sex, attempts at and actual penetration of the vagina or anus.

Child sexual abuse does not *always* involve sexual contact. A child may be forced to look at the genitals of another person, or the person may ask the child to undress or expose parts of his or her body. The force may involve threats, bribery, or taking advantage of the child's intellectual, psychologic, or sexual immaturity.[18]

Child sexual abuse is quite different from normal physical contact between an adult and a child. Table 10-1 presents the characteristics of the two types of contacts. As demonstrated in the table, normal physical contact between an adult and a child usually involves a healthy, affectionate, and playful expression of love. In contrast, sexual abuse between a child and an adult involves using the child for gratification of the adult. In normal physical contact the child is respected and the relationship is affec-

**Table 10-1. Normal physical contact vs sexual contact between adult and child**

| Normal adult-child physical contact | Child sexual abuse contact |
| --- | --- |
| Healthy, affectionate, and playful activity | Child is used for adult's gratification |
| Child is respected, loved | Child is love object or sex object |
| Child is usually happy, nonthreatened | Child may be entrapped, enticed, or threatened |

tionate; in sexual abuse contact the child is perceived as a love object or sex object. Within the framework of healthy or normal physical contact the child generally feels happy and nonthreatened by the experience. In a sexual abuse experience, the child may be entrapped, enticed, or threatened into sexual contact.[15]

Approximately one half of all reported child sexual abuse cases are the result of *incestuous* relationships.[21] Incest is defined as "sexual relations in a kinship pattern that prohibits marriage by law."[13] A wide variety of incestuous relationships exists: brother-sister, mother-child, father-child, uncle-child, and grandparent-child. For the purpose of discussion, incestuous behavior involving children is sometimes broadened to include *intrafamily sexual abuse* so that parent figures can be included in the discussion. Reported sexual abuse cases also include adults who are step-parents or are involved in a dating relationship with one of the child's parents. Although not kin, these parent figures represent parental authority to the child.[19]

The cases of intrafamily sexual abuse that are most often reported in the literature are the father-daughter incestuous relationships. Mother-child incest seems to be rarely reported.[13] The American Humane Association estimates at least 5,000 cases of father-daughter incest in the United States per year. In communities with active referral and treatment centers statistics exceed these estimates. For example, the Child Sexual Abuse Treatment Program in San Jose, California, has reported more than 200 father-daughter incest cases per million population per year. Projecting this number to the national population, estimates are 50,000 cases of father-daughter incest per year.[15]

## SCOPE OF THE PROBLEM

Reported child sexual abuse is not limited by race, economic status, or neighborhood.[19] The incidence of child sexual abuse is difficult to assess, but most professionals are now aware that sexual abuse of children occurs more often than previously recognized.[23] Child sexual abuse is considered a major social problem, an issue that is only being recently addressed by professional caregivers, families of abused children, concerned legislators, and community members.

No accurate national statistics exist on child sexual abuse; statistics that do exist

Table 10-2. Incidence of sexual assault reported to Sexual Assault Center, Harborview Medical Center, Seattle, Washington, 1979

| Sex | Request for services | | |
| --- | --- | --- | --- |
| | Male | Female | Total |
| Age by sex | 95 | 430 | 525 |
| 0-4 years | 14 | 59 | 73 |
| 5-8 years | 36 | 88 | 124 |
| 9-12 years | 26 | 93 | 119 |
| 13-16 years | 18 | 187 | 205 |
| Age unknown | 1 | 3 | 4 |

Reprinted with permission of the Sexual Assault Center (SAC), Harborview Medical Center, Seattle, Washington.

reflect only *reported* cases. Reasons for vague statistics on child sexual abuse include the following: (1) social taboos that view child sexual abuse as socially deviant often deter persons with the problem from seeking help; (2) intrafamily sexual abuse commonly goes unreported and is often kept secret; (3) most children (40 to 50%) who are sexually abused never tell anyone; (4) not all the child abuse statutes (laws) of the states in this nation include laws related to child sexual abuse; (5) state registries do not necessarily list child sexual abuse as a separate offense from child abuse; and (6) sometimes cases reported to the police do not get recorded or included with child sexual abuse statistics.

Information on the incidence of child sexual abuse is primarily obtained from reported cases, private research surveys, and data collected from sexual abuse treatment centers. Most researchers assume that a large amount of child sexual abuse goes undetected or unreported, and they consider the reported incidence of child sexual abuse to be "only the tip of the iceberg." Some authorities believe child sexual abuse is widespread, involving 200,000 to 300,000 children a year. Statistics from one study indicate that 1 in 4 children will be involved in some form of inappropriate sexual behavior.[7] Based on current information, statistics indicate that 1 out of 4 women will have been sexually abused by the time she reaches the age of 18.[10]

Some cities reflect a higher reporting rate for child sexual abuse cases. However, higher rates of reported child sexual abuse do not necessarily mean a higher incidence of such abuse; the higher rates may reflect a greater public awareness or greater social service or legal system visibility. For example, Table 10-2 depicts 1979 statistics on child sexual assault for a center in Seattle, Washington, whose professional staff did massive public education efforts and developed treatment programs to which they invited referrals.

As the data in the table show, the center received a total of 525 referrals for 1979; the largest number, 430 (or 82%), were female child victims (this is consistent with reported national data of a higher incidence of sexual abuse in females)[1]; and when the data are separated by age, most victims referred to the center were between the ages of 13 to 16 years.

## FACTS AND MYTHS

Misconceptions about child sexual abuse exist in society as do myths about rape. (See Chapter 1 for a complete discussion of myths related to rape victims.) As more professional caregivers, researchers, legislators, and community members collect data and examine facts, many long-held myths about child sexual abuse are being refuted. It is important that professional nurses know both the facts and the myths about child sexual abuse because this knowledge base aids the delivery of professional nursing care to child victims and their families.

Myths and facts about child sexual abuse can be categorized according to (1) relation to the offender, (2) relation to the child victim, and (3) relation to the sexual abuse. This section presents common myths about child sexual abuse and the corresponding facts. We emphasize that the current "facts" related to child sexual abuse are biased because they represent information based only on *reported* cases rather than all cases of child sexual abuse. Unfortunately, no facts about child sexual abuse can be collected from unreported cases. Despite the biased nature of available information, common myths related to child sexual abuse can be refuted based on facts from reported cases.

## Myths related to the offender

Table 10-3 summarizes current myths and related facts that concern the offender in child sexual abuse cases. The myth that offenders are "dirty old men," dangerous or insane men who grab children and molest them is not supported by facts on reported child sexual abuse cases.[7] Insanity is defined by Webster as "such unsoundness of mind or lack of understanding . . . as removes one from criminal or civil responsibility." Therefore child sexual abuse is viewed as a *criminal* (illegal) act for which the offender is *held responsible* rather than as a psychiatric problem. Child sexual abuse is not a diagnostic category within the Diagnostic and Statistical Manual (III) of the American Psychiatric Association. The child sexual abuse offender is aware of his acts and their illegality—that is, he is not "out of touch with reality" or "deranged." However, most clinicians who do therapy and research with child sexual abuse offenders generally consider such persons to be emotionally disturbed and suffering from severe personality dysfunction in many aspects of their lives. Perpetuation of the myth that the offender is "insane" or "deranged" is related to society's abhorrence of the crime and its need to arrive at an acceptable explanation for such an intolerable deed. (Belief in myths as a response to cognitive dissonance created by violent or abusive crimes is discussed in Chapter 3.) Steps in the thought process that result in belief in myths about the offender are as follows:

1. Child sexual abuse is awful.
2. No one in his or her right mind (no sane person) would sexually abuse a child.
3. Therefore child sexual abuse offenders are insane.

By viewing a person as "insane," one is able to objectify the offender and not see him as someone known, loved, or perceived as responsible (such as father, stepfather, brother, uncle) under the assumption that known, loved, and responsible men do not commit such horrible deeds. For some people it is easier to cope with an intolerable reality (abuse or violence) by believing that only someone not responsible (insane) for

Table 10-3. Myths and facts about sexual offenders of children

| Myths | Facts |
|---|---|
| "Dirty old men," "insane men," or pedophiles commit child sexual abuse. | Sexual offenders of children are usually adult males between the ages of 21 and 30, are not insane, and are not limited to pedophiles. |
| Offenders are nonwhites from lower social classes and poor neighborhoods. | Offenders come from all socioeconomic classes, races, and neighborhoods. |
| Sexual offenders of children are strangers to their victims. | Offenders are usually persons known to the child, such as a family member, neighbor, or friend of the family. |
| Offenders seek sexual gratification from children who seductively precipitate their own victimization. | Offenders use sexual behavior to meet nonsexual needs, such as relief from feelings of low self-esteem and powerlessness. |

his behavior would commit such an act. The net effect of such logic is to deny that child sexual abuse could happen (or is happening) in one's own home, among neighbors, friends, or relatives.

The same type of logic used in arriving at the mythical notion of offenders being insane is used when one concludes that only pedophiles commit child sexual abuse. The general public often regards a pedophile as someone "really weird," which usually translates as a "stranger or someone unknown" who molests children. Once again, the logic permits one to remove the possibility of the crime as an act that occurs at home or with trusted persons. Research generally describes child sexual abuse offenders in terms of one of two types: (1) fixated or (2) regressed.[3] A *fixated child sexual offender,* also called pedophile, is an adult who follows a persistent pattern of being primarily or exclusively attracted, since the time of adolescence, to children or persons significantly younger than himself. In contrast, a *regressed child sexual offender* is an adult who, prior to the offense or under usual circumstances, prefers sexual gratification with peers or adult partners but, under stress or a conflictual adult relationship, replaces the adult partner with a child as a focus of meeting his needs, interests, or desires. Contrary to myth, facts on *reported* child sexual abuse indicate that pedophiles are not responsible for most sexual abuse of children.[9]

As in rape, *motives* of the offender are primarily *power* or *aggression.* In a case of child sexual abuse where *power* is the motive, the offender reports feeling a sense of low self-esteem and powerlessness; he reports feeling secure, competent, and comfortable relating to and getting needs met by a child because he can control the relationship. In child sexual abuse where *aggression* is the motive the offender reports a release of pent-up, accumulated tension through physical and/or psychologic violence. An aggressive child sexual offender may report (1) that merely overpowering the victim is insufficient to decrease intolerable feelings states such as low self-esteem, depression, loneliness, and inadequacy or (2) that hurting the child was not his intent but necessary to attain his goal. The victim of an aggressive offender is frequently a child who has also resisted the offender—for example, a prepuberty child who elects to be with peers rather than the abuser and is forced into compliance with the offender's demands (see discussion of myths below).

Recent clinical data indicate that the offender is a male who also maintains consenting adult heterosexual relationships. The male offender generally has the following characteristics:

1. *Sex.* Over 95% of the reported cases of child sexual abuses are committed by men. Reported cases of women molesting children are rare.
2. *Age.* Most male offenders are between the ages of 21 and 30 years of age. The second most frequent age for offenders is between the ages of 11 and 21 years.
3. *Social status.* Child sexual offenders come from all socioeconomic classes, races, and neighborhoods. They may be upper class and socially prominent, or they may be lower class and socially isolated. No specific class, race, or ethnic background differentiates child sexual offenders.
4. *Relationship to victim.* The offenders are usually persons known to the child. In 80 to 90% of the cases, the offender is a family member, neighbor, or friend of the family.

5. *Psychologic status.* Although child sexual abuse offenders are often emotionally disturbed and suffer from personality dysfunction in many aspects of their lives, current research does *not* report the offender as being "insane" or "out of touch with reality."[3,8,13,19]

## Myths related to the child victim

Table 10-4 presents facts about the victims of child sexual abuse. *Any child* is a potential victim of sexual abuse. As demonstrated in the table, both male and female children are victimized, but sexual abuse is reported to occur more frequently among young girls.[21] Reported child sexual abuse cases show the average age of girl victims to be between 11 and 12 years. A common myth is that the abuse is a one-time occurrence. But often the abuse has lasted for several years and it is only at 11 to 12 years of age that the child victim discloses the abuse.[7] Factors relating to disclosure are discussed under victim responses later in this chapter.

Child sexual abuse victims are *not* concentrated by socioeconomic status, race, or neighborhood. Finally, the National Institute of Mental Helath has reported that 66% of child (ages 2 to 12) sexual abuse incidents were commited during daylight or dusk, usually in unsupervised activities that are a routine part of the child's life such as playing, coming home from school, or taking a walk.[21]

## Myths related to the sexual abuse

Recent evidence indicates that child sexual abuse is usually nonviolent and involves nonforcible contact between the child victim and the offender. Most often the sexual abuse does not involve a physical trauma to the child or forcible penetration of the vagina, rectum, or mouth. The sexual contact usually involves mutual stroking, fondling, masturbating behaviors, disrobing, and handling of genitals. The offender may use the fingers to penetrate the child's vagina or rectum. When penetration does occur, the child's mouth, the largest orifice, is often selected so that genital-oral contact (fellatio or cunnilingus) is the most often reported nature of sexual activity.[24]

Groth describes two types of child sexual abuse: (1) sex-pressured offenses and (2) sex-forced offenses. The *sex-pressured abuse* the offender tries *enticement or entrapment* to pressure the child into sexual contact. Enticement occurs when the offender tries to persuade or convince the child to consent to sexual contact. Entrapment occurs when the offender puts the child in a position of obligation or indebtedness. The offender who uses sex pressure bribes or rewards the child with attention, gifts (money, candy), or approval. This type of offender does not use physical force; he gains sexual control

**Table 10-4. Child sexual abuse victim facts**

| | |
|---|---|
| Age | |
| At onset | 6 to 9 years of age |
| At time of disclosure | 11 to 12 years of age |
| Sex | Most cases are female (90%) |
| Socioeconomic status (SES) | All levels of SES |
| Race | All races |
| Neighborhoods | All neighborhoods |

of the child by "developing a willing or consenting sexual relationship."[13]

In *sex-forced abuse* the offender *intimidates or physically overpowers* the child. Since most children hold adults as authority figures or more powerful persons, the child involved in this type of abuse feels relatively helpless and fears the offender. The offender responsible for sex-forced abuse often does not want to hurt the child, but he will use whatever force or physical aggression is necessary to attain his goal of the sexual act.[13]

The myths surrounding intrafamily sexual abuse are refuted by facts from reported cases. Predominant myths include:

1. *Incest is a one- or two-time occurrence.*

   FACT: Reported incest cases have usually been going on for an average of 2 years prior to discovery. The element of secrecy plays an important part in the sexual relations. Sexual abuse generally begins when a child is between 6 and 9 years old and often continues for many years.

2. *Incest involves a single child in the family.*

   FACT: Incestual relationships are usually not confined to one but often involve other children in the family. Most often the oldest daughter is abused by her father or stepfather and, in cases where there are other children, subsequent daughters or sons may also be abused.

3. *Mothers are always aware of what is going on.*

   FACT: Sometimes the mother of the sexually abused child is uninformed of the assault. If the mother does become aware of the assault, she may remain silent for several reasons. Physical abuse by the father or parent figure and fear of rejection may stop her from acting; or lack of economic and emotional support from the abuser or significant others may also be a factor. The mother may perceive silence as the only mode of survival in the family. Mothers may suspect something is going on within the family, but they are often afraid to find out for sure what is happening between family members or do not know where to get support or help for the family problem. Some mothers are unable to acknowledge the abuse related to their own difficulties with emotional and/or economic dependence on the abuser.

4. *Most sexually abused children want to and will leave home to escape the abusive situation.*

   FACT: Most sexually abused children do *not* want to leave home. However, the children do wish the abuse to cease. Intrafamily sexual abuse is often only disclosed inadvertently or after the child has acquired enough independence to seek outside help.

5. *Incest occurs only in lower socioeconomic families.*

   FACT: Incest affects all families regardless of socioeconomic level. The lower socioeconomic families may be more likely to come to the attention of law enforcement agencies or health care systems. In lower socioeconomic levels persons are also more likely to ask for social service help, and staff will report the case. Families in higher socioeconomic levels seek help from physicians in private practice, clergy, or relatives who do not report incest cases as readily.[14]

## VICTIM RESPONSE

There has been limited research about the effects of sexual abuse on the child. Since children react differently depending on their particular situation, general statements regarding the child victim's response are impossible.[19] Therefore this section attempts to (1) describe variables that have been reported in the literature as affecting child victim responses and (2) report stress reaction responses that have been observed in clinical studies of sexually abused children. Professional nurses are encouraged to assess each child victim as a *unique individual* who is responding to circumstances particular to his or her situation.

Characteristics that are considered to be related to child victim responses include (1) the age and developmental status of the child, (2) the child's role in the abusive situation, (3) the disclosure of the incidence, (4) the child's relationship to the offender, and (5) the reactions of the child's family.[19] Reported child sexual abuse cases demonstrate that children do *not* initiate the sexual abuse and that children do *not* seduce offenders into sexual contact.

In child sexual abuse *the offenders are responsible for the sexual abuse contact.*[19] Children agree to go along with sexual relations for various reasons,[7] including their level of cognitive understanding or personality development. The child's age or developmental status makes the child incapable of using adult judgment to make a decision relating to consent and sexual activity. Young children (less than 6) may sense or know that sexual activity between them and an adult is "wrong," but they may believe or can be convinced by the offender that the norm of the family or community is to engage in sexual activity.[4] Other young children are unsure, ambivalent, or powerless in relation to an adult authority figure who pressures them or convinces them to engage in sexual activity.[18] Some children are rewarded for sexual contact through material goods (money, candy, games), social activities (movies, carnivals, sports games) or adult approval and affection. For other children the sexual encounter begins in a nonsexual manner, and the child is cognitively unaware that sexual activity is to follow.[4] The following clinical example demonstrates how a child with a limited understanding of sexuality interpreted and handled sexual contact.

### CLINICAL EXAMPLE

Susan (age 6) and Kathy (age 10) were attending a Saturday matinee together when a man sat beside Susan. During the movie Susan became aware that the man had put his hand on her leg and, over time, was moving it up her leg until he was under her dress and touching her thighs. Susan began to feel uncomfortable and glanced over at the man, who seemed to be intently watching the movie. Susan became confused and wondered to herself, "Does that man know he has his hand on me? Maybe he does not realize his hand is up my dress." The man proceeded to try to feel under Susan's panties, at which time Susan knew something was unusual—she began to feel strange body sensations and thought the man should not be touching her "private place." Susan finally became so uncomfortable that she asked Kathy to exchange seats with her. (Susan did not share with Kathy her reason for the seat exchange.) As Susan began to move, the man slowly withdrew his hand; he did not move from his seat. In her new seat Susan felt more comfortable and thought to herself, "Kathy will know what to do if that man touches her." Susan could not concentrate fully on the remainder of the movie because she kept peeking through the darkness to see if the man was touching her friend Kathy. After the movie Susan did not say a word to anyone about the incident.

The above clinical example demonstrates how a child with a limited concept of sexuality is not yet fully aware of the implications of the sexual contact and therefore keeps it a secret. The child does not consent to sexual activity, but her confusion and lack of knowledge contribute to her "participation" as an unwilling victim. The child's solution to increasing discomfort was *not* to disclose the event but to remove herself from the situation. Unfortunately, Susan put her older friend in a vulnerable position for sexual abuse.

Enticed or entrapped victims and children who have derived pleasure from sexual contact may not report the event because they misperceive themselves as willing participants and expect to feel guilty if the abuse is discovered.[19] Pressure to keep the sexual activity a secret is generally experienced as psychologic fear. Burgess and Holmstrom describe the following fears that bind children to secrecy: (1) fear of punishment, (2) fear of not being believed, (3) fear of being blamed, and (4) fear of abandonment or rejection.[4]

Burgess and Holmstrom report their observations and impressions of child victim responses by relating the victim responses to the type of sexual abuse. They have identified three categories of victim response based on the type of sexual abuse:[4]

1. *Rape trauma syndrome* is characterized by two phases: (a) an *immediate phase* in which the victim experiences shock and disbelief; physical reactions, including sleep and eating pattern disturbances, and symptoms specific to the body area assaulted; emotional reactions of extreme anxiety and fear; and thoughts about the rape, which the victim attempts to block; and (b) a *long-term reorganization process* noted by changes in life-style, dreams and nightmares, and phobias. Rape trauma syndrome is a time-limited, stress response syndrome that typically follows a forcible sexual assault or abuse. (See Chapter 4 for a detailed discussion of rape trauma syndrome.)

2. *Accessory-to sex* consists of the inability to consent to or not consent to sex because of the victim's stage of personality or cognitive development. The child is placed in a pressured sex situation that results in the responses of the syndrome. A person in a power position pressures the child into sexual activity and pressures the child to keep the activity secret. The result of these pressures influences a child victim's responses and produces stress reactions (discussed later in this chapter).

3. *Sex-stress situation* is an anxiety reaction in response to a situation in which the parties consented to sex but something subsequently "went wrong." The person most anxious about the situation usually discloses its occurrence, with the reporting party usually being (1) parents anxious about a child's sexually active life-style, (2) an anxious "partner" in the (sexual) relationship, or (3) authorities who intervene in the situation. Sex-stress situations are of two types: (1) mutual agreement or (2) contracting for sex.

Burgess and Holmstrom note that many children have *silent reactions*.[4] Silent reactions are characterized by the victim keeping sexual activity a secret from everyone. Reasons for keeping the contact a secret include the following: (1) the offender may threaten to harm, implicate, or discredit the child if the activity is disclosed; (2) the offender may be watching or observing the child to guarantee that the child keeps the secret; and (3) the child may feel loyalty to the offender.

Adolescents (youths between the ages of 13 and 18 years) are usually more conscious of sexuality. Reported incidence, type of attacks, and dynamics of sexual abuse appear different for the adolescent than for the younger child, and they often involve acts of rape. The National Institute for Mental Health has found that 55% of adolescents "were raped on weekends, away from home, often at social affairs."[21] The rape act for adolescents has been reported as longer, involving more force (roughness, slapping, beating, and choking), and including more penal-vaginal intercourse than in child cases.[21] Adolescent sexual abuse victims show reactions that are based on their age and level of physical, psychologic, and social development. Because the adolescent is usually more conscious of sexuality, feelings of guilt, shame, being "soiled," or humiliation may occur after a sexual abuse.[6]

The nature of the relationship between the child and the offender needs to be assessed because it may influence the child victim's response. Sgroi considers that the closer the emotional tie between the child and perpetrator, the "more emotionally traumatic the situation is likely to be for the child." For example, the child may not want to get a relative, friend, or neighbor "in trouble" by disclosing the sexual abuse.[6]

Family responses may also affect the child victim's response to sexual abuse. Initial parental reactions are assessed for the degree of support and concern toward the child. (The variable of family support is explored in the next section of this chapter.)

No one knows for sure how a child will react after a sexual abuse episode. However, based on reported cases, Table 10-5 presents common stress reaction indicators of child sexual abuse. The immediate responses of children are divided according to (1) physical indicators, (2) psychologic indicators, and (3) social indicators. Some of these signs and symptoms may also be indicative of other stressors in the child's life and thus can complicate attempts to assess the presence of child sexual abuse.

### Physical indicators

Physical indicators are signs of physical trauma, bodily injury, pain, or somatic symptoms. Indicators of sexual abuse of the female child include swelling, redness, or bruising of tissue around the vagina (labia minora), which indicates that the child has been penetrated; vaginal discharge, which indicates that the child may have a venereal disease; and pregnancy.[25] Fig. 10-1 depicts body areas frequently subjected to trauma in sexual abuse of the female child.

In the male child subjected to forceful suction of the penis (through fellatio), there may be bruises, redness, or cuts on the shaft or glans of the penis. Bleeding from the urethra suggests that the abuser may have inserted a foreign object. Three days postassault the boy may have a discharge. This may indicate that he has a sexually transmittable disease.[25] Fig. 10-2 depicts body areas frequently subjected to trauma in sexual abuse of the male child.

**Table 10-5. Common stress reaction indicators of child sexual abuse**

| Physical indicators | Psychologic indicators | Social indicators |
| --- | --- | --- |
| Physical trauma to body | Regressive behaviors | No desire for social interaction |
| Complaints of pain | (wanting to be held, thumbsucking) | Poor peer relationships |
| Sleep disturbances | Withdrawal behaviors | Disruptive classroom behaviors |
| Genital injury | (shy, isolated) | Inattention or truancy at school |
| Loss of appetite | Fears | Avoidance of social activities |
| Vaginal or penile discharge | (being alone, going to sleep) | Seductiveness |
| Concerns about pregnancy | Irritability | Inappropriate expressions of affection |
| Difficulty urinating | Short tempered | |
| | Crying | |

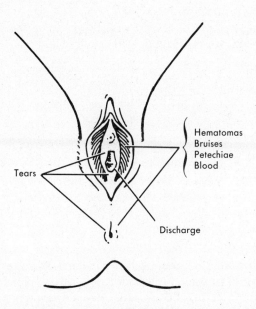

**Fig. 10-1. Physical indicators of sexual abuse in the female child.**

Modified with permission from Paul, D.M.: The medical examination in sexual offenses, Med. Sci. Law **15**:3, 1975.

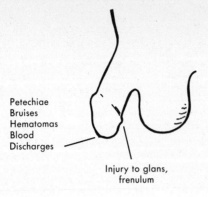

Petechiae
Bruises
Hematomas
Blood
Discharges

Injury to glans,
frenulum

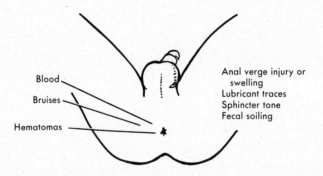

Blood

Bruises

Hematomas

Anal verge injury or
    swelling
Lubricant traces
Sphincter tone
Fecal soiling

**Fig. 10-2. Physical indicators of sexual abuse in the male child.**

Modified with permission from Paul, D.M.: The medical examination in sexual offenses, Med. Sci. Law **15**:5, 1975.

### Psychologic indicators

Psychologic indicators depend on the child's developmental level and usual style of reporting or handling distress.[21] For example, some children may exhibit regression, which is defined as a return to younger, earlier childhood patterns of behavior. Regressive behaviors include thumbsucking, bed-wetting, asking for help in toileting, wanting to be held, or clinging to parents. Other children may exhibit withdrawal—a need to be alone or away from people. Withdrawing behaviors include staying inside, refusing to play with friends, shying away from touching, or running away. Fears are common psychologic responses of children to sexual abuse. Children may fear going to bed, sleeping alone, being around an adult or a male person, going to school, or being away from a parent. Other psychologic indicators include irritability, short-tempered behavior, and crying. Since the psychologic symptoms mentioned above can indicate stressors other than sexual abuse, accurate assessment is a complex matter.

## Social indicators

Like psychologic indicators, social indicators depend on the child's developmental level and usual style of coping with stress. The sexually abused child may want no social interaction or, on the other hand, may want someone always present because of fear of being alone. Poor peer relationships may develop in response to sexual abuse. For example, the child may choose not to play with friends or go to usual social or school activities (movies, football games, playground activities). Classroom behaviors that have been reported include (1) avoidance of gym class, (2) inattention to studies, (3) preoccupations, or (4) increase in physical complaints to the school nurse. Sexually abused children may respond in unusual ways around adults. For example, some children show a preoccupation with sex and may try to express affection in inappropriate ways such as touching the genitals of the adult. Adolescents may act seductive or rebellious, run away, turn to prostitution, abuse alcohol or drugs, or skip school.

Little is known about the long-term effects of child sexual abuse. Studies reported in the literature do not follow child sexual abuse victims for many years. Studies of child victims of intrafamily sexual relations indicate a variety of long-term reactions, depending on the child's unique circumstances and life situation. Reported long-term reactions to incest include guilt, early marriage, low self-esteem, depression, confusion over identity, and a sense of isolation. Other child victims of incest seem able to progress toward adulthood without reporting any consequences of the sexual abuse.[19] A causal effect or direct relationship between the child's sexual abuse and long-term physical and psychologic reactions or behavior influences has not yet been scientifically proved. Further empirical research on the long-term effects of child sexual abuse on the physical, psychologic, or social behaviors of adults is indicated before professional nurses can make general conclusions regarding the long-term effects of child sexual abuse.

Like adult reactions following a rape (see Chapter 4), most stress reactions of child sexual abuse are time limited. These stress reactions are considered *normal signs of psychologic upset*.[19] Many authorities take the position that it is "in the best interest of the child to assume that sexual abuse experiences are potentially harmful."[15]

## FAMILY RESPONSE

Burgess and Holmstrom support the fact that the reactions of the social network may facilitate or further complicate the child's reaction to disclosing the sexual activity.[4] The child's social network is made up of those persons who have emotionally close relationships to the child. (Social network theory is discussed in Chapter 5.)

This section describes findings in the literature that are related to family member responses to the disclosure or discovery of child sexual abuse. Generalizations based on reported findings or clinical studies *cannot* be made because the research efforts and clinical studies of family response are limited. As with child victim responses, professional nurses are encouraged to assess *each family* as to its particular response to child sexual abuse.

Families are often thrown into a crisis state when child sexual abuse is discovered. The period of crisis normally lasts for about 6 to 8 weeks after disclosure or discovery of the event. Families report feeling rage, guilt, confusion, or helplessness. Feelings of the family toward the child often include disbelief and blame.[6] DeFrances has described parental reactions in three ways: (1) child-oriented, (2) self-oriented, and (3) offender-oriented.[10]

### Child-oriented family response

Child-oriented families can positively support the child or negatively blame the child for the sexual abuse. *Positive child-oriented responses* focus on concern for the child—that is, concern for what the child has undergone and what the child is undergoing.[19] *Negative child-oriented responses* include blaming the child for what has happened, being angry with the child for doing something "wrong," pressuring the child to talk about the experience, or overprotecting the child.[6]

### Self-oriented family response

Self-oriented responses center around concern for what others will think about the sexual abuse and the family members. Public humiliation is a primary concern of self-oriented families. Another self-oriented response is to look within the family for someone to blame—for example, the mother, who the family may consider responsible for protection of the child.[19]

### Offender-oriented family response

Offender-oriented responses include blame and anger directed at the offender. Sgroi has described family responses as varying according to the nature of the perpetrator's relationship with the child. Child sexual abuse by a perpetrator outside the family "generates far less emotional trauma for everyone concerned, even though the likelihood of physical trauma is greater."[23] Child sexual abuse by an "intrafamily perpetrator" generally involves a high degree of disturbance for all family members.

When sexual abuse occurs within the family, reactions to disclosure of the abuse can vary depending on the family's functional level.[23] Family reactions to disclosure include:

1. Failure of the mother to deal with the child's sexual abuse
2. Rejection of the child
3. Divided family loyalty
4. Blaming the child
5. Increasing occurrences of violence

Even if it means rejecting the child, mothers sometimes choose not to deal with intrafamily child sexual abuse. As discussed earlier in this chapter, the mother's response pattern may reflect her own emotional or economic dependency on and attachment to the offender.

When the perpetrator is blamed for the intrafamily abuse, the result is often marital disruption through divorce or forceful removal of the perpetrator from the home. Another influence on responses related to intrafamily abuse is divided loyalty: Should the family be loyal to the child and bring the offender (a family member) to the attention of the law, *or* should the family be loyal to family ties and keep the abuse "a family secret," believing that it is not a concern for outside attention?[5]

## SOCIETAL RESPONSE

Almost every society has cultural taboos against child sexual abuse and incest. According to these taboos, it is socially inappropriate and deviant for an adult to subject a child to sexual experiences. Sexual abuse violates existing societal sanctions regarding the ways children learn about human sexuality.[13] Social taboos against incest influence the reporting of such offenses. For example, the "sanctity" of the family and social mores that hold that children are the property of their parents make it difficult for other members of society, such as neighbors or professional caregivers, to enter family systems to stop or prevent intrafamily sexual abuse.[19]

Societal concern about child sexual abuse has just recently come to public notice. Yet the problem of child sexual abuse has always existed, and according to many authorities it shows increasing magnitude.

Societal responses to child sexual abuse are intense, ranging from utter disbelief to anger and distress. The sexual abuse of children is generally never talked about or believed by most people. Those members of society who respond with disbelief would like to believe the myth that child sexual abuse is rare. Some members of society surround child sexual abuse with other myths; for example, they believe that if child sexual abuse occurs, the offender is "a dirty old man" or a deranged person. (Myths related to child sexual abuse were discussed earlier in this chapter).

Other societal responses involve failing to realize that children are *victims* of sexual abuse and not suspects in its perpetration or occurrence. Societal responses to incest cases include focusing on the relationship of the adults rather than trying to understand the impact on the child victims.[17] It can be generally stated that the "universal revulsion" toward child sexual abuse is rarely connected to an understanding of the social problem.[19]

Sexual abuse has been determined by society to be a "sex crime" and is punishable under the law. Society has laws related to rape, fondling, molestation, exhibitionism, and sodomy. Any sexual relations between adults and children are also forbidden by law.[7] In 1974 the Federal Child Abuse Prevention and Treatment Act was passed; it established some guidelines for reporting different types of child abuse. Some states required the reporting of child sexual abuse; other states considered the reporting a matter of court or individual decision.[19] Now all states require the reporting of child sexual abuse.

Laws related to child sexual abuse vary from state to state in definition and detail. For example, in New York there are a total of nine counts for sex offenses: rape (relating to sexual intercourse), sodomy (relating to deviate sexual intercourse), and sexual abuse (relating to sexual contact such as touching the genitals). Sexual abuse is considered a misdemeanor, which is a minor offense punishable by fines or short-term imprisonment, rather than a felony, which is a major offense punishable by imprisonment.[17]

Penalties for incest range from simple fines to long-term imprisonment. In some states incest is not in the sexual offense category but in part of the laws related to the marital relationship.[17] Laws against incest originally developed over concern for the production of biologically defective offspring, which was thought to result from sexual intercourse between persons of the same kinship. More recent social thinking and state laws reflect a belief that sexual relations between children and family members is psychologically detrimental to the personality development of the child.[26]

Some social communities are exploring ways of developing programs to assist or protect the child who reports child sexual abuse.[17] Most communities have two social systems to work with children and families of child sexual abuse: health care systems and legal systems. Health care systems include hospital settings, child abuse treatment centers, and pediatric clinics, all of which have similar goals: to maintain the physical and psychologic well-being of the child and the family. The legal systems that have been set up to work with children and their families include police departments, criminal investigation offices, and the judicial court systems. The goals of the legal system agencies include determining if a crime has been committed, prosecuting offenders, and ensuring availability of professional caregivers for the child and the family.

### Health care systems

When sexually abused children and/or their families seek help from health care services, nurses are aware that they have the following rights:

1. To be treated with respect and dignity, with an appreciation of their age, emotional maturity, and intellectual maturity
2. To be protected from further abuse
3. To receive comprehensive medical and psychologic services from sensitive, trained, child-oriented personnel
4. To have the benefit of thorough and complete collection of evidence to enable court prosecution of the alleged offender
5. To be informed of legal services that are available, including the possibility of pursuing a criminal or civil suit
6. To have access to continued physical and psychologic services as they are available in the community, particularly with experts in victimology[8]

The type of professional health services available may vary within social communities. For example, some communities now provide family counseling in child abuse centers that allow the members of intrafamily sexual abuse to remain together rather than removing the child from the home. Other types of health care services include initial interviewing of the child and the family, medical management of the child, and psychologic management of child and family. (Health care services are described in detail later in this chapter.)

### Legal systems

This section describes the legal system services that are available to children and their families and stresses the need for coordination of social service systems that are concerned with children and families of child sexual abuse. Today every state has a child abuse and child neglect law that *requires* persons to report suspected cases of child abuse.[15] Despite the fact that all states have child abuse statutes, only 42 states include the offense of *child sexual abuse*. Of these 42 states only 3 states have defined child sexual abuse under their child abuse and neglect statute.

In each state at least one agency has statewide responsibility to receive and investigate reports of suspected child abuse. The receiving agency decides whether or not sexual abuse has occurred. In some cases the court may make a final decision. If the court decides sexual abuse has occurred, several actions are possible: (1) the court may order that the child be removed from the home; (2) the court may mandate the family to participate in a treatment program; or (3) the court may bring criminal charges against the offender. Since the majority of child sexual abuses are not reported, very few offenders are prosecuted for their offense or receive therapeutic treatment. Conviction is unlikely because child sexual abuse is difficult to prove.[15]

Estimates show that over 80% of child sexual abuses are reported to police departments. The ways in which the crime is reported to police include (1) a direct report, (2) an indirect report, (3) a referral report, and (4) a proactive report. A *direct report* is made by the child who recognizes that "something bad has happened" and turns to the police as a source of help. A child who reports directly to the police is usually willing to give information and can talk about the incident. An *indirect report* is often received from a parent or parent figure. The child sometimes does not comprehend the nature of the act, and time may have lapsed between the event and the child's disclosure to the parent. The *referral report* involves a social service or agency representative who calls the police to make a report of suspected or disclosed sexual abuse. The referring person, usually from a hospital or school, becomes aware of the sexual abuse while dealing with another problem. A *proactive report* is one in which the police, while investigating a complaint, discover that there is a sexual abuse or an incestuous situation.[17]

The function of the police officer is to establish rapport with the child and collect information related to the reported crime. Police officers also try to solicit the cooperation of the child's parents whenever possible. Besides responding to the child and the family, police officers generally assume other responsibilities: (1) coordinating care with the hospital or child abuse treatment center; (2) determining if a sex crime has been committed; (3) obtaining a description of the offender; (4) communicating with the prosecutor's office and police departments regarding the situation, including crime and offender description; (5) collecting necessary evidence for criminal proceedings and taking the evidence to a laboratory for analysis; (6) recording how the child victim looks and any observations related to the crime; and (7) searching the scene for evidence and checking on witnesses. Some prosecutors' offices have specialists available to assist police officers in sex crime investigations. Coordination between these departments facilitates a thorough investigation of the reported crime.[17]

Some authorities believe that the coordination of social services concerned with victims of child sexual abuse will lead to better treatment services and to more offender arrests and convictions.[19] For example, the coordination of police officer and prosecutor services might decrease the number of interviews to which the child is subjected and could lead to better coordination in areas of the criminal investigation. One suggestion for coordination between police officers and hospital staffs includes having the police inform the hospital about the type of case being brought into the emergency department to ensure the availability of professional caregivers. In turn, the hospital staff would collect evidence properly and inform the police of the outcome of their examination so the police officers could proceed with criminal investigations. Keefe suggests the following areas to be addressed in the coordination of social services: (1) social service agency staff should inform others in the field of their capabilities to avoid role conflict; (2) better coordination could lead to a detection of gaps in service and to community efforts to fill them; and (3) the coordination of services could lead to consistent goals: the physical and psychologic well-being of the child.[17]

## NURSING INTERVENTIONS

Nurses who work with children and families of child sexual abuse get involved at various points in the abuse situation. For example, nurses who work in emergency departments may get involved when the police officer informs the hospital staff that he is bringing a suspected child abuse victim to the emergency room. School nurses may get involved much earlier in the abuse situation by detecting child sexual abuse based on reported classroom behaviors from a concerned teacher or from the physical complaints of a child victim. Community health nurses also identify or detect child sexual abuse through home visits.

Professional nurses who attempt to help children and their families with child sexual abuse keep in mind the ultimate goal of nursing intervention: *to deliver quality care in the best interest of the child.* Nursing interventions with child victims are specifically directed at (1) assessing the child victim's situation in an attempt to understand individual circumstances, (2) knowledge-based clinical skills that relieve the physical, psychologic, and social stressors and do *not* add to any existing trauma for the child or family, and (3) referral for ongoing treatment or counseling as necessary.

Within the limitations of a chapter, it is difficult to explore *all* possible roles for professional nurses related to the care of child abuse victims and their families. However, basic guidelines and goal-directed nursing interventions are presented here to provide professional nurses with a solid framework for directing their nursing care. We have selected interviewing child victims, the medical management of the child, and the psychologic management of the child's parents as essential information to convey to nurses who work in areas of child sexual abuse. Nurses who require additional skills or information are encouraged to refer to the Annotated Suggested Readings at the end of this chapter.

### Interviewing the child

Many people, including professional nurses, believe the myth that a child's accusations of sexual abuse are exaggerations, misunderstandings, or far-fetched fantasies. Facts based on reported cases show that children seldom lie about child sexual abuse. Children who report child sexual abuse are generally speaking from experience and report only what happened. The element of secrecy is a significant factor in the disclosure of child sexual abuse. Children respond to threats and bribery and are often not able to share their experience of sexual abuse. Some children lack the physical, psychologic, or sexual maturity to understand what is happening to them or to explicitly convey their dilemma.[4]

Interviewing the child is a sensitive process during which information is gathered related to the sexual abuse. The initial interview is *not* a police investigation to determine if a crime has been committed. The purpose of the initial interview is threefold: (1) to determine if the child is physically injured, (2) to assess the child's psychologic status, and (3) to assess the child's safety.[11]

Some children are remarkably open about the sexual abuse, often because they are not aware of the seriousness of the crime. Other children find it very difficult to discuss what has happened to them, particularly in the presence of their parents or other adults viewed as rejecting or disapproving. Before proceeding with any interviewing, it is necessary for the nurse to first obtain the parents (or guardian's) consent. Often it is helpful to separate the child from the parents or parent figures because this involves less direct threat to the child for revealing information.[11]

When sexual abuse is suspected or reported, nurses must interview the child in a competent, professional manner. Special skills or techniques are necessary for this type of interviewing. For purposes of this discussion the initial interview can be divided into three areas: (1) establishment of credibility and an alliance, (2) verbal techniques of interviewing, and (3) other expressive techniques of interviewing. Background information for professional caregivers to consider when interviewing child victims of sexual abuse is presented on p. 390.

### Establishing credibility and alliance

The nurse begins to establish credibility by telling the child that he or she has talked with other children who have had problems. In developing an alliance with the child, the nurse (1) lets the child know that the nurse is there to help and (2) tells the child that nurse will be honest. Honesty is particularly important because the child may have been deceived in the abuse situation. The nurse develops a trusting relationship with the child by mentioning specifically who will know about their conversation and what information will be divulged. The following guidelines help the nurse establish a positive alliance with the sexually abused child:

1. Be patient and kind to the child. Allow the child to express feelings without prying. Have a sincere attitude of concern and understanding for what the child has experienced.
2. Respond to disclosure in a calm, professional manner. Quiet, unhurried conversations convey calmness. Children are sensitive to nonverbal responses to disclosure.
3. Help the child feel comfortable in surroundings that are frequently strange. Give clear explanations and answers to questions related to instruments and procedures.

### Verbal techniques of interviewing

Verbal methods of interviewing usually move from the least to the most threatening subject matter for the child. For example, it is helpful to discuss less threatening topics with the child such as school or a favorite television program in a nondirective fashion so that rapport can be established with the child. Next the nurse can return to inquiring about what happened when the child was in the abusive situation. It is important that the nurse convey genuine concern for the child by asking, for example, if the child hurts anywhere.[8] Although verbalization of the abuse is generally considered helpful, no child should be forced to verbalize when seemingly unable to do so.

Language is an important element in the initial interview because it is important that the nurse try to *use phrases or terms that are familiar to the child*.[11] Otherwise the child may become frustrated and the initial alliance may not be established. For exam-

# INTERVIEWING CHILD VICTIMS:
## BACKGROUND INFORMATION*

The following issues affect the child's ability to give a history of sexual assault and influence the cooperativeness of victim and family.

## I. Child's developmental level

A child's cognitive, emotional and social growth occurs in sequential phases of increasingly complex levels of development. Progression occurs with mastery of one stage leading to concentration on the next.

*Cognitive*—Preconceptual, concrete, intuitive thinking in the young child gradually develops toward comprehension of abstract concepts. Time and space begin as personalized notions and gradually are identified as logical and ordered concepts.

*Emotional*—The young child perceives her/himself egocentrically with little ability to identify her/himself in a context. S/he is dependent on the family to meet all needs and invests adults with total authority. The child often reflects the emotional responses of the parents. S/he gradually shifts to greater reliance on peer relationships and emotional commitments to people outside the family.

*Behavioral*—The young child is spontaneous, outgoing and explosive with few internal controls and only a tentative awareness of external limits. S/he has a short attention span. A child most often expresses feelings through behavior rather than verbally. As the child grows, s/he develops internal controls and establishes a sense of identity and independence. Peers and other adults have increasing influence on behavior.

## II. Sexual assault

Characteristics of the assault affect the child's emotional perception of the event and to a great extent determine the response. The closeness of the child's relationship to the offender, the duration of the offense, the amount of secrecy surrounding the assault, and the degree of violence are the factors which have the greatest impact on the child's reaction. The child may very well have ambivalent feelings toward the offender or be dependent on him for other needs.

## III. Response to child

The child is fearful of the consequences of reporting a sexual assault. The response to the family support system and official agencies will directly affect the resolution of the psychological trauma and her/his cooperativeness as a witness. The child fears s/he will be disbelieved or blamed for the assault and almost always is hesitant about reporting.

---

*Reprinted with permission of the Sexual Assault Center, Harborview Medical Center: Interviewing child victims: guidelines for criminal justice system personnel, October 1979 (325 9th Avenue, Seattle, WA 98104).

ple, the nurse could use such words as *tummy* or *wee wee* that the child uses for parts of the body and genital areas.

## CLINICAL EXAMPLE

Sarah, a pediatric nurse in a children's hospital, is assigned to interview Julie, a 4-year-old white female who is brought into the hospital by her distressed mother. The mother reports just discovering that a 14-year-old neighbor boy has been fondling Julie by convincing the child that such an activity is part of a "doctor-patient game" in which Julie plays the part of the patient. The nurse assesses that Julie does not fully understand the sexual nature of the abuse and seems confused by her mother's anxiety.

| Interaction | Analysis |
|---|---|
| *Nurse:* Your mother is a little concerned about the game you play with Steven (neighbor boy). | Tries to relieve the child's anxiety and gives simple explanation of mother's behavior. |
| *Julie:* I play sick; Steven is my doctor. | |
| *Nurse:* I am Sarah, a nurse, and I would like to know how you play. | Establishes a relationship. Gives name and brief, simple explanation of role. |
| *Julie:* It's easy. Do you want to play with me and Steven? | |
| *Nurse:* Not right now, but I would like you to tell me or show me how you play the game. Do you think you can do that? | Does not try to force the child to talk. Continues to build alliance. Enlists child's help. |
| *Julie:* I'll try. | |
| *Nurse:* Good, here are two dolls. Let's pretend that the girl doll is you and that the boy doll is Steven. | Allows playing because it meets child's physical and social needs and allows her to talk less guardedly. |

In the above clinical example the nurse recognized that the mother's anxiety was a potential stressor for the child. The nurse gave the child a simple explanation for the mother's behavior before reviewing the circumstances of the assault. Determining the child's developmental status and capabilities, the nurse used verbal techniques to elicit the child's help in learning the "game." Because the child was familiar with playing games, she was willing to try to teach the nurse how to play. The use of dolls to demonstrate the activity helped the child talk about and portray what happened to her in the abuse situation. The material on pp. 392-396 presents helpful guidelines developed by the Sexual Assault Center, Harborview Medical Center, in Seattle, Washington, for use when conducting a verbal interview with child sexual abuse victims.

*Text continued on p. 397.*

## GUIDELINES FOR VERBAL TECHNIQUES OF INTERVIEWING CHILD SEXUAL ABUSE VICTIMS*

### INTERVIEWING CHILD VICTIMS

### I. Preparing for interview

Prior to interviewing the child, obtain relevant information from parents/guardian, and if applicable, Child Protective Services caseworker, physician, and/or Sexual Assault Center/Rape Relief counselor.

A. Explain your role and procedures to above personnel, and enlist their cooperation.
B. Determine child's general developmental status: age, grade, siblings, family composition, capabilities, ability to write, read, count, ride a bike, tell time, remember events; any unusual problems: physical, intellectual, behavioral, knowledge of anatomy and sexual behavior; family terminology for genital areas.
C. Review circumstances of assault (as reported already by child to other person): what, where, when, by whom, and to whom reported; exact words of child; other persons told by child; how many have interviewed child; child's reaction to assault; how child feels about it and what, if any, behavioral signs of distress (nightmares, withdrawal, regression, acting out) have occurred.
D. Determine what reactions and changes child has been exposed to following revelation of the asault(s): believing; supportive; blaming; angry; ambivalent; parents getting a divorce; move to a new home.

### II. Beginning the interview

A. Setting—The more comfortable for the child, the more information s/he is likely to share.
1. Flexibility—A child likes to move around the room, explore and touch, sit on the floor or adult's lap.
2. Activity—Playing or coloring occupy child's physical needs and allows her/him to talk with less guardedness.

*Reprinted with permission of the Sexual Assault Center, Harborview Medical Center: Interviewing child victims: guidelines for criminal justice system personnel, October 1979 (325 9th Avenue, Seattle, WA 98104).

3. Privacy—Interruptions distract an already short attention span, divert focus of interview, and make self-conscious or apprehensive child withdraw.
4. Support—If the child wishes a parent or other person present, it should be allowed. A frightened or insecure child will not give a complete statement.

B. Establishing a relationship
   1. Introduction—Name, brief and simple explanation of role, and purpose: "I am the lawyer (or legal person) on your side, my job is to talk to children about these things because we want them to stop happening."
   2. General exchange—Ask about name (last name), age, grade, school and teacher's name, siblings, family composition, pets, friends, activities, favorite games, TV shows (it often helps to share personal information when appropriate, e.g., children, pets).
   3. Assess level of sophistication and ability to understand concepts—Does child read, write, count, tell time, know colors or shapes, know the day or date, know birthdate, remember past events (breakfast, yesterday, last year); understand before and after; know about money; assume responsibilities (goes around neighborhood alone, stays at home alone, make dinner, etc.)?

## III. Obtaining history of sexual assault

A. Preliminaries
   1. Use language appropriate to child's level; be sure child understands words. (Watch for signs of confusion, blankness, or embarrassment; be careful with words like incident, occur, penetration, prior ejaculation, etc.)
   2. Do not ask WHY questions ("Why did you go to the house?" "Why didn't you tell?") They tend to sound accusatory.

*Continued.*

## GUIDELINES FOR VERBAL TECHNIQUES OF INTERVIEWING CHILD SEXUAL ABUSE VICTIMS—cont'd

3. Never threaten or try to force a reluctant child to talk. Pressure causes a child to clam up and may further traumatize her/him.

4. Be aware that the child who has been instructed or threatened not to tell by the offender (ESPECIALLY if a parent) will be very reluctant and full of anxiety (you will usually notice a change in the child's affect while talking about the assault). The fears often need to be allayed.

   "It's not bad to tell what happened."

   "You won't get in trouble."

   "You can help your dad by telling what happened."

   "It wasn't your fault."

   "You're not to blame."

5. Interviewer's affective response should be consonant with child's perception of assault (e.g., don't emphasize jail for the offender if the child has expressed positive feelings toward him).

6. Ask direct, simple questions as open-ended as allowed by child's level of comprehension and ability to talk about the assault.

B. Statement

1. WHAT

   "Can you tell me what happened?"

   "I need to know what the man did."

   "Did he ever touch you? Where?"

   "Have you ever seen him with his clothes off?"

   "Did you ever see his penis (thing, pee pee, wiener) get big?"

   "Did anything ever come out of it?"

   Once basic information is elicited, ask specifically about other types of sexual contact.

   "Did he ever put it into your mouth?"

   "Did he ever make you touch him on his penis?"

2. WHO

   Child's response here will probably not be elaborate. Most children know the offender and can name him, although in some cases the child may not understand relationship to self or family. Ascertain from other sources what is the exact nature/extent of the relationship.

3. WHEN

The response to this question will depend on child's ability, how recently assault happened, lapse between last incident and report, number of assaults (children will tend to confuse or mix separate incidents). If the child is under six, information regarding time is unlikely to be reliable. An older child can often narrow down dates and times using recognizable events or associating assault with other incidents.

"Was it before your birthday, the weekend, Valentine's Day?"

"Was it nighttime or daytime?"

"Did it happen after dinner, 'Happy Days,' your brother's bedtime?"

4. WHERE

The assault usually occurs in the child's and/or offender's home. Information about which room, where other family members were, where child was before assault may be learned.

5. COERCION

What kind of force, threat, enticement, pressure was used to insure cooperation and secrecy?"

"Did he tell you not to tell?" "What did he say?"

"Did he say something bad would happen or you would get in trouble if you told?"

"Did the man say it was a secret?"

C. Assessing credibility and competency

1. Does child describe acts or experience to which s/he would not have normally been exposed? (Average child is not familiar with erection or ejaculation until adolescence at the earliest.)

2. Does child describe circumstances and characteristics typical of sexual assault situation? ("He told me that it was our secret"; "He said I couldn't go out if I didn't do it"; "He told me it was sex education.")

*Continued.*

## GUIDELINES FOR VERBAL TECHNIQUES
## OF INTERVIEWING CHILD
## SEXUAL ABUSE VICTIMS—cont'd

3. How and under what circumstances did child tell? What were exact words?
4. How many times has child given the history and how consistent is it regarding the basic facts of the assault (note times, dates, circumstances, sequence of events, etc.)?
5. How much spontaneous information can child provide? How much prompting is required?
6. Can child define difference between truth and a lie? (This question is not actually very useful with young children because they learn this by rote but may not understand the concepts.)

IV. **Closing the interview**

A. Praise/thank child for information/cooperation.
B. Provide information
   1. Child—do not extract promises from child regarding testifying. Most children cannot project themselves into an unknown situation and predict how they will behave. Questions about testifying in court or undue emphasis on trial will have little meaning and often frightens the child (causing nightmares and apprehension).
   2. Parent—Produce simple, straightforward information about what will happen next in the criminal justice system and approximately when the likelihood of trial, etc.
C. Enlist cooperation—Let them know who to contact for status reports or in an emergency, express appreciation and understanding for the effort they are making by reporting and following through on process.
D. Answer questions, solicit responses.

## Expressive techniques of interviewing

Less verbal children may find more comfort in describing what has happened to them through methods that permit them to act out or draw the traumatic experience through play or artwork. Two expressive methods used to interview child sexual abuse victims are drawing pictures and play therapy. In the interview process the nurse provides the less verbal child with colored paper and magic markers, and the nurse asks the child to draw three pictures: (1) a picture of his/her family and home, (2) a picture of him/herself, and (3) what happened that brought the child to the hospital.[3] These drawings are then labeled and submitted as evidence of information gathered about the abuse. Drawings provide the nurse with a stimulus for further exploration of the events surrounding the child's sexual abuse. In the example below, the child (age 9) talks about her drawing, which is part of the account of her sexual victimization.

CLINICAL EXAMPLE

*Nurse:* Who is the man in the picture?
*Child:* Oh, he's the babysitter.
*Nurse:* Where is Mommy?
*Child:* She is next door playing cards with the neighbors.
*Nurse:* What is happening with you and the babysitter?
*Child:* We were playing "snuggles."
*Nurse:* How do you play "snuggles"?
*Child:* Well, I sit on his lap and he holds me, wraps me up in his arms. Then after awhile he starts to touch me.
*Nurse:* Where does he touch you?
*Child:* Here (pointing to genitals) and here (pointing to breasts).
*Nurse:* I see. And what does he say to you about touching you?
*Child:* Sometimes he says that he only plays "snuggles" with his *most favorite* child, so I feel special. Sometimes he says he won't come back if I don't play with him, and I don't want him to go away.

In the above clinical example the nurse helped the child talk about what happened in her sexual victimization. The child described to the nurse a situation of sex-pressured abuse. She was *enticed* into the transaction with the babysitter by his presentation of the abuse as an activity he shares only with a *favorite* child and *entrapped* to comply with his wishes because of her fear of losing him if she refused. The child also talked about the acts of sexual abuse by pointing to where the babysitter touched her. For some children drawings take away the pressure of verbalizing and provide a means to talk about what has happened. The nurse is not responsible for diagnosing or interpreting drawings. Sometimes an expert in children's art therapy is consulted for diagnostic or interpretive assessments. However, the nurse can examine the drawings for their general portrayal of a child's state of psychologic stress and resultant disorganization (see Burgess and others, 1981, cited in Annotated Suggested Readings.) Art therapy is used more often by some treatment centers in follow-up care than during the immediate interview in the emergency department.[3] However, the technique of art therapy is useful (particularly if a child is not verbal) at most points in assessment and intervention.

Play therapy with puppets and dolls is another expressive method nurses use to help children talk about or portray in play what has happened in the abuse situation. It is important that anatomically correct dolls be used for this intervention. Action toys, dollhouses, and hand-sized dolls are used by sexually abused children to project their feelings and to convey what happened to them during the sexual abuse. Some nurses and mental health professionals prefer to use play-therapy expressive techniques in follow-up care. The use of puppets and dolls requires a cooperative child, good rapport with the clinician, and a degree of comfortable intimacy that often may not be developed in one short-term intervention interview.[11] When used in follow-up care, the play-therapy approach has been found to be very helpful for children.

### Medical management

The medical examination ascertains any injury the child may have sustained as a result of sexual abuse. Such injury may include scratches or bruises, hematomas, lacerations, and injuries to the head, scalp, back, neck, torso, and extremities. Bruises may

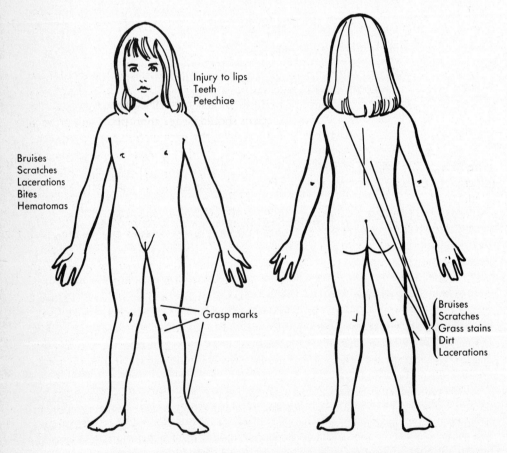

Injury to lips
Teeth
Petechiae

Bruises
Scratches
Lacerations
Bites
Hematomas

Grasp marks

Bruises
Scratches
Grass stains
Dirt
Lacerations

**Fig. 10-3. Trauma and foreign substance sites assessed in sexually abused children.**

Modified with permission from Paul, D.M.: The medical examination in sexual offenses, Med. Sci. Law **15:**1, 1975.

not appear on the initial examination because they take time to become visible. The nurse is advised to see the child within a day or two of the sexual abuse to examine for bruises that may have been sustained in the child's efforts to escape, to resist forceful spreading of the legs, or to avoid being grasped and restrained. Photographs of these injuries are obtained for later use in legal proceedings as evidence of abuse to the child.[25] Fig. 10-3 depicts common injuries children sustain and the areas of the body the nurse and physician closely evaluate in a medical examination.

A careful description of the genital anatomy, an examination of the child's clothing, and tests for the presence of sperm also need to be included in the examination. Evidence is collected according to the same protocol discussed for hospital care of the rape victim (see Chapter 6). A Johnson Rape Evidence Kit* provides prepackaged materials that facilitate collection of evidence. Results of the medical examination are to be labeled and well documented. Any significant statements made by the child or family members should also be documented. Medical records and evidence collected are then managed according to local agency and legal procedures.[24]

### Positioning for examination

Professional caregivers attempt to minimize the anxiety and discomfort involved in the medical management of child sexual abuse. The intent is to decrease trauma, not compound it. Thus the necessary procedures should be well explained to both the child and the parents. The child's explanations should be age appropriate and given in terminology the child can understand. Generally, the examination moves from the least threatening to the most threatening and invasive procedures.[11] The presence of parents or guardians during this procedure should be considered optional; it is usually determined by the child's age and comfort as well as the hospital's protocol for child sexual abuse examinations.

When positioning a child for examination, it is important for the nurse to be aware of positions used during the sexual victimization that might be upsetting for the child. For example, if the child was sexually victimized while being held in a frog-leg position, this position might increase the child's stress state if used for the examination; in such a case an alternate position would be indicated. Positioning for examination of the external genitalia varies according to the child's age and level of comfort. An infant can be examined on the mother's lap and in a frog-leg position (see Fig. 10-4). Older children are examined in a lithotomy position with their feet flat on the table. The child's feet can be gently lifted for examination of injury to the external genitalia (see Fig. 10-5). Stirrups are not used because they are beyond the child's reach, do not fit, and are uncomfortable.

The child is more comfortable, less anxious, and less frightened when encouraged to participate in the examination process. For example, the nurse can encourage the child to elevate herself or himself on the elbows so that the child can observe the collection of evidence and assessment of external trauma. Mirrors can be given to the child or held in place for seeing "what is going on down below." The use of drapes or sheets that block the site being examined or block eye contact with the professional

---

*Kits are prepared by Sirchie Laboratories, Morristown, N.J.

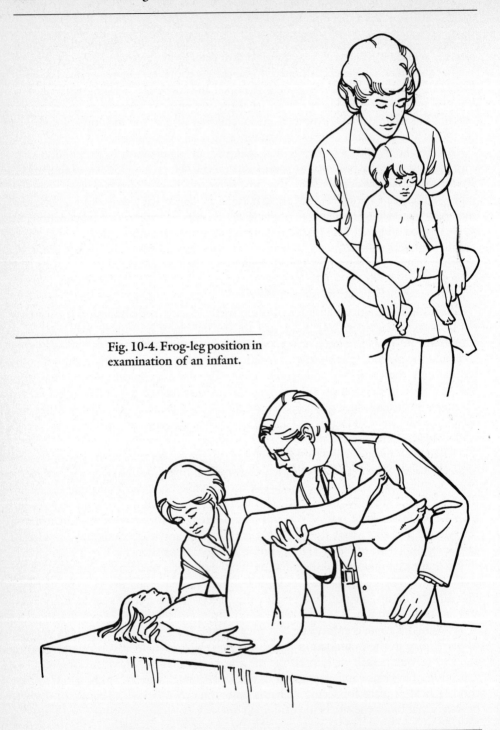

Fig. 10-4. Frog-leg position in examination of an infant.

Fig. 10-5. Lithotomy position in examination of an older female child.

staff should be avoided. If children can help hold the evidence collected, they will be distracted from intense anxiety, which becomes redirected toward participating in their care and trusting the nurse. If swelling, redness, lacerations, and blood are found upon examining the labia majora, labia minora, urethra, and anus, the physician is to be notified to complete further examination. Young females evidencing condyloma acuminata, vaginal discharge, or herpes genitalis are to be highly suspected as victims of sexual abuse, and arrangements for follow-up referral and treatment should be considered.[11]

The internal vaginal examination should be undertaken only when indicated by evidence of penetration, genital trauma, or insertion of a foreign object into the vagina; bleeding; extensive abdominal trauma; or a history of sexual activity. When there is little to no trauma, there is no need for this examination. Some agency protocols recommend the use of anesthesia for a child under the age of 12 to prevent further physical and psychologic trauma from an internal vaginal exam. However, the examination can usually be completed without sedation and minimal psychologic trauma if it is done gently and with understanding and if the child is encouraged to participate in the procedure.[27] The child should be reassured that the physician will proceed slowly and not hurt him or her further. If the nurse is relaxed about the procedure, this attitude will be communicated and comforting to the child. The child should be prepared for each step of the examination procedure to experience a sense of control by knowing "what comes next." For example, the nurse may tell the child: "The doctor is going to look at the outside of your bottom to see that it didn't get hurt either and if there is anything we can do to help you heal if it looks like you got hurt there. If you feel uncomfortable, let me know so we can slow down and help you." The nurse should let the child know that any discomfort experienced will be temporary and that "a little bit of discomfort now" will assure that the child's body is healthy.

Positioning for the internal vaginal examination depends on the age of the child. An infant or young child can be examined in the frog-leg position while sitting on the mother's lap. The hymen can be examined by putting the index fingers on the labia major and laterally spreading the labia apart while pressing downward toward the floor[11] (see Fig. 10-6). Examination of the hymen in an older child can be accomplished by the use of a knee-chest position, which eliminates the need for using a speculum in conducting the examination[11] (see Fig. 10-7).

With the child in a knee-chest position the vagina and cervix can be examined while the child rests with arms folded on the table under the head. The child can usually hold a knee-chest position for several minutes without undue discomfort, and the examination can be more easily completed than if the child were lying flat on the table. An otoscope is adequate for visualization of trauma to the area or the presence of foreign matter. The examiner may find that the help of an assistant in spreading the child's buttocks facilitates the examination process.[11]

The condition of the hymen can be described by the use of one of four basic phrases: (1) "the hymen is present, intact, and free of evidence of trauma"; (2) "the hymen is present, intact, and shows evidence of old scarring"; (3) "the hymen is present and recently ruptured"; or (4) "the hymen is absent."[27] If no trauma is present and the hymen is intact, the internal examination can be discontinued.

Speculum examinations are completed on young females who are sexually active or

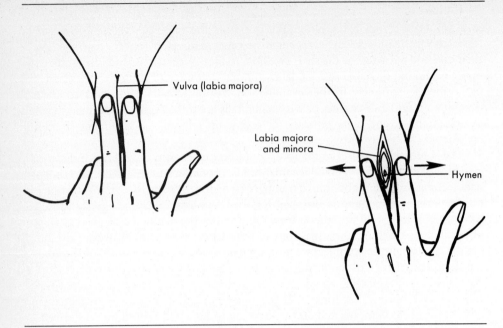

Fig. 10-6. Examination of the hymen in the female child.

if the offender has attempted to have intercourse with the victim. A well-lubricated pediatric speculum is used for the examination, and the child should be told to "bear down" when the speculum is being inserted. Although young children may engage in sexual explorations and experimentation, considered by some to be age-appropriate behavior, it cannot be assumed that these young children understand their bodies. The examination procedures need to be explained to children in simple terminology, and children can be encouraged to participate in the exam process. For example, the child can be instructed to elevate herself on her elbows to observe her genitalia in a mirror provided by the nurse. The nurse can explain to the child different parts of the body. The child can be asked to point to traumatized body structures and to describe what discomfort she is experiencing. If the physician encounters difficulty in inserting a pediatric speculum, the speculum should be removed quickly after a quick observation of the vaginal vault is made.[11]

Tests completed from an internal vaginal examination are the same as those completed in the hospital care of a rape victim (see Chapter 6). Swabs, smears, and slides are prepared to diagnose venereal disease, gonorrhea, and the presence of sperm by an acid phosphatase test. Oral specimens are also collected. Prophylactic treatment may be instituted for venereal disease.

A rectovaginal examination is the last procedure done to rule out trauma that is secondary to a vaginal assault or a direct result of sodomy. The abdomen is palpated and, in the female child, the cervix is located. If the child has reached menarche, then the ovaries can also be felt. The rectal examination is completed by the physician. Swabs are taken to test for gonorrhea, sperm, and acid phosphatase.

A procedural guide for child sexual abuse examination that outlines tests to be

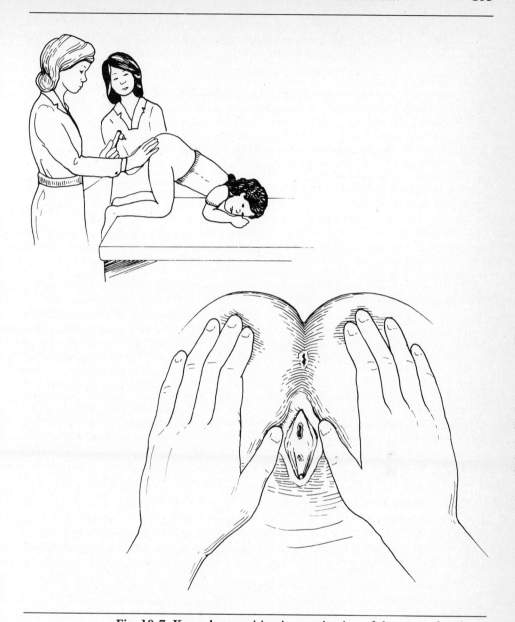

**Fig. 10-7. Knee-chest position in examination of the young female.**

From Chinn, P.L., and Leonard, K.B.: Current practice in pediatric nursing, vol. 3, St. Louis, 1980, The C.V. Mosby Co.

completed has been developed by Children's Hospital, Pittsburgh, Pa., and has been printed in Appendix Q.[9] With the increase in reported sexual abuse, professionals offering health care to child/adolescent victims have developed protocols for emergency room care of victims. The emergency room protocol for child/adolescent patients developed by the Sexual Assault Center, Harborview Medical Center in Seattle, Washington, has been reprinted in Appendix R. In completing the sexual assault examination, evidence of trauma is recorded on an illustration such as the Traumagram (See Appendix S). Finally, as in the care of rape victims, the nurse will find a checklist of evidence collection procedures helpful in completing the examination. One evidence collection checklist developed by the Sexual Assault Center, Harborview Medical Center in Seattle, Washington, has been reprinted in Appendix S.

### Psychologic management of the child's parents

Parents of sexually abused children may react by not believing the child, by believing the child but feeling unable to directly acknowledge or deal with the abuse, or by becoming extremely upset and reacting irrationally. The parents of sexually abused children are indirect victims of the abuse.

Understanding the sequence of events during the crisis period (6 to 8 weeks after disclosure of the event) enables the professional nurse to take into consideration the number of stressors impacting on a family after disclosure or discovery of child sexual abuse: (1) a trip to the hospital for a physical exam by a physician; (2) police involvement because sexual abuse is a crime; (3) concern for privacy and fear that neighbors or community members will learn of the event; (4) decisions about pressing charges or involvement in other criminal or court proceedings; and (5) child abuse and child neglect civil proceedings in incest cases.

In the health care system nurses help parents of child sexual abuse cope with the crisis. The following guidelines are some general ways in which nurses can provide parents with information or support:[12,14]

1. Encourage parents to believe the child unless allegations are proven false. Encourage parents not to jeopardize the child's trust in them.

2. If the parental attitude is not destructive, invite one parent to be with the child during the physical exam. (Policy on this matter will vary according to geographic regions and hospitals.) If the parent is unable to be present for the examination, the professional nurse offers a thorough explanation of the findings, stating where any physical trauma was noted and the child's general state of health.

3. Teach parents about signs and symptoms of venereal disease, urinary tract infections, or any other physical symptoms that may be normal and natural following child sexual abuse. Reassure the parents that any cultures or laboratory tests that were taken will be reported to them if there is any cause for concern.

4. Assess the family's coping reactions and their flexibility in handling the crisis. Explain what parents might expect in terms of short- or long-term "normal" reactions from their child and from themselves. Identify the need for short- or longer-term counseling with the parents, and refer the family for continued management if necessary. Providing parents with information on "normal reactions" also assists in limiting the extent to which they may otherwise overprotectively scrutinize the child's behavior and activities.

Centers for child sexual abuse assist parents through counseling or educational services to better understand the problems and to help their child following sexual assault.[6] In San Jose, California, a self-help group called Parents United was formed by individuals and families who have experienced child sexual molestation. The purpose of this group is to provide assistance to such families, particularly during the initial crisis period following child sexual abuse.[20]

Parents often want to be helpful to their child but are not always familiar with *how to be helpful* or what to expect from the child or agencies involved in handling cases of reported child sexual abuse.[19] Nurses who work with families following child sexual abuse assess family responses to the event and determine interventions that are most helpful in facilitating the family's response through the crisis period.

Parental response to child sexual abuse by a stranger is usually less complex than if the parents know the attacker or if he is related to the family. The following discussion of psychologic management of the child's parents is divided into three sections: (1) sexual abuse by a stranger; (2) sexual abuse by a person known to the family; and (3) sexual abuse by an immediate family member (incest).

### Sexual abuse by a stranger

Cases of nonviolent sexual abuse by a stranger can be treated with crisis intervention techniques.[17] The crisis intervention model emphasizes (1) gaining a realistic perception of the event, (2) developing or supporting healthy coping mechanisms, and (3) providing situational support. Within a short time the child and the family return to a functional, healthy state of equilibrium. (See Chapter 7 for a complete discussion of the crisis intervention model.)

Parents who react negatively to the child and who demonstrate behaviors that show an inability to give support to the child are usually referred immediately for continued counseling. Weeks recommends the following advice to parents whose children have been sexually abused by a stranger:

1. Discuss the incident with the child in an open, calm, and understanding manner. Judgmental remarks inhibit children from speaking openly and honestly.
2. Children should be allowed to discuss the incident rather than to "forget about it." Be careful not to probe or ask too many questions. Allow the child to discuss the incident at the child's comfort level.
3. The incident *is a crisis* for the family and the child, but lasting effects are not usual in sexual abuse cases by a stranger.
4. Children may react more to the parental responses than to the sexual abuse situation. Taking their cues from parents, children will attach significance to the event based largely on their parents' responses.
5. Children will show "normal" stress reaction patterns after the abuse. Regressive, withdrawn, or fearful behaviors should be handled with reassurance and understanding.
6. If any lasting effects of stress are noted in the child (more than 6 to 8 weeks), the parents should seek counseling or consultative services.[28]

### Sexual abuse by a person known to the family

Counseling techniques used with parents of children who disclose a sexual abuse by a perpetrator known to the family depend on the parental response to the disclosure. For example, some parents may think that the child fabricated or fantasized the situation because the parents trust the perpetrator and cannot believe such an abuse would happen. Other parents may feel anger toward the perpetrator or guilty for allowing the perpetrator to be alone with the child. Weeks suggests these general guidelines for parents in this type of sexual abuse situation:

1. Parents should be careful to obtain an accurate story from the child. If for some reason the parents doubt the child's story, they would be wise to monitor the child's interaction with the individual and never allow the child to be alone with the suspected offender.

2. Parents should discuss the child's story with the accused offender, making sure that the child is not present. The intent is not to prove the story's validity, but to put emphasis on the future relationship of the offender and the child. The parents send a clear message that the offender will not be allowed to visit the child alone at any time. In cases of sexual abuse by a person known to the family, the child is informed about visiting rules and the parents might suggest psychiatric evaluation for the offender.

3. The child should be taken for immediate physical and psychiatric assessment related to the sexual abuse.

4. The parents can explain to the child that the offender "is a nice person, but his actions with you are wrong."[28]

The following clinical example demonstrates nursing intervention with a family who knew the person who committed the sexual abuse. The nurse's response depends on the parental response to the disclosure.

### CLINICAL EXAMPLE

Tracy is a 10-year old black female who attends a school near her home. Tracy's teacher, known by her parents for years, has been sexually molesting young girls in the school (about 5 or 6 of them), including the victim. One day Tracy came home and told her mother that she wanted to change schools. The mother insisted that Tracy tell her what was going on, and the child divulged details of sexual abuse.

Tracy's mother brought her into the emergency room and requested a medical examination for her daughter. The following interaction took place with the emergency room nurse.

| Interaction | Analysis |
|---|---|
| *Mother:* I can hardly believe this. My husband and I have known Jim (the teacher) for years! | |
| *Nurse:* It's hard to believe that this sort of thing can happen, especially by someone you know. | Provides information and recognizes that denial and doubt are normal reactions to first hearing of sexual abuse by someone known to the family. |
| *Mother:* But I have no reason to doubt Tracy's story. She would not make up a thing like this. . . . Could she? | |

| Interaction | Analysis |
|---|---|
| *Nurse:* Children usually do not make up things like this. | Encourages mother to believe the child and not to jeopardize the child's trust in her. |
| *Mother:* I can't think of any reason she would make this up. No, it's true. . . . This is terrible. | |
| *Nurse:* Tracy will get the best possible care right now. It was wise of you to bring her in for an examination. | Gives mother positive recognition for health care decision. Also provides reassurance and establishes an alliance. |
| *Mother:* What will they do to her? Can I be with her? | |
| *Nurse:* The physician will give her a thorough physical exam and check for signs of sexual abuse. You can be with Tracy if you want. | Gives simple explanation and invites mother to be with child during the physical exam. Allows way for mother to be helpful. |
| *Mother:* Thank you. I want to be with her; she needs me. | |

As demonstrated in this clinical example, the initial family reaction to hearing about sexual abuse by someone known to them is disbelief and shock. Some parents initially doubt the child's report and send a message to the child that they do not believe the child's account. Because children rarely make up a story of sexual abuse, the wise parent seeks immediate physical and psychologic assessment of the sexual abuse. The nurse assesses the family's coping reactions and helps them by providing information and support.

### Sexual abuse by an immediate family member

The psychologic management of incestuous relationships is complex. The professional nurse addresses each situation before deciding on nursing intervention strategies. The child and family are generally referred (or court ordered) to family counseling (if available). It is believed by some professionals that to remove the father or child from the home does not help the child or the family.[25]

The occurrence of father-daughter incest generally reflects an overall pattern of family dysfunction.[12] For example, incest may be one symptom of an overall family pattern of child abuse.[17] All family members and their intrarelationships need to be assessed to understand the intrafamily structure and dynamics.

Motivational intents underlying intrafamily sexual abuse varies with reported cases. Literature reports the following intents in intrafamily sexual abuse: (1) retaliation by husband to wife's unfaithfulness (real or imagined), (2) a sense of entitlement by a parent to their children (sexual property), (3) loneliness and the need for closeness and relatedness, and (4) isolation and depression.[19]

Although masked by a social facade of stability and contentment, intrafamily sexual abuse symptoms are termed *dysfunctional*—that is, they represent a high degree of family disruption and poor interpersonal relationships. The key factor in father-daughter incest is often the husband-wife relationship, which is described as "strained or nonexistent" and characterized by "a great deal of underlying hostility [which] may be present on both sides."[19] Groth reports finding the "marital relationship between husband and wife to be characterized by dependent attachments on the part of one or both parents . . . unspoken expectations met with frustration, and immature needs [that] sabotage the marital relationship."[13]

Parental sexual abuse is rarely violent. The sexual contact may include fondling, forced masturbation, oral-genital contact, or vaginal or anal intercourse. The offender has needs (warmth, love, sexual gratification), feels inadequate or frustrated in obtaining them from his adult spouse/partner, and seeks out his child. The child does not usually reject the father's request for sexual relations for one or more reasons: (1) he or she may be in search of love and caring; (2) he or she may be flattered by the father's attention; (3) he or she may submit to the authority of a parent figure; (4) he or she may be unaware that sexual relations with the father are unusual; (5) he or she may fear rejection or other types of abuse.[22]

If the disclosure of intrafamily sexual abuse leads to further disruption or if a member leaves the family, psychologic management involves counseling of the remaining family members to help them cope with the multiple stressors. Long-term counseling with parents of intrafamily sexual abuse has many goals:

1. To assess the family's level of dysfunction and determine intrafamily structure and the dynamics involved in the sexual abuse
2. To assess the motivational intents underlying the incestuous relationship
3. To rework and stabilize the husband-wife relationship through couples therapy
4. To offer group therapy separately for the offender, the mate-spouse, and the victim to work through (a) predisposing and precipitating conflicts that are acted out by the maladaptive sexual abuse behavior and (b) the impact of the abuse on the family

## PREVENTION

The prevention of child sexual abuse can be approached in two ways: (1) increased public awareness to the problem and (2) educational campaigns. The general public needs to know that the problem of child sexual abuse exists.[15] Many professionals and society members are unaware, fail to recognize, or deny the reality of child sexual abuse.

Public awareness of child sexual abuse is beginning to grow for several reasons: (1) national and local media—such as radio, television, educational pamphlets, and newspapers—are giving more attention to the topic of child sexual abuse; (2) increased attention regarding rape victims and more sexual assault legislation at the federal and state levels has heightened public awareness to the problem of child sexual abuse; (3) greater public attention to the issues related to child abuse has drawn attention to the specific problem of child sexual abuse; (4) more professional caregivers have shown an interest in the problems related to child sexual abuse; (treatment centers for offenders, victims, and families of child sexual abuse are being started in many cities); and (5) greater societal discussion of child abuse and sexuality issues among lay people and professionals has drawn more public attention to issues related to child sexual abuse.[7]

Educational campaigns are directed at professional caregivers, teachers, parents, and children. Professional caregivers and teachers learn to disseminate information about the problem of child sexual abuse, to detect signs of child sexual abuse, and to refer cases of suspected child abuse for physical and psychologic treatment. Education campaigns directed at parents make them aware of the possibility of child sexual abuse, which may happen to children "near and dear" to them. In "A Message to Parents about Child Sexual Abuse," Children's Hospital National Medical Center in Washington, D.C., describes the following preventive measures that parents can take in relation to child sexual abuse: (1) telling children that their bodies are "private" and to seek help immediately if any person or persons attempts to do things to their bodies; (2) cautioning children about playing alone in isolated places; (3) sending clear expectations about when children are to be home from school; and (4) teaching children how to get help in case of emergencies.[6]

Children usually learn about sexuality through guidance from parents or teachers. As guidelines, children generally learn that (1) sexuality is normal; (2) sexual behavior is intimate and private; and (3) persons should *never* engage in sexual activity against their wishes. Attempts to initiate child sexual abuse preventions programs in elementary and secondary schools are generally directed toward female students. Since a large number of rapists and sexual offenders of children are young males (see Chapter 2), prevention programs can also reach potential offenders if they are directed toward male students. Educational programs aimed at prevention of child sexual abuse help children develop an increased awareness of "good" touch from "bad" touch, of strange or dangerous sexual situations that may involve someone they know, inform children who suffer from sexual abuse that their experience is not "normal," and direct sexually abused children to where they can go for help.

Helping older children and adolescents prevent child sexual abuse, professional nurses can explain that many cases of child sexual abuse occur under certain circumstances, such as hitchhiking, babysitting, dating, in the home, and on the street. The older child's and adolescent's recognition of a potentially dangerous situation is his or her best defense and protection against child sexual abuse. The following preventive measures have been recommended:

1. *Hitchhiking.* Educational programs generally recommend a safer way to travel, such as buses, cars, carpools, or even walking. If the child or adolescent is determined to hitchhike, then the following suggestions are offered: never hitchhike alone; see if someone is hiding in the back seat; and do not accept a ride from someone who has changed direction just to pick you up.
2. *Babysitting.* Be sure you know the people you are sitting for, or get a reliable reference. A parent or friend should have the address and telephone number where you are sitting and the expected time of return. Make sure of transportation to and from the house.
3. *Dating.* Try to find out something about your first date prior to making the date. If at all possible double-date, or at least go places where there are other people. Avoid being alone with someone you do not know well. Always keep someone informed of where you are going on the date, who you are with, and when you expect to return.

## SUMMARY

Existing research and literature related to child sexual abuse is limited. The numbers of reported child sexual abuse cases and the research studies related to the subject provide information that cannot be generalized to all situations of child sexual abuse. Yet professional nurses draw on this information to obtain an overall picture of the problem. They learn to critically review reported facts and research studies, noting how terms such as *child* or *sexual abuse* are defined. When professional nurses learn the facts of child sexual abuse, many wonder how they could have believed the myths about the crime. An understanding of the facts and the scope of the problem help nurses become aware that child sexual abuse is widespread and that a large number of cases go undetected and unreported.

Reported cases of child sexual abuse provide nurses with general information about child victim responses and family reactions that follow disclosure or discovery of the abuse. Characteristics of a child's reaction are related to (1) the child's age and developmental status, (2) the child's role in the abusive situation, (3) the disclosure of the incident, (4) the child's relationship to the offender, and (5) the reactions of the child's family. Families are often undergoing a period of crisis after the discovery of child sexual abuse. Feelings of rage, guilt, blame, or confusion are directed three ways: (1) toward the child, (2) toward the family, and (3) toward the offender. When sexual abuse occurs within the family, the reactions of the child and the family reflect the level of family dysfunction. Nurses are encouraged to assess each case as a unique situation since children and families respond to particular circumstances related to the abuse.

Societal responses to child sexual abuse cover a wide range—from utter disbelief to distress. Health care systems and legal systems are present in most communities to assist sexually abused children and their families. The responses of health caregivers and legal staff often reflect the many myths held in the wider community regarding child sexual abuse. Educational campaigns and coordination of community social systems can lead to better treatment services and better criminal investigations.

Nurses who intervene to help children and families in the aftermath of child sexual abuse keep the *child's interest* as their focus. They assess the child's particular situation, intervene to relieve physical and psychologic distress, and, if necessary, refer the child or family for further treatment or counseling. The initial interview with the child requires special skills for establishing credibility and alliance as well as the use of verbal and other expressive techniques (such as art therapy or play therapy). The medical management of the child includes specialized clinical skills for ascertaining injury while minimizing the child's anxiety and discomfort. Nurses who intervene to support parents following their child's sexual abuse aid parents in understanding and handling their own feelings about what has happened while helping them learn how to support their child.

The prevention of child sexual abuse is directed at increasing public awareness of the problem and educating the general populace about it. Professional caregivers and educators can learn to detect and report suspected cases of child sexual abuse. Parents can learn preventive measures that help their children decrease their risk of sexual abuse. Children can learn healthy sexual behaviors; they can be taught to discriminate between abnormal or inappropriate sexual contacts and healthy sexual behaviors.

Professional nurses with an interest in child sexual abuse may feel encouraged by the recent increase in public awareness and social services related to child victims, families of child victims, and treatment offered to offenders. Yet the field of child sexual abuse offers much opportunity for increased nursing activity. Suggested areas for expansion of nursing roles include (1) educating the public and professional sectors about the facts, incidence, and indicators of child sexual abuse; (2) developing programs that treat child victims and their families; (3) developing, organizing, and coordinating community services to better meet the needs of child victims and their families; and (4) conducting and publishing clinical research about child sexual abuse.

## Learning activities

### EXERCISE 1: Child sexual abuse myth-fact awareness

*Directions:* Indicate which of the following statements are true or false by placing an "X" in the appropriate column.

### Survey statements*

| True | False | |
|------|-------|---|
| ___ | ___ | 1. A total stranger who is weird, dangerous, or a "dirty old man" is the greatest potential threat to a child. |
| ___ | ___ | 2. Sexual abuse is an isolated incident. |
| ___ | ___ | 3. Sexual abuse does not happen "out of the blue"; it is predictable. |
| ___ | ___ | 4. Sexual abuse is not a rare and extreme offense; it is a common problem. |
| ___ | ___ | 5. Sexual abuse is usually a violent attack that hurts children physically. |
| ___ | ___ | 6. Children who are sexually abused often do not tell their parents/guardians about being molested. |
| ___ | ___ | 7. Children initiate or precipitate sexual abuse (directly or indirectly) by seducing, fantasizing, or exaggerating such activity. |
| ___ | ___ | 8. Most sexually abused children will not leave home to escape the abusive situation. |
| ___ | ___ | 9. Mothers always know about and give explicit or implicit approval for sexual abuse within their own families. |
| ___ | ___ | 10. Incest victims come from low socioeconomic families. |
| ___ | ___ | 11. Nurses are required by law to report child sexual abuse. |
| ___ | ___ | 12. Most sexual offenders of children are convicted of the crime. |

*Answers to these statements are listed at the end of the Learning Activities for this chapter.

### EXERCISE 2. A family affair*

*Purpose:* The following exercise is intended to help the nurse open discussion and clarify values about elements specifically related to child sexual abuse. It is designed to assist nurses in sharing values with one another.

*Directions:* Read the account below and privately rank the four characters according to their behavior: one (the family member having the most objectionable behavior) through four (the family member with the least objectionable behavior). Next divide the class/nurses into small groups and arrive at one set of answers. Finally, have the small groups compare their answers and rationale for ranking of characters. The following account is an actual case history.

### Case history

David and Arlene Johnson and their two children, Janis, 12, and Jim, 8 live in a suburb of Minneapolis, where they have been for 15 months. During their 15-year marriage, the Johnsons have moved 7 times, living in 4 different cities. Each of their moves has been prompted by a new and better job promise for Dave.

Arlene and Dave met while he was in the army and she was finishing high school. They married 3 months later, had a child 9 months later, and subsequently spent 3 years in the service.

Dave has always had the decisive role in the family and maintained tight control over his wife and two children. He came from a family with eight children—where he was the oldest and carried a tremendous amount of responsibility for his younger siblings. His father was an alcoholic and was very abusive of all the family members. After Dave's son, Jim, was born and even though Arlene felt a third child would be desirable in the future, Dave had a vasectomy. He had no desire to be "burdened" with the size of family that he grew up in and didn't care about what Arlene desired.

Arlene grew up in a family where she was the only child. She was always resentful of her mother and father for refusing to have any more children and hated the pressure they placed upon her as well as the constraints on her time. In fact, one of the reasons she married Dave shortly after she met him was to escape the tyranny she felt existed in her own home. She also felt that since Dave grew up in such a large family, he would naturally want a lot of his own children. When Dave had his vasectomy, she felt like a child again; a partner in a marriage where she had no decision-making power. About this

*We wish to thank Linda Metropolis, M.A., Parents United/Parents Anonymous (Suite 240M, 300 6th Avenue Buildings, Pittsburgh, PA 15222) for compiling the case history and altering the identities and data to protect the anonyminity and confidentiality of the family.

time, she became very anxious about her young son and eventually overprotective. All of her time was spent cuddling and tending to the needs of Jim. This behavior continued to the exclusion of Janis.

Dave's reaction to Arlene's response to his vasectomy was to turn to Janis to get back at his wife. He felt Arlene was clinging to Jim in order to get him angry, and he was going to do his best to make Arlene angry. The house became like a battleground with Arlene and Jim on one side and Dave and Janis on the other.

Dave's attention to Janis continued to the exclusion of his son and his wife. He was very unwilling to share the parenting responsibilities, and he started taking Janis with him wherever he went. About the time Janis became five, Dave started to get into bed with her and rub up against her. This was to be just their secret; something special he was sharing with her. He soon had her touching his penis while he was rubbing between her legs. As this continued and she became more inquisitive, Dave told her that if she said anything to her mother he would leave the house and never return. He had also convinced Janis that her mother didn't love her and would only be mad at Janis if she found this out.

After these sexual encounters with Janis, Dave always felt very guilty and angry with himself and he swore that he would never do it again. This contributed to the poor relationship and lack of communication he had with his wife at this time. He often channeled this anger at his wife as well as at his job. From the time of the beginning of the abuse until the eventual disclosure, Dave went through three different jobs and a number of different locations. He became very indifferent to his wife and his job performance. He knew what was bothering him, yet he didn't know how to stop this compulsive behavior.

The sexual contact between Dave and Janis continued for years. About the time Janis was 11 she knew these interactions were terribly wrong, but she felt that there was nothing she could do about it. Her grades in school were failing, and she became very much preoccupied with thinking about how to get out of the home. Every time her father came into the room and molested her, she would get physically sick. She started experiencing severe stomach cramps and even started wetting the bed. Her mother remained very distant and didn't tend to Janis's symptoms. She never offered Janis a chance to get close, and, in fact, Arlene was very much jealous of Janis and blamed her for the poor relationship she had with her husband.

When Janis was 12 and entered a new school, she encountered a guidance counselor who took a lot of interest in Janis and her poor performance in school. Ms. Phillips befriended Janis and eventually was confided in about the relationship with her father. That same day, Ms. Phillips called the police and arranged with Child Welfare to allow Janis to come home with her. In the early afternoon, the police came to the school and spoke with Janis in the company of the guidance counselor. Later that afternoon they went to Janis's house and confronted the mother, who was so badly shaken that she had to be taken to the hospital. She said that she knew he was no good but she didn't think he could hurt her "baby" so greatly. Dave was arrested when he came home that day and reluctantly made a confession.

Most objectionable family member (1) _____

(2) _____

(3) _____

Least objectionable family member (4) _____

### EXERCISE 3. Professional roles for nurses (May be done individually or in groups)

#### A. Assessment model

You are asked to develop an assessment model for child sexual abuse to be used by pediatric nurses working in two settings of a children's hospital: (1) the emergency department and (2) the outpatient clinic. Both services accept referrals and walk-ins for treatment. Include in the model *both* early detection skills and skills for reported cases of child sexual abuse.

#### B. Treatment model

A community mental health center needs to establish a treatment service for *children* and *families* of child sexual abuse. You are called for consultation on this project. What recommendations would you make about the following issues?
1. Goals of treatment
2. Theoretic model for treatment
3. Specific approaches based on selected theoretic model

#### C. School prevention project

A school has asked you to create a puppet show that teaches first- and second-graders (6-, 7-, and 8-year-olds) how to protect themselves from child sexual abuse. How would you respond to the following issues and questions? (Responses can be shared for discussion.)
1. Who's role is it to teach children prevention of child sexual abuse? (parents, teachers, community?)
2. What elements are essential for children to understand relevant to prevention of child sexual abuse?

3. Can children really understand sexual abuse prior to its occurrence?
4. What developmental needs, tasks, and emotions of these young children might influence their response to child sexual abuse?
5. What might be the reactions of parents to this project?

*Optional:* Create and perform the show for your peers for constructive criticism.

### D. Parental concern group

You are asked to speak to a parents' group about child sexual abuse. To facilitate your preparation, you ask the group to submit their questions or concerns *prior* to your speaking engagement (this also gives you the opportunity to prepare your answers!). Based on current theoretic and research data, how would you respond to the following list of parental concerns?

1. How can I protect my child from sexual abuse?
2. How can I talk to my children about sexual abuse without scaring them?
3. How do children react to sexual abuse?
4. How should I respond if my child says he or she has been abused?
5. Do child victims of sexual abuse recover from the physical or emotional damage?

---

### Answer key for Exercise 1: Child sexual abuse myth-fact awareness

True: 3,4,6,8,11
False: 1,2,5,7,9,10,12

---

### REFERENCES

1. Berliner, L.: Sexual misuse. In Holley, K.C.: Sexual misuses of children: tools for understanding, Tacoma, Wash., 1979, Pierce County Rape Relief.
2. Breen, J.L., Greenwald, E., and Gregori, C.A.: The molested young female: evaluation and therapy of alleged rape, Pediatr. Clin. North Am. **19:**717, 1972.
3. Burgess, A.W., and Groth, N.A.: The sexually abused child: a seminar, Pittsburgh, 1979. Sponsored by Pittsburgh Action Against Rape, University of Pittsburgh School of Nursing, and the Parental Stress Center.
4. Burgess, A.W., and Holmstrom, L.L.: Accessory to sex: pressure, sex and secrecy. In Burgess, A.W., and others: Sexual assault of children and adolescents, Lexington, Mass., 1978, Lexington Books.

5. Burgess, A.W., Holmstrom, L.L., and McCausland, M.P.: Child sexual assault by a family member: decisions following disclosure, Victimology **2:**236, 1977.

6. Child Protection Center—Special Unit, Children's Hospital National Medical Center: A message to parents about child sexual abuse, Washington, D.C., 1979.

7. Child Protection Center—Special Unit, Children's Hospital National Medical Center: Public concern and personal action: child sexual abuse, Washington, D.C., 1980.

8. Child Protection Center—Special Unit, Children's Hospital National Medical Center: Child sexual abuse victim assistance project, Washington, D.C., 1979. Brochure.

9. Davis, H., Hughes, S.E., and Harger, J.H.: Sexual abuse and rape protocols, Children's Hospital of Pittsburgh. Prepared in consultation with Interagency Task Force on Rape-Related Services, Pittsburgh Action Against Rape, Center for Violent Crimes, and Pittsburgh Law Enforcement Agencies, Pittsburgh, Pa., 1980.

10. Gagnon, J.: Female child victims of sexual offenses, J. Soc. Problems Vol. 13, 1978; and Coleman, P.: Incest: family treatment model. In Holley, K.C.: Sexual misuses of children: tools for understanding, Tacoma, Wash., 1979, Pierce County Rape Relief.

11. Gorline, L.L.: The nurse and the sexually abused child. In Chinn, P.L., and Leonard, K.B., editors: Current practice in pediatric nursing, St. Louis, 1980, The C.V. Mosby Co.

12. Gorline, L.L., and Ray, M.M.: Examining and caring for the child who has been sexually assaulted, MCN **4:**110, March/April, 1979.

13. Groth, A.N.: Pattern of sexual assault against children and adolescents, Lexington, Mass., 1978, Lexington Books.

14. Halpern, S., Hicks, D., and Crenshaw, T.L., editors: Rape: helping the victim, Oradell, N.J., 1978, Medical Economics Books.

15. Institute for Law and Social Research: Highlights of interim findings and implications: basic facts about child sexual abuse, Washington, D.C., 1978.

16. Justice, B., and Justice, R.: The broken taboo, New York, 1979, Human Sciences Press.

17. Keefe, M.L.: Police investigation in child sexual assault. In Burgess, A.W., and others: Sexual assault of children and adolescents, Lexington, Mass., 1978, Lexington Books.

18. King County Rape Relief: "He told me not to tell," Seattle, Wash., 1979.

19. MacFarlane, K.: Sexual abuse of children. In Chapman, J.R., and Gates, M., editors: The victimization of women, vol. 3, Beverly Hills, Calif., 1978, Sage Publications.

20. Parents and Daughters and Sons United, Inc.: The run: official newsletter of the Santa Clara County Chapter **14:**1, 1979.

21. Rape Crisis Center of Syracuse, Inc.: Rape: awareness and prevention for educators, Syracuse, N.Y., 1980.

22. Sexual Assault Center, Harborview Medical Center: What to do if your child has been sexually molested, Seattle, Wash., 1978.

23. Sgroi, S.M.: Child sexual assault: some guidelines for intervention and assessment. In Burgess, A.W., and others: Sexual assault of children and adolescents, Lexington, Mass., 1978, Lexington Books.
24. Sgroi, S.M.: Comprehensive examination for child sexual assault: diagnostic, therapeutic and child protection issues. In Burgess, A.W., and others: Sexual assault of children and adolescents, Lexington, Mass., 1978, Lexington Books.
25. Simrel, M.S., and Lloyd, D.A.: Medical corroborating evidence in child sexual abuse/assault cases, Washington, D.C., 1980, Child Protection Center—Special Unit, Children's Hospital National Medical Center.
26. Swift, C.: Sexual exploitation of children in the United States, paper presented to Subcommittee on Domestic and International Scientific Planning, Analysis and Cooperation, Washington, D.C., Jan. 11, 1978.
27. Warner, C.: Rape and sexual assault: management and intervention, Rockville, Md., 1980, Aspen Publications.
28. Weeks, R.B.: Counseling parents of sexually abused children, Med. Aspects Hum. Sex. **10:**43, August 1976.

## ADDITIONAL REFERENCES

American Humane Association, Children's Division: Sexual abuse of children: implications for case work, Denver, 1969.

Bender, L., and Blau, A.: The reaction of children to sexual relations with adults, Am. J. Orthopsychiatry **7:**500, 1937.

Berliner, L.: Child sexual abuse: what happens next? Victimology **2:**327, 1937.

Burgess, A.W., and Holmstrom, L.L.: Interviewing young victims. In Burgess, A.W., and others: Sexual assault of children and adolescents, Lexington, Mass., 1978, Lexington Books.

Burgess, A.W., and Holmstrom, L.L.: Sexual trauma of children and adolescents, Nurs. Clin. North Am. **10:**551, 1975.

Burgess, A.W., and Holmstrom, L.L.: Rape trauma syndrome, Am. J. Psychiatry **131:**981, 1974.

Giarretto, H.: Hank . . . and . . . the impact of intervention, Human. Psychol., Fall 1978.

Giarretto, H.: Humanistic treatment of father-daughter incest. In Helfer, R.E., and Kempe, C.H., editors: Child abuse and neglect: the family and the community, Cambridge, Mass., 1976, Ballinger Publishing Co.

Greenberg, N.H.: The epidemiology of childhood sexual abuse, Pediatr. Ann. **8:**289, 1975.

Groth, A.N.: Sexual abuse of children. In Groth, A.N., with Birnbaum, J.: Men who rape: the psychology of the offender, New York, 1979, Plenum Press.

Groth, A.N., and Burgess, A.W.: Motivational intent in the sexual assault of children, Criminal Justice Behav. **4:**253, 1977.

Henderson, D.J.: Incest. In Freedman, A.M., Kaplan, H.I., and Sadock, B.S., editors: Comprehensive textbook of psychiatry, ed. 3, Baltimore, Md., 1980, Williams & Wilkins.

Holley, K.C.: Sexual misuses of children: tools for understanding, Tacoma, Wash., 1979, Pierce County Rape Relief.

Kliman, A: Crisis: psychological first aid for recovery and growth, New York, 1978, Holt, Rinehart & Winston.

Lukianowicz, N: Incest, Br. J. Psychiatry **120**:301, 1972.

Maisch, H.: Incest, New York, 1972, Stein & Day Publishers.

Meiselman, K.C.: Incest, San Francisco, 1978, Jossey-Bass, Inc.

Molnar, G., and Cameron, P.: Incest syndrome: observations in a general hospital psychiatric unit, Can. Psychiatr. Assoc. J. **20**:373, 1975.

Paul, D.M.: The medical examination in sexual offenses, Med. Sci. Law **15**(3):154-163, 1975.

Peters, J.J. Children who are victims of sexual assault and the psychology of offenders, Am. J. Psychotherapy **30**:398, 1976.

Queen's Bench Foundation: Sexual abuse of children: a guide for parents, San Francisco, 1977.

Rascovisky, M.W., and Rascovisky, A.: On consummated incest, Int. J. Psychoanal. **31**:42, 1956.

Sexual Assault Center, Harborview Medical Center: Sexual abuse within the family: the problem, treatment philosophy, goals, service, Seattle, Wash., 1977. Mimeograph.

Shamroy, J.A.: A perspective on childhood sexual abuse, Social Work **25**:128, March 1980.

Summit, R., and Kryso, J.: Sexual abuse of children: a clinical spectrum, Am. J. Orthopsychiatry **48**:237, 1978.

Tilelli, J.A., Turek, D., and Jaffi, A.G.: Sexual abuse of children, N. Engl. J. Med. **302**:319, 1980.

## ANNOTATED SUGGESTED READINGS*

Berliner, L., and Stevens, S.: Special techniques for child witnesses. In Schultz, L.G., ed.: The sexual victimology of youth, Springfield, Ill., 1979, charles C Thomas, Publisher.

  The authors describe child molesting as often being a compulsive behavior. The offender, if not prosecuted, will undoubtedly continue the abuse. Observations of the negative effect of criminal proceedings on the child are presented. The article presents some general information about child development and child molestation. It also suggests some strategies for accommodating the child witness in criminal justice system proceedings.

Blumberg, M.L.: Collateral therapy for the abused child and the problem parent, Am. J. Psychotherapy **33**(3):339, July 1979.

  Child abuse is described as a manifestation of a family *in* crisis. Any therapy should involve the child, the abusing parent, and other persons in a still-intact family. The role of the child, the psychologic effects on the child, and the generational perpetuation of the problem are also discussed.

Burgess, A.W., and others: Sexual assault of children and adolescents, Lexington, Mass., 1978, Lexington Books.

*We wish to thank Doris Mikell, R.N., M.S.N., for contributing to this list of readings.

This book provides specific treatment approaches for personnel who work with children and adolescent victims of sexual abuse. The major themes are (1) the human dimension of sexual assault victims, (2) community program planning, and (3) interagency cooperation.

Burgess, A., McCausland, M., and Wolbert, W.: Children's drawings as indicators of sexual trauma, Perspect. Psychiatr. Care **19**(2):50, 1981.

The authors discuss the use of children's drawings by nurses to assess and intervene in child sexual abuse cases. They present drawings of child victims that illustrate acute rape trauma syndrome and ongoing sexual victimization. The drawings are discussed as a means of gaining access to the child's unexpressed thoughts, feelings, and reactions and of reducing pressure on the child to verbalize. The use of victim counseling with rape trauma and of victim therapy with ongoing sexual victimization is also described.

Gorline, L.L.: The nurse and the sexually assaulted child. In Chinn, P.L., and Leonard, K.B., editors: Current practice in pediatric nursing, vol. 3, St. Louis, 1980, The C.V. Mosby Co.

This chapter defines sexual assault, particularly of the young female, and describes the anatomy and physiology of prepubertal female genitalia. The author also explains methods for assisting the child through the social, legal, and health care systems and describes techniques for interviewing the pediatric client.

Justice, B., and Justice, R.: The broken taboo, New York, 1979, Human Sciences Press.

This book, based primarily on the author's own study of 100 incest cases, explores the occurrence of incest, the dynamics of the problem, and what can be done about it. The indicators and effects of incest are also presented as the authors emphasize the need to explore this social problem.

Lieske, A.: Incest: an overview, Perspect. Psychiatr. Care **19**(2):59, 1981.

The author presents an overview of literature and research findings on incest. Four areas of discussion include (1) causative factors, (2) incestuous family dynamics, (3) psychologic effects of incest, and (4) treatment of the incestuous family. The article offers a comprehensive introduction to the subject matter for readers unfamiliar with literature and research on child sexual abuse.

MacFarlane, K.: Sexual abuse of children. In Chapman, J.R., and Gates, M., editors: The victimization of women, vol. 3, Beverly Hills, Calif., 1978, Sage Publications.

The author offers definitions of child sexual abuse information relating to the scope and dynamics of the problem and the effects on the victims, primarily female. Societal responses of the criminal justice, health, and other social service systems are also presented along with recommendations for change.

Rathbone-McCuan, E., and Pierce, R.: Intergenerational treatment approach: an alternative model of working with abusive/neglectful and delinquent prone families, Family Therapy **5**(2):121, 1978.

Child sexual abuse is approached through a general framework of abuses to children. Societal responses to child abuse are described. The authors present a theoretic model that implies an intergenerational transference of behavioral and attitudinal predispositions for child abuse. The operational model emphasizes an assessment of all significant family members—including child, abusing parent, and grandparent. A clinical illustration demonstrates the model.

Sgroi, S.M.: Sexual molestation of children, Children Today **4**(3):18, 1975.

The author advocates the need for professional involvement in the problem of sexual abuse of children. Social sanctions related to child sexual abuse are presented along with reasons that this problem is largely unaddressed: lack of recognition of the problem, failure to obtain adequate medical corroboration, and reluctance to report.

Tilelli, J., and others: Sexual abuse of children, New Engl. J. Med. **302**(6):319, 1980.

This article describes a review of hospital records of children who came into a hospital over an 18-month period with the complaint of sexual assault or abuse. The authors use collected data to look at antecedent conditions, common situational variables, clinical management, and use of the medical record as a legal document.

Weeks, R.B.: Counseling parents of sexually abused children, Med. Aspects Hum. Sex. **10**:43-44, Aug. 1976.

The author describes counseling principles with parents of a sexually abused child and stresses the importance of parental responses in influencing the child's short- and long-term reactions to the trauma. Parental advice is divided into three areas, depending on the relationship to the offender.

# APPENDIX A

# Sample consent forms for medical examination and photography

**Consent for medical examination***

Date: _____ Time: _____

_____
Name of patient

Brought by: _____

_____
Address

Birthdate: _____

### AUTHORIZATION FOR RELEASE OF INFORMATION

I hereby authorize _____ to supply copies of
(hospital name)
the Evidentiary Report form including any laboratory reports, specimens, evidence and/or clothing immediately upon completion, to the Police Department and the Office of the District Attorney having jurisdiction.

_____
(Signature of patient)

_____
(Date)

_____
(Signature of parent or guardian)

_____
(Date)

_____
(Signature of witness)

_____
(Date)

_____
(Name and signature of examining physician)

_____
(Date)

Distribution: Copy 1: To be transferred with evidence
Copy 2: Hospital record

*Reprinted with permission of the Pennsylvania Coalition Against Rape (PCAR), Harrisburg, Pa., 1979.

**Consent for photography\***

I, _____ , hereby grant permission to be photographed while a patient of Harborview Medical Center. I understand that these photographs will become part of my medical record.

_____
Patient's signature

_____
Hospital number

_____
Parent or guardian

_____
Date

Witness: _____

Witness: _____

Date: _____

\*Repinted with permission of the Sexual Assault Center, Harborview Medical Center, Seattle, Wash.

# Rape kit contents and hospital-prepared rape kit

**Rape kit contents\***

Assuming the emergency room is properly equipped, the following items are essential:

- 3 Tubes with a set of 2 swabs each
- 1 Tube with anticoagulant for blood samples
- 2 Envelopes for debris collection
- 2 Envelopes, each containing an orange wood stick for fingernails
- 2 Envelopes, with 1 comb each for head and pubic hair combings
- 2 Envelopes, for standard head and pubic hairs
- 1 Envelope with non-chemically sterilized gauze pad for saliva sample
- 5 Slides with frosted ends in containers
- 3 Labels for swab tubes
- 2 Labels for evidence
- 1 Control swab

\*The rape kit contents listed above were approved as standard items by the Interagency County Task Force on Rape-Related Services, Pittsburgh, Pa., Feb. 21, 1979. The items required may vary from county to county and state to state. Reprinted with permission.

### Contents for hospital-prepared rape kit*

CONTENTS:  8 Envelopes (paper)
1 Purple-top tube for 5cc whole blood sample
3 Test tubes
7 Swabs
5 Slides in containers (cardboard containers or plastic slide box)
6 Gummed labels (4 for tubes; 2 extra)
2 Combs
2 Orange sticks
1 Sterile gauze pad (4" × 4")
Paper bags for clothing

To assemble the rape kit, follow the instructions listed below:

1. Use 2 envelopes. Label 1: *Fingernail scrapings: right hand*
Patient's name _____
Date _____
Collected by _____
Label 1: *Fingernail scrapings: left hand*
Patient's name _____
Date _____
Collected by _____
Put an orange stick in each envelope.
2. Use 2 envelopes. Label 1: *Head hair combings*
Patient's name _____
Date _____
Collected by _____
Label 1: *Pubic hair combings*
Patient's name _____
Date _____
Collected by _____
Put a comb in each envelope.

*Reprinted with permission of the Interagency County Task Force on Rape-Related Services, Pittsburgh, Pa., 1979.

**Contents for hospital-prepared rape kit\*—cont'd**

3. Use 2 envelopes. Label 1: *Head hair standards*
     Patient's name _____
     Date _____
     Collected by _____
   Label 1: *Pubic hair standards*
     Patient's name _____
     Date _____
     Collected by _____
4. Use 1 envelope. Label:  *Saliva sample*
     Patient's name _____
     Date _____
     Collected by _____
   Put sterile gauze pad in envelope.
5. Use 1 envelope. Label:  *Debris collection*
     Patient's name _____
     Date _____
     Collected by _____
     Body origin _____
6. Put in paper bag:      The above 8 labeled envelopes
                          3 Test tubes
                          7 Swabs
                          1 Purple-top tube
                          5 Slides in containers
                          6 Gummed labels
7. Extra paper bags for clothing should be stored with the rape kit.

# Emergency room supplies for rape examination*

### Rape kit contents

1. Appropriate "sexual assault" forms
2. Large paper bags for clothing
3. Labels (peel-and-stick variety)—about 20
4. 2 urine containers
5. 30 ml NaCl in a container
6. 10 cotton-tipped swabs
7. 10 red-topped blood tubes (used for collecting blood and whenever a stoppered test tube is needed)
8. Fingernail file
9. 2 paper envelopes (about 2″ × 3″)
10. Forceps (may be of the disposable variety)
11. Scissors (may be of the disposable variety)
12. Plastic comb
13. Large paper towel
14. Paper envelope (about 4″ × 6″)
15. 2 aspiration micropipettes
16. 2 bulbs to fit the pipettes
17. 6 glass slides with frosted ends
18. Slide container to accommodate 2 slides
19. Sharpened pencil
20. Cervical scraper for the Pap smear
21. 10 ml. syringe
22. 20 ml. syringe and needle (for blood drawing)
23. 2 sterile 2″ × 2″ gauze pads
24. Tourniquet
25. Prepping solution that does not contain alcohol; e.g., Zephiran Chloride (benzalkonium chloride)
26. 2 cover slips (glass)
27. Tongue blade
28. 4 rubber bands
29. Lubricant for the bimanual pelvic examination
30. A cardboard container for all the above

### Additional supplies in the room, but not necessarily in the kit

1. Camera and film
2. Wood's light (ultraviolet) (This is not essential, however.)
3. Vaginal speculum
4. Rubber gloves
5. Pap-smear fixative
6. 3 Thayer-Martin plates or 3 Transgrow® media

### Additional supply in the hospital, but not necessarily in the E.D.

1. Microscope

*From Braen, G. Richard: The rape examination, North Chicago, Ill., Abbott Laboratories. Copyright 1981 Abbott Laboratories. Reprinted with permission.

# APPENDIX D

# Medical report form for sexual assault

**Checklist for completing rape examination***

*Directions:* Check off the following items as they are completed before the patient is discharged.

- ___ 1. Identifying data
- ___ 2. Consent forms
- ___ 3. Brief gynecological history
- ___ 4. Nature of the assault
- ___ 5. General physical examination
- ___ 6. Pelvic examination
- ___ 7. Wet mount and test on specimens
- ___ 8. Evidence collection
- ___ 9. Receipt for the release of evidence to the police
- ___ 10. Mental status assessment
- ___ 11. Treatment
- ___ 12. Follow-up instructions
- ___ 13. Distribution of copies
  - ___ 1st copy - Medical Records
  - ___ 2nd copy - Police

THIS SHEET IS NOT TO BE INCLUDED AS PART OF THE PERMANENT MEDICAL RECORD AND SHOULD BE DISCARDED AFTER THIS FORM HAS BEEN COMPLETED AND REVIEWED.

*Modified and reprinted with permission of the Interagency County Task Force on Rape-Related Services, Pittsburgh, Pa., 1979.

## APPENDIX E

# Sexual assault form for hospital use only*

Patient's name _____ Birthdate ___/___/___

Date _____ Time _____ Physician _____

*Instructions*

The victim of sexual assault has just been through a frightening experience. In order to help her during the crisis, the emergency room personnel must take time to explain all treatments, procedures, laboratory tests and questions which are included in this form. Your interaction with the victim will affect how she copes with the assault.

A. *Brief description of patient*

_____

_____

Temp: _ Pulse: _ Respiration: _ Blood pressure: _____

B. *Personal health*

1. Allergic to any medications: Specify _____

   Other allergies _____

2. Presently taking any medications (including over the counter medications) or receiving any type of treatment? If so, specify _____

   _____

3. Any pre-existing health problems? _____

   _____

*Reprinted with permission of the Interagency County Task Force on Rape-Related Services, Pittsburgh, Pa.

C. *Gynecological history*
   1. Date of last menstrual period _____
   2. Did you have a tampon inserted at the time of assault?

      Yes _____ No _____

   3. Are you pregnant? Yes _____ No _____ If yes, how many weeks? _____

   4. Were you using a contraceptive at the time of the assault? _____

   5. Any recent gynecological problems? _____

   6. Date and time of last intercourse _____
D. *Tests*
   1. Pregnancy _____

   2. Venereal (sexually transmissible) diseases _____

      _____

   3. Other _____
E. *Diagnosis*

   _____

   _____

   _____

# Record of patient's description of sexual assault*

Copies: 1 Hospital record
       1 With evidence

Patient's name _____ Sex M _____ F _____

Date _____ Time _____ Birthdate _____/_____/_____

Signatures: _____ _____
             (Attending physician)          (Attending nurse)

Print names: _____ _____

Date and time of sexual assault: ___ ___ ___ Date _____ Time: AM/PM

## TO BE COMPLETED BY MEDICAL PERSONNEL

Patient's description of assault

1. Where did assault take place? (Examples: apartment, alley, parking lot, etc.)

   _____

   _____

   Address _____ Date _____ Time _____

2. Physically injured? _____ How? _____

   _____

   _____

3. Loss of consciousness at any time? _____

4. Any weapons involved? _____ Yes _____ No

   What kind? _____

5. Were restraints used? _____ Yes _____ No

   What kind? _____

6. Number of assailants? _____

*Modified and reprinted with permission of the Interagency County Task Force on Rape-Related Services, Pittsburgh, Pa., 1979.

7. Did assailant place or attempt to place his penis in your:

_____ Vagina    _____ Mouth    _____ Anus

†8. Have you consumed any drugs or alcohol before, during or after the assault by force or voluntarily?

| *Drugs:* (specify) | Before | During | After | Forced | Voluntarily |
|---|---|---|---|---|---|
| Explain: | | | | | |
| *Alcohol:* (specify) Explain | | | | | |

9. Did assailant ejaculate? _____ Yes _____ No _____ Not sure

Where (what part of body)? _____

_____

Use of a condom? _____ Yes _____ No

10. Did the assailant insert any foreign objects into your vagina, mouth or rectum?

Specify_____

11. Did you scratch the assailant? _____

12. Since the assault, have you:

| | | | |
|---|---|---|---|
| Douched_____ | | Defecated_____ | |
| Bathed_____ | | Changed clothes_____ | |
| Gargled_____ | | Eaten_____ | |
| Urinated_____ | | Drunk_____ | |

†Some settings omit this data on sexual assault forms as the findings may be used to "damage the character" of the victim at trial.

## APPENDIX G

# Evidence collection form in sexual assault cases*

Do all tests. Bathing, douching, gargling, urinating, defecating do not necessarily affect results of test.

| | | | |
|---|---|---|---|
| Clothing in paper bags | —— | Smears and swabs: | |
| Debris collection | —— |   Vaginal | —— |
| Foreign hairs: | |   Rectal | —— |
|   Pubic hair combing | —— |   Oral | —— |
|   Head hair combing | —— |   Other _____ | —— |
| Hair standards: | | Whole blood sample | —— |
|   Pubic hair | —— | Saliva sample | —— |
|   Head hair | —— | Fingernail scrapings: | |
| | |   Right | —— |
| | |   Left | —— |

*Reprinted with permission of the Interagency County Task Force on Rape-Related Services, Pittsburgh, Pa., 1979.

## APPENDIX H

# Physical examination record of injuries sustained in sexual assault*

|  | Location | Description |
|---|---|---|
| Bruises | | |
| Punctures | | |
| Lacerations | | |
| Abrasions | | |
| Redness | | |
| Swelling | | |
| Fractures | | |
| Teeth marks | | |
| Ligature marks | | |
| Burns | | |
| Stains | | |
| Blood | | |
| Foreign material on body | | |
| Have photographs been requested of any visible physical injuries? | | |

*Reprinted with permission of the Interagency County Task Force on Rape-Related Services, Pittsburgh, Pa., 1979.

*Continued.*

**PHYSICAL EXAMINATION** (Please diagram bruising, lacerations, or any other physical trauma sustained by patient)

1. Head:

2. Chest:

3. Breast:

4. Heart:

5. Abdomen:

6. Extremeties:

7. Neurologic:

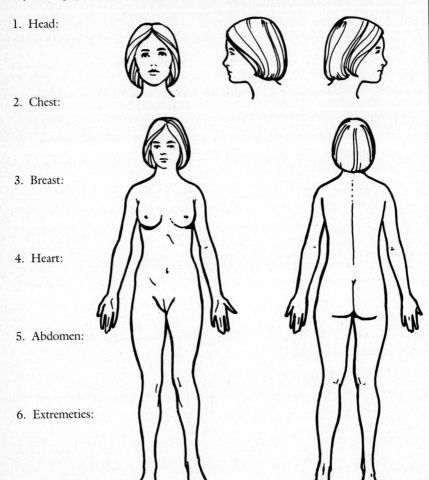

_____
Signature of physician

# Pelvic examination record of injuries sustained in sexual assault*

*Use water-moistened speculum.*

Pubic hairs matted by semen? _____ Any foreign material? _____

Include all signs of trauma (tears, bleeding, tenderness, edema, abrasion, parity, menstruation in simple, objective statements):

Vulva _____

Hymen _____

Vagina _____

Cervix _____

Uterus _____

Adnexae _____

Rectum _____

**Genitourinary:** Diagram and describe external trauma

*Reprinted with permission of the Interagency County Task Force on Rape-Related Services, Pittsburgh, Pa., 1979.

## APPENDIX J

# Record of wet-mount examination in sexual assault cases*

**Immediate laboratory examination of wet-mount slide** (list source affected area and check result).

| List source areas | Sperm present | Sperm absent | Sperm motile | Sperm nonmotile |
|---|---|---|---|---|
| Vagina | | | | |
| Anus | | | | |
| Mouth | | | | |

Wet mount: _____

Signature of physician

**Test on specimens:** (Check all tests completed and source of specimens.)

| Source | Sperm | Motility | Acid phosphatase | G.C. culture | VDRL | Pregnancy | Intoxication (drug screen) |
|---|---|---|---|---|---|---|---|
| Vagina | | | | | | | |
| Anus | | | | | | | |
| Mouth | | | | | | | |

*Reprinted with permission of the Interagency County Task Force on Rape-Related Services, Pittsburgh, Pa., 1979.

## APPENDIX K

# Treatment and follow-up protocol for nursing care of rape victims*

### TREATMENT AND FOLLOW-UP OF THE SEXUAL ASSAULT VICTIM

1. *Take the female patient's menstrual history and test for pregnancy.*
   A pregnancy test should be routinely performed whether the patient is menstruating or not. If the patient is at risk for pregnancy, she should be given a follow-up appointment for pregnancy testing. Such appointments should be made at the earliest possible time, depending upon the stage of the patient's menstrual cycle or any previous sexual intercourse, but no later than six weeks following the initial visit to the hospital. Where the Saxena (HCGRRA) test is available, an appointment can be made for 16 days after the alleged assault.

2. *Explain the pregnancy-prevention alternatives to the female, postpubertal patient.*
   The alternatives are:
   a. Waiting to determine whether or not the patient begins her next period or until such time as the results of a pregnancy test are known.
   b. Menstrual extraction, if next period is late.
   c. Diethylstilbestrol, provided the patient presented herself at the hospital within 72 hours after the alleged assault.
   d. Post-coital IUD, inserted within 5 days of suspected assault and retained for at least 7 days.

   Family planning services and supplies may be provided to eligible females of child-bearing age, who can be considered sexually active and who desire them, in accordance with the laws and regulations of the federal government and New York State. HOWEVER, no person can be compelled or coerced to accept such services.

3. *Prescribe diethylstilbestrol (DES) only if the woman is at high risk for pregnancy and if it is felt that she whould have extreme difficulty dealing with a pregnancy resulting from the alleged assault.*
   a. Do not administer DES if more than 72 hours have elapsed since the alleged assault.
   b. Fully explain the short-term and possible long-term consequences of DES. Patients who receive DES and subsequently become pregnant increase the possibility that their female offspring will develop vaginal cancer. Advise her that, if she becomes pregnant despite the DES, she should immediately seek counsel with a physician regarding the advisability of an abortion. If a patient is absolutely opposed to abortion, do not prescribe DES.
   c. Dosage of DES is 25 mg twice a day for 5 days.
   d. Prescribe an antinauseant such as Compazine to be used if necessary.

---

*Reprinted with permission of the Rape Crisis Service of Planned Parenthood of Rochester and Monroe County in New York.

4. *After doing baseline testing for venereal disease, advise the patient of the dangers and modes of transmission of venereal disease. Schedule follow-up appointments to test for gonorrhea (one week) and syphilis (four to six weeks).*
   a. Prescribe prophylactic antibiotic therapy *only* if it is felt that the patient would have difficulty keeping follow-up appointments. However, follow-up appointments should still be scheduled, particularly as a precaution against the occurrence of a penicillin-resistant form of gonorrhea.
   b. Dosages for VD (syphilis) prophylaxis (for adults) are as follows:
      (1) Procaine penicillin (4.8 million units I.M.), with probenicid (1 gram by mouth). In younger children 50,000 units per kilogram is adequate for procaine penicillin. (See discussion below.)
   **or** (2) Ampicillin (50 mg/kg, to a maximum of 3½ gm p.o. in one dose), with probenicid (1 gm p.o.).
   **or** (3) Tetracycline (1.5 gm p.o. in one dose and 0.5 gm q.i.d. for 4 days—total of 9 gm). *This is the treatment of choice in most places* (emphasis added).
   c. Dosages for gonorrhea prophylaxis are as follows:*
      (1) For adults and children over 100 pounds (45 kg) or more:
         (A) Aqueous procaine penicillin G (APPG): 4.8 million units injected intramuscularly at two sites, combined with 1.0 gm of probenecid given orally.
      **or** (B) Tetracycline hydrochloride: 0.5 gm orally four times per day for five days for a total dose of 10.0 gm. A single-dose therapy method is ineffective for all tetracyclines. Tetracycline is effective for patients allergic to penicillins including ampicillin and amoxicillin.
      **or** (C) Ampicillin: 3.5 gm orally combined with 1.0 gm of probenecide given orally. This treatment regime is not as effective as other treatment regimens recommended.
      **or** (D) Amoxicillin: 3.0 gm orally combined with 1.0 gm of probenecid orally. This treatment regime is not as effective as other treatment regimes recommended.
      **or** (E) Spectinomycin hydrochloride: 2.0 gm in one intramuscular injection. This treatment regime is effective for patients allergic to penicillins, including ampicillin and amoxicillin, probenecid, or intolerant of tetracyclines.
5. *Follow-up appointments should include the following: gonorrhea (one week), syphilis (six weeks), pregnancy (at the latest six weeks). Psychiatric follow-up should also be considered.*
   If the victim is under 16, an appointment should be made with the pediatrician, nurse-practitioner, or family physician on the following day, even if Child Protection team (a child specialty team of the agency) has been involved.
6. *The Guide to Medical Services Following Sexual Assault (in Spanish, English or other languages) should be completed by hospital personnel and given to the patient or relative of patient before she leaves the hospital.*

---

*Atlanta Center for Disease Control: Newest treatment schedules for gonorrhea, March, 1979, pp. 121-127, U.S. Department of Health, Education, and Welfare.

# Resources and services for sexual assault victims

## GENERAL RESOURCE LIST*

Complete *written* lists of the following information for your community. The resource list can be posted or readily available in work settings for reference or distribution to victims.

A. Rape Crisis Center—name and address
  1. Hotline number
  2. Office Number
B. Police
  1. City police, phone number
  2. County police, phone number
  3. Sex Squad (if a special squad in your community, phone number)
  4. University police, phone number
C. City Police Stations
  1. List names and phone numbers of police stations in your city, county, borough, or township
  2. Refer readers to the phone book under POLICE for other phone numbers
D. County Crime Lab—phone number
E. Legal
  1. District attorney's office
  2. Neighborhood legal services
  3. Neighborhood legal services child advocacy unit
  4. Juvenile shelters
  5. City human relations commission
  6. United States Equal Employment Opportunity Commission
  7. State human relations commission
  8. State action hotlines
F. Medical
  1. Hospitals (city—phone numbers)
  2. Health clinics—address, phone number and hours
    a. Nurse practitioners
    b. County health department
    c. Women's center
    d. Birth Right
    e. Free clinics

---

*Modified from Pittsburgh Action Against Rape, Pittsburgh Pa., 1980.

      f.  Planned Parenthood
      g.  Family practice offices
      h.  Reproductive clinics
      i.  Women's health services

G.  Counseling
1.  Psychiatric–mental health nurse clinical specialists
2.  Feminist consultants
3.  University counseling programs
4.  Catholic social services
5.  Drug abuse centers
6.  Alcoholics Anonymous
7.  Parents Anonymous
8.  Free clinics
9.  Mental health/mental retardation community counseling centers
10.  Women's center
11.  Family and children's services
12.  Planned parenthood
13.  Gay counselors/agencies
    Briefly include a description of the type of service offered, fee scale (e.g., sliding or otherwise, short- or long-term services offered), qualifications of counselors (e.g., students, certified), and if located in more than one area.

H.  Crisis Counseling Lines
1.  Mental health crisis
2.  Child abuse hotline
3.  Parents Anonymous
4.  Teenage runaway number

I.  Domestic Violence
1.  City women's center and shelter
2.  Community action programs

J.  Miscellaneous
1.  Child welfare office
2.  Community action groups for safer neighborhoods
3.  Karate women's centers

K.  Resource People—name and phone number
1.  Legal
2.  Counseling
3.  Community
4.  Public relations
5.  Nursing
6.  Hospitals
7.  University

L.  Other Rape Crisis Centers in the State

# SERVICES AVAILABLE FOR VICTIMS OF SEXUAL ASSAULT*

## Venereal disease test sites

Free venereal disease tests may be obtained at:

_____(name)_____ County Health Department

Address
Phone number
Hours of service
Listing of locations of these test sites (for example, may be 4 of 5 sites).

## Pregnancy test sites

Free pregnancy tests may be obtained at:

_____(name)_____ County Health Department

Address
Phone number
Hours of service

List site locations and/or phone numbers where the victim may call (e.g., in Pittsburgh, Pa., there are 23 health clinics. It is suggested to the victim that she call the location nearest her).

List of Other Test Sites—for example:
Birth Right                   Women's center
Planned Parenthood            Women's health services

## Advocates

Advocates have specialized skills for helping victims of sexual assault. Their skills include crisis intervention techniques, counseling, and a detailed knowledge of medical and legal procedures. They will help you with any immediate needs such as transportation, temporary housing in a safe place, notification of authorities, and calling a family member or friend. They are also aware of the special problems which confront victims of a violent crime. An advocate will be available when you need her.

_The hospital._ At the hospital, the advocate will provide emotional support and an explanation of hospital procedure. She will stay in the emergency room during the medical examination and evidence collection, if you wish her to do so.

_The police interview._ Since this can be a frightening experience for one who has just been sexually assaulted, the advocate will explain police procedures and the reasons for some of the puzzling questions. She will help you over the rough spots.

_The legal system._ While the detective will explain the legal process, the advocate, with her own first-hand knowledge of the system, can help you understand what is expected of you and how you can best work with the police and district attorney in prosecuting your assailant. An advocate will accompany you to all the legal proceedings.

---

*Reprinted with permission of the Interagency County Task Force on Rape-Related Services: A handbook for victims, Pittsburgh, Pa., 1979.

_Continued._

## Important Names and Phone Numbers

Rape crisis center name(s) _____

Address _____ Phone _____

Advocate's name _____

Agency _____ Phone _____

Doctor's name _____

Hospital _____ Phone _____

Police officer's name _____

Police department _____ Phone _____

Detective's name _____

Police department _____ Phone _____

Assistant district attorney's name _____

Phone _____

# Follow-up care instructions for sexually assaulted patients*

A. You have been given the following medication:
   1. _____ Purpose _____
                        Dosage _____
   2. _____ Purpose _____
                        Dosage _____

B. Instructions: _____
_____
_____

C. It is recommended that you have:
   1. Gonorrhea testing done two weeks after the assault. Date _____
   2. Syphilis testing done six weeks after the assault. Date _____
   3. Pregnancy testing done six weeks after the assault.
      Yes ___ No ___

D. Please call your physician or clinic if you experience:
   1. Signs of infection such as fever, pain, sores, discharge, etc.
   2. Urinary symptoms such as frequent urination, pain on urination, or difficulty urinating.
   3. Unusual vaginal bleeding.
   4. A missed menstrual period.

E. Venereal disease tests have been done. For testing results telephone
   _____ on _____ .
      (number)             (date)

F. The policeman handling your case is _____
   from the _____ police department.

G. The nurse handling your case is _____
   and s/he can be reached at _____ (phone number).

*Modified and reprinted with permission of the Interagency County Task Force on Rape-Related Services, Pittsburgh, Pa. 1979.

# After-care protocol for nursing care of rape victims*

After-care instructions generally include the components listed below.

1. Directions for home care, including the use of the prescribed medications as well as signs to watch for related to injuries sustained.
2. Instructions for what to do if bruises or other injuries or symptoms become apparent.
3. Recommended medical follow-up for examination and further treatment related to trauma.
   a. Explain methods of pregnancy prevention.
   b. Remind her to return for removal of stitches, if she has had them.
   c. Advise her to return for evaluation of wound-healing even if she was given tetanus toxoid.
4. Specific times, locations, and phone numbers of community agencies, clinics, and/or private physicians available for follow-up examinations and tests for venereal disease and pregnancy; recommended follow-up periods are usually:
   a. Gonorrhea at two weeks.
   b. Gonorrhea, syphilis, and pregnancy at six weeks.
5. An appointment schedule, such as the one below, is completed and given in writing to the victim:†

Medical appointments: Date _____ Time _____
    Place _____
                 Date _____ Time _____
    Place _____
Police appointments: Date _____ Time _____
    Place _____
District attorney: Date _____ Time _____
    Place _____
Court hearings: Date _____ Time _____
    Place _____
Counseling appointments: Date _____ Time _____
    Place _____

---

*Reprinted with modifications with permission of the Rape Treatment Center, Santa Monica Hospital Medical Center.
†Reprinted with permission of the Interagency Task Force on Rape-Related Services: A handbook for victims, Pittsburgh, Pa., 1979.

6. Name and phone number of the crisis intervention counselor who saw the patient at the hospital.
    a. Patient is told he/she will be contacted within 24-48 hours after disposition; emotional and physical status will be assessed and any additional services appearing to be indicated will be recommended.
    b. Several telephone numbers are obtained where patient may be reached for follow-up. Victims frequently move or have their telephone numbers unlisted.
7. Names, locations, and phone numbers of agencies and services available in the community to meet the patient's other medical, legal, psychological, or advocacy needs (see Appendix L). Resources listed need to be:
    a. Geographically and financially accessible to patient.
    b. Immediately available and responsive to crisis needs of sexual assault patients.
8. With the patient's consent, the hospital should assist with making arrangements for follow-up care to insure that the patient obtains the recommended services. Make a definite appointment date, time and location.
9. A written copy of the after-care plan is placed in the patient's permanent medical record.
10. Patient is given:
    a. Copies of all consent forms.
    b. After-care instructions (including resources and referrals).
    c. Needed medications (or prescriptions for same).

## APPENDIX O

# Receipt for release of evidence to police*

On _____ at _____, I, _____,
  (date)        (time)              (hospital employee)

gave the following items to _____
                                      (police officer)

of the _____
                         (police department)

_____ Clothing

_____ Laboratory specimens

_____ Other _____

Signed _____
                 (hospital employee)

Signed _____
                 (police officer)

*Reprinted with permission of the Interagency County Task Force on Rape-Related Services, Pittsburgh, Pa., 1979.

# Study guide: the rape examination*

This is a brief outline of the steps in a complete rape examination. There is no system that holds up for all times and in all places, so there may be alterations needed to comply with the local authorities.

| Test | Material needed | Procedure | Comments |
|---|---|---|---|
| History | Appropriate "sexual assault" forms | See text. | See text. |
| Photography of clothing | 1. Camera<br>2. Film | Photograph the patient in the clothes in which she allegedly was attacked. | Omit this step if the patient is not wearing the clothes in which she was attacked, or if the police already have obtained these photographs. |
| Clothing collection | 1. Paper bags<br>2. Labels | Handle clothing as little as possible. Place each item in a separate paper bag and affix a completed label. | Plastic bags may promote molding of secretions and seminal stains. |
| Physical examination | Appropriate "sexual assault" forms | See text. | See text. |
| Photography of wounds | 1. Camera<br>2. Film<br>3. Label | Photograph any signs of trauma. Remove the undeveloped film from the camera. Affix a completed label. | If "instant" (e.g., Polaroid®) pictures are used, affix a completed label to the back, and affix the picture to the record in a sealed envelope. Diagrams may be used instead of photography. |
| Urine for pregnancy test and drug screen | 1. Two urine containers<br>2. Labels | Routine urine collections. Affix completed labels to both samples. | Discourage defecation and perineal wiping. Collect urine at this point so the pelvic examination can be done on an empty bladder. |
| Removal of dried seminal stains from the skin | 1. NaCl<br>2. Cotton-tipped swabs<br>3. Paper envelopes<br>4. Labels | Moisten a swab with NaCl and gently rub the stain from the skin. Place the swab in a paper envelope, seal it, and affix a completed label. | This will be sent to the crime laboratory to check for semen and acid phosphatase. See text for a description of dried seminal stains. |

*Braen, G. Richard: The rape examination, North Chicago, Ill., Abbott Laboratories. Copyright 1981 Abbott Laboratories. Reprinted with permission.

Note: A complete bimanual and speculum examination need not be done on a child or on an inexperienced woman in whom it might produce additional severe pain or emotional trauma. Specimens can be obtained by a moist swab or pipette in these cases.

Note: At the very minimum, vaginal contents should be submitted for these tests:
  (1) Swab and wet mount for the presence of sperm with a note as to the number and motility.
  (2) Two air-dried slides.
  (3) A Pap smear.

*Continued.*

| Test | Material needed | Procedure | Comments |
|------|-----------------|-----------|----------|
| Fingernail scrapings | 1. Fingernail file 2. Glassine envelope 3. Label | Scrape beneath the fingernails and place the debris in the envelope. Affix a completed label. | This will be checked by the crime laboratory for foreign skin, blood, etc. |
| Wood's light check of the pelvic area | Wood's light (ultraviolet) | With the patient in the lithotomy position and the room lights off, observe the pelvic area for spots of fluorescence. | Semen has a bright bluishwhite fluorescence, while urine, feces and pus are less brilliant. This step may be omitted if a Wood's light is not available. |
| Pubic hair trimming | 1. Forceps 2. Scissors 3. Glassine envelope 4. Label | Trim any hair thought to be matted with semen, place it in the envelope, and affix a completed label. | This will be sent to the crime laboratory for a check for sperm and acid phosphatase. |
| Pubic hair combing | 1. Plastic comb 2. Large paper towel 3. Envelope (4″ × 6″) 4. Label | Place one edge of the paper towel under the buttocks of the patient (who is in the lithotomy position) and use it to catch any foreign material while combing the mons pubis. Fold the comb into the towel and place both into the envelope. Affix a completed label. | Foreign material (pubic hair, etc.) obtained may be checked against the suspect and the scene of the crime. A positive identification of a suspect by a pubic hair is impossible. It may, however, identify the race and the hair color of the rapist. |
| Aspiration of vaginal contents | 1. Vaginal speculum 2. Gloves 3. Aspiration pipette 4. Bulb for pipette 5. Test tube and stopper 6. Label | Insert a water-lubricated speculum into the vagina and check for signs of trauma. If secretions are present, aspirate them, place them in a test tube, seal it, and affix a completed label. | If no secretions are present, go on to the next step. Aspirated secretions will be tested for motile sperm, acid phosphatase, blood group antigens, and sometimes a sperm precipitin test to see if the sperm was of human origin. |
| Swab of the posterior fornix of the vagina | 1. NaCl 2. Cotton-tipped swab 3. Test tube and stopper 4. Labels 5. Two glass slides with frosted ends 6. Container for the slides 7. Pencil | Moisten the swab with NaCl and squeeze out any excess against the inside wall of the test tube. Liberally wipe the posterior fornix. Smear two glass slides, and air dry them. With a pencil, label the frosted end with the patient's name and hospital number. Place the slides in their container when dry and seal it with a completed label. Place the swab in the test tube, seal it, and affix a completed label. | The swab will be checked for motile sperm, acid phosphatase, blood group antigens, and sometimes for sperm precipitins. One glass slide will be stained by the laboratory for sperm, and the other will be checked for acid phosphatase. |

| Test | Material needed | Procedure | Comments |
|------|-----------------|-----------|----------|
| Vaginal washing | 1. NaCl, 10 ml<br>2. Aspiration pipette<br>3. Bulb for pipette<br>4. Test tube and stopper<br>5. Label | Irrigate the vaginal vault with 10 ml NaCl, aspirate the fluid, place it in a test tube, seal it, and affix a completed label. | Avoid the cervix while washing the vagina (see text). This will be checked for motile sperm, acid phosphatase, blood group antigens, and sometimes for sperm precipitins. |
| Pap smear | 1. Two clean slides<br>2. Cervical scraper<br>3. Pap fixative<br>4. Label | Routine. Affix a completed label. | This is both good medicine and part of the medicolegal exam. Stained sperm are frequently found by the pathologist. |
| Cervical gonorrhea culture | 1. Thayer-Martin plate or Transgrow® medium<br>2. Cotton-tipped swab<br>3. Label | Routine. Affix a completed label. | |
| Bimanual pelvic examination | 1. Gloves<br>2. Lubricant | Routine. | |
| Perianal examination | 1. Cotton-tipped swab<br>2. Test tube and stopper<br>3. Label | Look for signs of trauma and lubrication. If a lubricant is present, remove some with a cotton-tipped swab, place it in the test tube, seal it, and affix a completed label. | Lubrication is not commonly found. Be careful not to contaminate the anorectal area with vaginal contents from the gloved hand which has just been used to do a bimanual pelvic examination in the preceding step. |
| Rectal gonorrhea culture | 1. Thayer-Martin plate or Transgrow® medium<br>2. Cotton-tipped swab<br>3. Label | Routine. Affix a completed label. | |
| Rectal washing | 1. NaCl, 10 ml<br>2. 10 ml syringe<br>3. Test tube and stopper<br>4. Label | With the patient in the lithotomy position, place the *hub* of the NaCl-filled syringe into the anal opening and irrigate the rectum. Wait for 1 to 5 minutes and aspirate, again with the hub of the syringe. Place any liquid in a test tube, seal it, and affix a completed label. | If anal intercourse has occurred, evidence of sperm and acid phosphatase may be recovered by this method. If the patient denies anal intercourse, omit this step. |

*Continued.*

| Test | Material needed | Procedure | Comments |
|---|---|---|---|
| Pharyngeal gonorrhea culture | 1. Thayer-Martin plate or Trans-grow® medium<br>2. Cotton-tipped swab<br>3. Tongue blade<br>4. Label | Routine. Affix a completed label. | This step is included if the patient allegedly was forced to perform oral sex, or if the physician suspects pre-existing pharyngeal gonorrhea. |
| Saliva for se-cretor status | 1. Sterile 2×2 gauze pad<br>2. Forceps<br>3. Test tube and stopper<br>4. Label | Using the forceps, place the gauze pad in the patient's mouth and have her saturate it with saliva. With the forceps, place the pad in the test tube, seal it, and affix a completed label. | This is a test for the secretion of blood-group antigens in the saliva (see text). Care must be taken not to contaminate the specimen with antigens from a nurse or physician. If the forceps were used earlier to remove matted pubic hair cuttings, another sterilized pair should be used. |
| Blood samples | 1. Three red-topped tubes<br>2. Tourniquet<br>3. Prepping solution not containing alcohol<br>4. Gauze pad<br>5. 20 ml syringe and needle<br>6. Labels | Routine. Affix a completed label to each tube. | These will be sent for a VDRL, drug and alcohol screen, and blood typing. At some institutions, a fourth blood sample for pregnancy testing may be drawn. |
| Microscopic examination for sperm motility | 1. Samples of vaginal aspirate, vaginal swab, vaginal washing, or rectal washing<br>2. Microscope<br>3. Slides<br>4. Cover slips | Prepare a wet mount with a drop of the sample to be tested, and observe for motile sperm. Record the findings. | If RBC's obscure the field, add one drop of SediStain®. This will stain the sperm bright blue with little loss of motility. The use of a drop of glacial acetic acid will render the sperm completely immotile while lysing the RBC's. |
| Consolidation of the samples | 1. Empty box from the rape examination kit<br>2. Label | Place all the samples destined for the police in the box and affix a completed label. Samples destined for the hospital laboratory should be handed personally to the pathologist or senior technologist. A written chain of evidence should be initiated. | All samples obtained are worthless unless a proper routine for labeling and the "chain of evidence" is followed. |

# Procedural guide for child sexual abuse examination*

| Oral-genital contact | Genital contact | Anal penetration | Vaginal discharge |
|---|---|---|---|
| **PROTOCOL I: Prepubescent seen > 72 hours** | | | |
| 1. Obtain throat swab for GC culture | No evidence of injury or penetration. | †1. Rectal exam & stool quiac | 1. Swabs (can use 2 at a time) |
| 2. Obtain baseline VDRL, FTA | Evidence consistent with penetration (absent hymen, healing tears) | 2. Rectal swab for GC culture | a. Gram stain for GC, if + Rx for GC |
| | 1. Urinalysis for occult blood | 3. Baseline VDRL, FTA | b. GC culture |
| | †2. Gyne consult within a week | | c. Wet prep for trichomonas if + Rx with Flagyl |
| | 3. Swab for GC culture | | 2. Urinalysis |
| | 4. Baseline VDRL, FTA | | 3. Baseline VDRL, FTA |
| | 4. Instruct to return if develops vaginal d/c | | |

Postpubescent > 72 hours - same applies except schedule for gyne consult and pelvic exam within a week, consider pregnancy test.

*Protocols I and II modified by H.W. Davis, M.D. (Children's Hospital, Pittsburgh, Pa.), from Pascoe, D.J.: Management of sexually abused children, Pediatr. Ann. **8**(5): 52, Table 1, May 1979, Copyright © 1979, Insight Publishing Co., Inc.

†If child shows evidence of recent tears or has abnormal abdominal exam, consult general surgery for consideration of EUA.

*Continued.*

## PROTOCOL II: Prepubescent seen < 72 hours

| Orogenital contact | Genital contact | Anal penetration |
|---|---|---|
| 1. Wood's lamp, if + get skin scrapings | Evidence consistent with vaginal penetration | 1. Wood's lamp, if + get skin scrapings |
| 2. Swabs—use 2 at a time | No evidence of penetration | 2. If external tears seen: |
|   a. For wet mount for sperm | 1. Urinalysis for occult blood |   a. Consult general surgery for possible EUA |
| ‡b. For 2 air-dried slides | 2. Wood's lamp, if + get skin scrapings |   b. If EUA done, collect evidence then |
|   c. For GC culture | 3. Swabs of introitus, use 2 at a time | 3. Swabs: use 2 at a time |
| 3. Baseline VDRL, FTA |   a. For wet mount for sperm | Must be done before rectal examination. |
| | ‡b. For 2 air-dried slides |   a. For wet mount for sperm |
| |   c. For GC culture | ‡b. For 2 air-dried slides |
| | 4. Baseline VDRL, FTA |   c. For GC culture |
| | | 4. If no tears: |
| | |   a. Rectal exam |
| | |   b. Stool guiac, if + consult general surgery |
| | | 5. Baseline VDRL, FTA |

*Genital contact (Evidence consistent with vaginal penetration):*
1. Urinalysis for occult blood
2. Wood's lamp, if + get skin scrapings
3. If external tears seen:
  a. Surgical consult for possible EUA
  b. If EUA done, collect evidence then
4. Vaginal swabs: use 2 at a time
  a. For wet mount for sperm
‡b. For 2 air-dried slides
5. Baseline VDRL, FTA

### Post pubescent < 72 hours

1. Same obtains but should have gynecology consent for pelvic exam when seen.
2. Stage of menstrual cycle should be determined and pregnancy prophylaxsis given if needed and desired.

‡1 slide is for gram stain; 1 goes to the coroner's lab along with the 2 swabs which should be placed in a dry culture tube.

# ADDITIONAL SPECIMENS NEEDED IN RAPE CASES (Seen within 72 hours)

NOTE: Specimens may be obtained by the physician or a nurse.

All containers used in evidence collection should be paper and must be labeled with:

1. Patient's name
2. Type of specimen
3. Body site
4. Date and time
5. Initials of collector

1. *Clothing.* If the patient is wearing the same clothes, they should be collected along with debris as this may provide valuable clues regarding the assailant. The patient should disrobe while standing on a towel or sheet. Each article including the towel or sheet should then be placed in a separate paper bag. Avoid shaking the articles. Each bag is then labeled and sealed.

2. *Fingernail scrapings.* These may provide bits of skin, fiber and debris from the assailant. Scrapings from beneath the nails or nail clippings should be obtained. Specimens from each hand should be collected over separate sheets of paper, and placed in separate paper envelopes, sealed and labeled.

3. *Hair samples*

   a. Any loose or suspected foreign hairs should be collected, placed in an envelope and labeled.
   b. Comb pubic hairs onto a sheet of clean paper, fold, place in an envelope with the comb, label and seal.
   c. Gently pull a small clump of the patient's pubic hair (12 hairs are needed), place on clean paper, fold, put in envelope and label standard pubic hair.
   d. Comb and obtain head hairs as in *b* and *c*.

   NOTE: *b* and *c* are obviously unnecessary in prepubescent patients.

4. *Blood sample.* 5 cc of blood in a purple-top tube should be drawn for blood grouping and enzyme typing.

# Emergency room protocol for child/adolescent patients

## INFORMATION FOR ALL INVOLVED WITH PATIENT

1. See immediately. Even though no physical trauma may be present, victims of sexual assault should receive high priority (immediately following acutely ill or injured patients).
2. Provide maximum support to parents as well as to the child/adolescent victim. Do not be judgmental or allow emotional responses (e.g., anger, outrage) to interfere with providing optimal care.
3. Only those DIRECTLY involved in care should talk with the patient; give the patient and parents your name and explain your role.
4. Do not discuss sexual assault cases with anyone without the consent of the parent or legal guardian and the patient, if an adolescent.
5. "Rape" and "sexual assault" are legal, not medical, terms. Do not use other than as "History of Sexual Assault."
6. The chart may be legal evidence. "Hearsay" statements from those who first see the child/adolescent may be admissible in court. All statements should be accurate, objective and legible.

## EMERGENCY ROOM PERSONNEL

1. Provide private facilities for the victim (ER 9 or the Quiet Room). Complete registration there.
2. Contact the ER physician immediately if there is evidence of moderate to severe physical trauma.
3. Obtain consent for care from the parents or legal guardian. If such consent cannot be obtained, contact the hospital administrator or the Juvenile Court for temporary consent. Examination of the adolescent should not be done without her/his consent unless a life-threatening emergency exists.
4. Contact social worker immediately.
5. If the assault occurred within the past 48 hours, contact the pediatric resident immediately. If the assault occurred more than 48 hours ago, the social worker will ascertain need for medical care.
6. The sexual assault tray and vaginal kit (containing Pedersen and pediatric specula) should be placed in exam room. (Check and replace items daily.)
7. Chaperone pelvic examination. A female chaperone (hospital employee) should be present for all pelvic examinations. Do not have the patient undress until just before the physical examination.

*Reprinted with permission of Sexual Assault Center, Harborview Medical Center, Seattle, Wash.

## SOCIAL WORKER

1. Assess immediate emotional needs of child and parents. Respond appropriately.
2. Confirm that the pediatric resident has been notified.
3. History: Obtain alone or in conjunction with the physician.
   a. Ascertain as much of the history as possible from parents or accompanying persons first, away from patient.
   b. See patient alone to obtain history (unless parent or other person is needed for support, i.e., in the very young child).
   c. Determine and use the patient's terminology for parts of the body, sexual acts, etc. Use aids, i.e., toys and picture books, as needed. Questions should be appropriate for age and developmental level.
   d. Obtain a directed history of the assault. Do not ask "why" questions, e.g., "Why did you go to his house?" Phrase questions in terms of "who, what, where, when," e.g., "Did the offender use oral, finger, penile contact to mouth, vulva, vagina, rectum?"; "How long ago did it happen?"; "Did penetration or ejaculation occur?"; "What kind of force, threat or enticement was used?"; "From whom did the patient seek help?".
   e. When the physician arrives, present history and impressions (out of patient's hearing) and complete history-taking conjointly.
4. Explain to patient and parents the reasons for questions asked, types of medical/legal tests needed, and possible treatment.
5. Obtain special consents, i.e., for photographs, release of clothing, release of information (specify to whom).
6. Assist with the physical examination, if indicated.
7. Discuss reporting to police and/or Children's Protective Service. Police may be contacted to come to the Emergency Room for an initial report.
8. Assessment and Counseling
   a. Assess behavior and affect. Ascertain support systems of patient and family. Do not return child home unless the environment is safe. Document changes in housing.
   b. Explain anticipated emotional problems. Give patient and parents SAC handout.
   c. Encourage consulting with the Sexual Assault Center.
9. Record on Sexual Assault Report from services offered to patient:
   a. Medical appointment for follow-up care.
   b. Ongoing counseling or advocacy by SAC.
   c. Children's Protective Service referral, when indicated. (Referral to CPS is legally mandated when the offender is a family member or when the home environment does not protect the child from further sexual abuse.)
   d. Referrals made to other agencies.
   e. Victim's compensation brochure, form, and brief explanation.

## PHYSICIAN

1. Medical History: Ascertain history from social worker and parents. Corroborate with patient. Do not needlessly repeat questions. Use "History of Sexual Assault" form #0245.
   a. Use vocabulary appropriate for age and developmental level. Use patient's words to describe and explain meaning if needed, i.e., "He put his 'thing' in me." (penis). Use picture books or toys as aids as needed.
   b. Ascertain activity post-assault: changes of clothing; bathing; douching; urinating; defecating; drinking.
   c. Obtain menstrual, contraceptive, VD history as needed.

d. Obtain pertinent medical history: chronic illnesses; allergies; etc.

e. Discuss VD prophylaxis, hormonal pregnancy prevention and abortion. Ascertain patient's feelings in these areas.

2. Approach to Examination

a. Be gentle and empathetic. Explain what you are doing in a calm manner and voice. Take time to relax the apprehensive patient.

b. If supportive, have parent stay with child during the examination. Allow the adolescent the option of having whom s/he wishes to be present.

c. Allow the patient to feel as much in control of his/her body during the exam as possible. Verbalize an understanding of his/her anxiety.

d. Use appropriate gowns and drapes to ensure modesty and decrease feelings of vulnerability.

e. Unless there is physical trauma which is apparent or must be ruled out, the complete examination does not need to be done (i.e., use of stirrups, speculum). All tests can be done with a glass pipette and cotton swabs.

   (1) A small child may lie across the mother's lap in a "frog-leg" position.

   (2) An older child may lie on the exam table in the same position.

   (3) An adolescent may lie on the table in the same position or in stirrups.

f. Use a REASONABLE approach. Use only those parts of the protocol appropriate for age of child and type of assault.

3. Physical Examination: Perform with hospital employee as chaperone.

a. General: Document emotional status; general appearance of patient and clothing.

b. Document areas of trauma on TRAUMAGRAM and describe in detail (see Table 11-9).

c. Examine areas involved in sexual assault, i.e., oral, vaginal, rectal, penile. Very carefully document even minor trauma to these areas. Photograph areas of trauma as indicated (per evidence collection checklist (see Table 11-10).

d. Ask patient to point with finger to exact area involved. Ask how much further offender penetrated.

e. Describe developmental level (Tanner Stage), external genitalia, type and condition of hymen and diameter of introitus.

f. Do exam as indicated by age of patient, type of assault and degree of injury. If injuries are extensive or cannot be determined due to lack of cooperation, consider examination and treatment under general anesthesia.

4. Medical Tests

a. Culture body orifices involved for gonorrhea. If history is uncertain, culture all orifices.

b. Obtain gravindex to rule out pregnancy as indicated.

c. Obtain VDRL baseline. May be deferred in the young child or apprehensive adolescent.

5. Legal Tests

a. UV light - semen fluoresces. Examine areas of body and clothing involved (in dark after visual adaptation).

   (1) Save clothing fluorescing for police (as per evidence collection checklist).

   (2) Swab body areas fluorescing with saline-moistened swabs. Place swabs in red-top tubes. (Follow evidence collection checklist—see Table 11-10).

b. Wet mount preparation:

   (1) Aspirate or swab areas of body involved (pharynx, rectum, vaginal pool). Saline-moistened swabs may be used; however, aspiration with a glass pipette after flushing area with 2cc of saline is preferred.

   (2) Place drop of secretions on glass slide, plus drop of saline; examine immediately.

(3) Physician should examine several fields under high power with light source turned down. Document presence or absence of sperm and number of motile/nonmotile seen per high power field.

  c. Permanent smears:

    (1) Physician will make two preparations. One slide will be a routine PAP from the endocervix and vaginal wall areas (may be deferred in child). The second slide will be a smear from the posterior vaginal pool, rectum, pharynx as indicated. Obtain in the same manner as the Wet Mount.

    (2) Put both slides promptly into the PAP bottle, back to back. DO NOT ALLOW TO AIR DRY. (Follow evidence collection checklist—see Table 11-10).

    (3) Physician will complete and sign PAP form noting "History of Sexual Assault; please do routine PAP and document presence or absence of sperm."

  d. Acid Phosphates:

    (1) Collect in same manner as for wet mount preparation.

    (2) Place saline-moistened swabs or secretions from pipette in red-top tube. (Follow evidence collection checklist—see Table 11-10).

  e. Other tests - as indicated or as police request (mainly to identify assailant), i.e., ABO antigens (collect as for acid phosphatase); fingernail scrapings; pubic hair combings.

6. Treatment

  a. Injuries—treat and/or consult with other specialties as indicated. Give tetanus prophylaxis as indicated by history; follow CDC-Public Health recommendations (available in ER).

  b. Pregnancy prophylaxis—may be given IF a vaginal assault occurred at midcycle, without contraception, and patient understands risks and side effects of estrogens to be given and is willing to have an abortion should pregnancy occur despite medication. *Do not prescribe* if there has been other unprotected intercourse during this cycle or any possibility of pre-existing pregnancy. Obtain a negative gravindex before instituting therapy.

    (1) Hormonal therapy—Estinyl: 2.5 mg b.i.d. for 5 days. (Prepacks in ER.)

    (2) Antinauseant therapy—Benedectin (ii h.s. as needed for nausea and vomiting). Give routinely to use as needed. (Prepacks in ER.)

  c. VD prophylaxis

    (1) Not given routinely but as indicated, e.g., high patient anxiety, possibility patient will not return for follow-up care, known disease, multiple rapists.

    (2) Therapy (over 12 years of age):

      (a) Probenecid 1 gm orally +Ampillicin 3.5 gm orally stat; OR

      (b) Probenecid 1 gm orally followed in 30 minutes by procaine penicillin G 4.8 million units IM; OR

      (c) If penicillin allergy, spectinomycin 4 gm IM OR tetracycline 500 mgm q.i.d. × 4 days.

    (3) Therapy (under 12 years of age): use age- and weight-appropriate dosages.

  d. Treatment for anxiety and/or difficulty sleeping—as indicated (rarely needed in children under 12 years; use age-appropriate dosage when given). Adult therapy as follows:

    (1) Mellaril 10 mgm one-half hour before sleep (may repeat once, if necessary; do not exceed 20 mgm/day. Give a 3-day supply (60 mgm); OR

    (2) Valium 5 mgm one-half hour before sleep (may repeat once p.r.n.). Do not exceed 10 mgm/day. Give 3-day supply (30 mgm).

7. Final Care

  a. Verbally express concern and availability for help as needed.

  b. Reinforce social worker information; reinforce that patient is physically intact and is not responsible for the assault/abuse.

  c. Discuss medical problems which may arise and encourage family to call as needed.

8. Final Diagnosis
   a. History of Sexual Assault.
   b. Presence or absence of sperm.
   c. Specific diagnosis of injuries, contusions, lacerations, etc.
   d. Other pertinent medical diagnoses.
9. Follow-up
   a. Pediatric clinic appointment in one week.
   b. Repeat gonorrhea cultures at follow-up visit; VDRL in 8 weeks; other as indicated.
   c. Consultation from other specialties as indicated.

# Traumagram and evidence collection checklist

**TRAUMAGRAM***

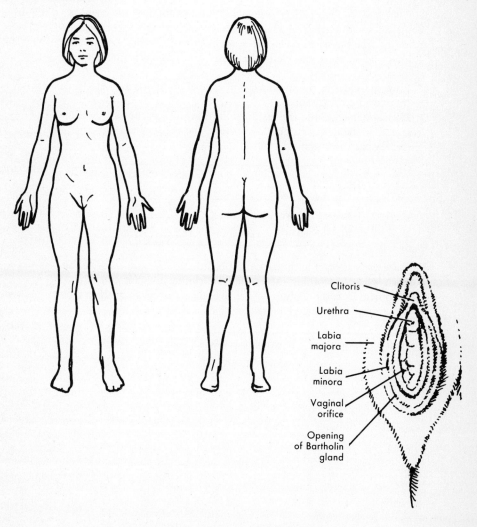

Clitoris

Urethra

Labia majora

Labia minora

Vaginal orifice

Opening of Bartholin gland

*Adapted from Traumagram of the Sexual Assault Center, Harborview Medical Center, Seattle, Wash.: *Progress Notes,* June 1977.

**Evidence Collection Checklist for Emergency Trauma Center Use***
(This accompanies the medical protocol for sexual assaults.)

**PAP smear**

A. RN/ERSW—Get cytology form from special folder on unit assistant's desk (these forms are already partially labeled for sexual assault cases). Stamp special cytology form and specimen labels with patient's name and hospital number and take into the exam room before starting the exam.

B. RN/ERSW—Etch patient's name and hospital number (or birthdate) on slides with electric engraver. Upon completion of the specimen collection, the physician doing the exam must write his/her name on the glass slides, using the electric engraver, and complete the cytology form.

C. Place the slides in the specimen bottle, label the bottle and attach the completed cytology form.

D. Place specimen bottle and cytology form in small paper sack. Seal the sack. Use stamp in ER, placed over seal. The person placing the specimen in bag must sign the seal.

Pap smear

Placed in sack by _____

Taken to lab by _____

Rec'd in lab by _____

E. Place the specimen in the locked cupboard.

F. Each weekday morning (M-F) the ETC clinical assistant will take the specimens from the cupboard and deliver them directly to the chief technician in the Cytology Laboratory.

*Reprinted from the Sexual Assault Center, Harborview Medical Center, Seattle, Wash., July 1978.

**Evidence Collection Checklist for Emergency Trauma
Center Use—cont'd**

**Acid phosphatase**

After obtaining specimen from patient:
A. RN/ERSW—Label red-top tube with patient's name and hospital number, place in designated envelope, date, and seal.
B. Physician—Sign evidence envelope over seal.
C. RN/ERSW—Place envelope in ER refrigerator until SAC personnel arrange transfer to police.

**Other evidence** (hairs, fingernail scrapings, foreign matter)

A. Same as Acid Phosphatase.

**Clothing**

A. ERSW/RN—Place in paper bag and seal with label showing patient's name and hospital number. Note on form that clothing was collected.
B. ERSW/RN—Fill out "Transfer of Specimen" section on form if clothing evidence is given to police in ER. Otherwise, leave near ER refrigerator until SAC arranges transfer to police. (Label bag "Sexual Assault Evidence—DO NOT REMOVE.")

**Photography**

A. ERSW/RN—Obtain witnessed signature from patient on Consent for Photography form.
B. ERSW/RN—Fill in photography information on form.
C. ERSW/RN—Place photographs in folder for SAC, along with Xeroxed copies of ER reports. (SAC will mount pictures for medical chart.)

## APPENDIX T

# Rape prevention strategies*

### PART I: PROTECTING YOURSELF AGAINST SEXUAL ASSAULT

Sexual assault is committed against women of all ages, incomes, and living arrangements.

According to reports by law enforcement and survey agencies, sexual assaults are committed much less frequently than all other crimes except homicide. It is therefore very unlikely that you will ever experience a real or threatened attack. It is also true, however, that all women must be aware of their actions and surroundings at all times in order to reduce chances of becoming a victim of any crime.

The following list of personal safety ideas has been formulated from publications of, and interviews with, many law enforcement agencies and experts on rape prevention. Perhaps you are familiar with some of these ideas; others may be new to you. In any case, they all deserve your careful consideration. While police, housing personnel, and neighbors may be helpful in deterring crime, your own skills in protecting yourself are far more important.

#### Personal safety ideas

*In Your Living Unit*

    I. Don't advertise living alone—
        a. Use initials on mailbox, in phone book; add dummy name
        b. If alone and the doorbell rings, call out, "I'll get it, John" as though someone is with you
        c. Draw shades, drapes at night
    II. House should always look and sound occupied—
        a. Use timers to turn on lights at night
        b. Use porch light
        c. Play radio
        d. Leave phone off hook if leaving home for considerable period during the day
        e. Notify neighbor if going away—ask to collect mail, papers, etc.
        f. Don't pin notes to door
        g. Keep a bathroom light on at night
    III. Essential hardware—
        a. Keep doors and windows locked
        b. Use peephole
        c. Change locks from former tenant
        d. Never hide key; give to a friend
        e. If key is lost, change cylinder
        f. Never put address on key ring

*From Davis, L.V., and Brody, E.M.: Rape and older women: a guide to prevention and protection, DHEW, NIMH, U.S. Government Documents Office, Washington, D.C., 1979, pp. 93-94, 131-136.

IV. Use of phone—
   a. Have phone near bed
   b. Have emergency numbers near phone in big letters so you can read them without glasses
   c. Never reveal personal information on phone: plans; that you live alone; your schedule; name or address; *any* personal information
   d. Report series of obscene calls to police
      1. Blow whistle into receiver
      2. Tap mouthpiece and say, "Operator—this is the call I wanted you to trace"
   e. Have friend check on you at specific time; verbal code to indicate if something is wrong
V. Valuables—
   a. Keep purse, radios, stereos, TVs out of window reach and visible view
   b. Engrave valuables with special security, social security, or driver's license number
   c. Deposit and keep money in bank
   d. Don't keep large amount of cash in home
VI. (This may sound unfriendly but) *Never* open door to stranger—
   a. Don't rely on chain for identification of visitors
   b. Require identification from everyone: utility men, maintenance men, police, repairmen, salesmen; ask them to pass ID under door; when in doubt, check with company by telephone
   c. If stranger requests use of phone, regardless of reason or "emergency," offer to make call for him while he waits outside of locked door
VII. If intruder is suspected—
   a. If awakened, pretend to sleep and stay in room
   b. Try to retreat without being seen
   c. If confronted, do not antagonize; observe description. Self-defense measures are appropriate only if you are certain of your advantage and skill or if loss of life appears imminent.
VIII. Know your neighbors—Work out procedure for alerting each other in case of emergency

*In a Building*
   I. Always have key in hand before you reach entrance
   II. Avoid deserted areas within building when alone—stairways, laundry, trash, and storage areas
   III. Avoid or use caution when getting into elevator with stranger—in elevator stand near control button and push for main floor or emergency if concerned
   IV. Don't overload yourself with bundles—Be prepared to drop them quickly if being followed
   V. If you think you're being watched when leaving apartment, shout to mythical companion, "Take the cake out in ten minutes, George!"
   VI. If apartment seems to have been entered, don't go in yourself
   VII. This may sound silly, but if accosted, yell "Fire," not "Help"—it will attract attention quickly

*On the Street*
   I. Whenever possible don't walk alone—
      a. Use buddy system or groups
      b. Don't shortcut through vacant lots or parking lots
      c. Stay away from doorways and shrubbery

    d. Walk near curb, facing traffic

    e. If car pulls next to you going the same way you are, reverse direction

    f. Avoid streets in unfamiliar neighborhoods

    g. Vary route in going to store, coming home

    h. If insecure on sidewalk and traffic permits, walk down the middle of street

II. Talking to strangers—

    a. Be very cautious when stranger asks directions or time or offers to carry your packages home

    b. Beware of individual who claims to have found money and wants to share it with you or who offers goods at low prices

III. Always look and be alert to surroundings—

    a. Don't walk through group of men; cross street or walk around them

    b. If approached, look for lighted windows; wave and shout upward as though someone at window is watching you

IV. Carry purse, papers, umbrella under arm or keep purse between body and bundles—

    a. Carry purse on side away from the street

    b. Carry minimum of cash

    c. Carry money in two places—shoe, bra, or hidden pocket

    d. Don't overload yourself with packages, keep hands free

    e. Don't hang bag on hook in public bathroom

    f. Keep bag tightly in grip in stores and market

    g. If you think someone might take purse, drop it in nearest mailbox; it will be returned to you

    h. Never wind purse-strap around wrist (if grabbed, you can be pulled down and injured)

    i. If someone tries for purse, throw it in street or turn it upside down and let contents fall out

    j. Insert comb in wallet with teeth up to prevent easy removal

    k. If purse is snatched, beware of phone call giving information where to retrieve it (call police for advice)

    l. If possible, do not carry a purse at all

V. Carry whistle—

    a. Put whistle on key chain, not around neck

    b. Have it available to blow when you feel threatened

VI. Know location of police call boxes, buildings with doormen on duty, all-night stores, and other sources of help along your route

VII. When going to visit, call ahead to tell how you are going, when to be expected

VIII. If accosted yell "Fire," not "Rape" or "Help"

IX. When brought home, have friend or taxi wait till you're inside and safe

*When Traveling*

    I. Travel with companion whenever possible

    II. When awaiting or riding public transportation, stand with feet apart in a balanced position

    III. At bus and subway stops, keep your back to the wall to avoid being approached from behind—

        a. Sit in front, near driver or conductor

        b. Always have token ready

        c. In subway, sit in populated car; avoid last car; get near conductor

        d. Use busy stop; avoid deserted ones

        e. If you suspect you are being followed, don't get off at normal stop; get off at busy stop, tell attendant in change booth

*While Banking*

    I. Bank by mail

    II. Deposit checks soon after receipt

    III. If you must walk, don't go alone and vary route and time of deposit

    IV. Put your cash away before leaving window

    V. Ask for direct deposit of checks by public assistance agency or other agencies involved

*In Your Automobile*

    I. Key in hand when approaching car—

      a. Keep car key on separate chain; separate from house keys

      b. Leave only ignition key with attendant

      c. Don't put name/address on keys

    II. Drive with doors locked and windows rolled at least three-quarters up

    III. Put packages on floor out of view

    IV. Don't pick up hitchhikers

    V. Always have at least one-fourth tank of gas in your car

    VI. Disabled car—raise hood; tie white cloth to aerial or doorhandle—

      a. Stay in car; do not get out

      b. Ask interested motorist to call police for you

    VII. At night—

      a. Always park in well-lit area

      b. Have friend escort you to car

      c. Always check back seat and floor before entering car; use flashlight at night if necessary

    VIII. If you notice a vehicle with person in distress, don't stop. Note location and stop at first phone to call police

    IX. Don't leave credentials or personal papers in car

You may notice as you read these tips that they are ideas that will help protect you from all types of crimes, not just sexual assault. There is a good reason for this. Statistics show that most sexual assaults against middle-aged and older women occur in the victim's own home and in connection with another crime, particularly burglery and robbery.

The main idea is to be aware, alert, and to prevent a potential assailant from having the opportunity to make you his next victim.

In addition to using these ideas for individual safety, many groups of neighbors have formally or informally organized in an effort to protect each other from victimization. Some examples of successful programs include buddy systems, neighborhood watches, lobby sitting, door monitoring, escort services, cooperative shopping, and many other activities.

In your community the agency to contact for guidance in planning and implementing a protection program is:

---

Remember, *every* woman is a potential victim of rape or other sexual offenses. The suggestions in this booklet deal with how to protect yourself and your neighbors from victimization. If you follow the suggestions for personal safety, chances are you will never be confronted with an attacker. If you are, however, the most important things to remember are:

1. Try to *remain calm* and *use your head. Escape* from the situation with the least amount of harm to yourself.

2. Be able to *identify* your assailant.

If a sexual assault occurs:

• Call the police immediately at _____ . Tell them what happened and how badly you are hurt.

- Avoid cleaning yourself or the area where the assault occurred. Physical evidence is essential for apprehension and prosecution of your assailant.
- Call a rape crisis center or other agency. (Insert name of local program.)

A volunteer will counsel you, and tell you what to expect and how they can help you. THEY UNDERSTAND. DON'T BE AFRAID TO CALL!

---

## PART II: COMMUNITY ORGANIZATION ACTIVITIES

*Within a Building*

I. Informal Activities
  - Residents' awareness of neighbors' habits and movements; calling police/management when a problem occurs
  - Informal checking on friends by telephone
  - Using panic buttons, freon horns to alert others
  - Front door monitoring and lobby sitting by residents
  - Buddy systems when using laundry rooms, basements, and other public areas

II. Formal Activities
  - Operation Identification[a]
  - Using panic buttons, freon horns to alert others with prearranged signals
  - Organizational structure/leadership pattern including floor captains and alternates
  - Scheduled front door monitoring, lobby sitting
  - Tenant watch
  - Tenant patrol of building
  - Escorting neighbors to laundry rooms, basements, and public spaces
  - Rape prevention/education programs
  - Crime prevention/education/training programs
  - Rental of one living unit to a police officer, at nominal rent, for on-the-premises protection
  - Transportation schedule posted conspicuously in lobbies, mailrooms, management offices
  - Doorman services
  - Security patrolling, guard services, tenant security guards
  - Security briefings for new tenants by management or tenants' council
  - Telephone reassurance services
  - Residential security counseling by police or police-trained community people, with hardware available at reduced prices (Installation could be done by volunteers from the community agency staffs.)

---

[a]Operation Identification is a program designed to deter burglars and facilitate identification of stolen goods. Personal possessions are permanently marked with an identifying number, often a social security number. This number is filed with the police department. A sticker can be displayed prominently on an outside door or window stating that this resident has participated in Operation Identification.

*In the Neighborhood*
  I. Informal Activities
   - Neighborhood or Town Watch[b]
   - Buddy system when traveling
   - Group shopping, banking trips
   - School crossing guards watching out for security of elderly
   - Drivers with citizens band radios reporting problems to police
  II. Formal Activities
   - Organized block program, either with a general focus or a crime prevention focus
   - Neighborhood patrols/walks by residents
   - Police Safety Corridors[c]
   - Escort services by screened and identifiable volunteers
   - "Safety Spots"[d]
   - Shopping assistance
   - Free banking services by mail or with volunteer assistance
   - Free delivery from local merchants, by reliable delivery persons
   - Improved transportation services, both public and private
   - Visible police patrolling
   - Police training for block watchers
   - Residential security counseling
   - Taxi patrol ("Cab Watch") reporting to police

---

[b]Neighborhood Watch or Town Watch is an informal or formal neighborhood security system in which persons familiar with neighborhood patterns watch occurrences and take action (e.g., call the police) when anything unusual happens. The watch can include a regular walk or patrol.

[c]Safety corridors are streets assigned by police for special patrolling in unmarked and marked police cars, ensuring "safe passage." Different streets can be designated on a rotating schedule, resulting in more territory being covered.

[d]A "Safety Spot" is a marked, designated merchant in a commercial area who agrees to render aid to a person in distress.

## APPENDIX U

# Resource films*

*A Crime of Violence: Rape and Sexual Assault,* 1977, Current Affairs, Division of Key Productions, Inc., 24 Danbury Road, Wilton, CT 06897. Producer: Russel-Manning Production, Inc., and Glenda Fischer-Epstein Productions for Current Affairs Films.

> ABSTRACT: This is a two-part filmstrip. Part 1 dispels myths that surround the crime of rape, shows the impact of myths on victims, discusses myths and facts, and defines sexual assault. Part 2 examines changes in sexual assault legislation, reasons victims do not report rape, role of rape crisis centers, approaches in medical care, family response to rape, and a variety of prevention/self-defense strategies.
>
> CRITIQUE: Suitable for junior and senior high school students, adult and civic groups, and a wide range of audiences from teenagers to the elderly. The filmstrip can be used at symposiums and workshops and as a tool to facilitate discussion.
>
> FORMAT: 20 min, color, filmstrip; automatic or manual operation; sound cassette. Discussion guide included offers pretest, discussion topics, and bibliography. Rental: $7.50; purchase; $57.50.

*Acquaintance Rape Prevention,* 1978, Association Films, Inc., 1111 N. 19th Street, Suite 404, Arlington, VA 22209 (distributor for NIMH). Producer: National Center for the Prevention and Control of Rape.

> ABSTRACT: The four vignettes in this film depict: misperceptions and stereotyped sex-role behaviors on a date that can lead to rape; a group of high school students after a football game; a teenage party; and a woman alone on the road after her car has broken down. Each vignette triggers a series of events that begin by a casual encounter and end in a rape-threatening situation. The audience is led to challenge rape myths and stereotyped sex-role behaviors; to recognize acquaintance rape and the interpersonal dynamics involved; and to identify the link between assertiveness and rape prevention.
>
> CRITIQUE: Suitable for junior and senior high school students and for colleges and organizations that provide rape prevention education programs to teenagers and young adults. This film can be used with coed groups.
>
> FORMAT: 16 mm, color, sound; each of the four films averages 6 to 9 min. Program guide and display poster; teacher's film guides; 30 student fact sheets; discussion posters; role-playing cards. Five-day free loan distribution through the National Center for Rape Prevention and Control.

*A Community Fights Rape,* 1978, MIT Teleprograms, Inc., 3710 Commercial Avenue, Northbrook, IL 60062, (800) 323-5343. Producer: CBS News.

> ABSTRACT: The film portrays a three-pronged effort by police, hospitals, and the community in San Jose, California, to attack the problem of rape. The "CBS News Magazine" program depicts the collaborative effort of the three groups to refute rape myths and taboos and to initiate programs sensitive to victim needs. This group effort resulted in a 100% increase in reporting and an 88% increase in arrests.

---

*Prices subject to change as affected by inflation and marketing by producers. For most films previews are available without cost.

CRITIQUE: Emphasizes the importance of community collaboration by concerned groups and its resulting effectiveness.

FORMAT: 16 mm, color. Rental: $40.00; purchase: $250.00.

*A Question of Consent: Rape,* 1979, Motorola Teleprograms, Inc., 4825 N. Scott Street, Suite 23, Schiller Park, IL 60176, (800) 323-5343.

ABSTRACT: The focus of this film is the court process, which attempts to blame the victim for the assault. Depicted is the defense attorney's strategy and basic techniques in defending the rapist. The victim is a single woman assaulted by her neighbor. The film clarifies why rape victims need emotional support from nurses, counselors, police, medical personnel, and family as well as the prosecutor in preparing for and testifying in court.

CRITIQUE: Suitable for communicating to general audiences the nature of a victim's experience in court. It is particularly useful for nurses who counsel victims through the court process and for the general public, who serve as jurors in rape cases.

FORMAT: 20 min, 16 mm, sound/color film or ¾″ U-matic videocasette.

*Better Safe than Sorry,* 1978, Film Fair Communications, 10900 Ventura Boulevard, Studio City, CA 91604.

ABSTRACT: This film presents situations in which children encounter strangers in potentially dangerous circumstances: loitering; car rides; hitchhiking; being followed; alone at home when a stranger calls. Subject areas include safety, guidance, and child molestation. Emphasis is on strangers, not persons known to children, and thus does not accurately portray the most dangerous perpetrators of child sexual abuse. The producers believe that the subject of sexual abuse by someone known or by a family member is better handled on an interpersonal level. The film can be stopped for discussion of situations depicted.

CRITIQUE: Can be used for primary, elementary, and junior high levels. The film also can be shown to parents' organizations to facilitate discussion of threatening situations for children and to civic groups for planning prevention programs.

FORMAT: 16 mm, color film, sound, 14½ min; teacher discussion guide. Rental: $25.00; purchase: $220.00.

*Beware the Rapist,* 1979, Sid Davis Productions, 1046 Robertson Boulevard, Los Angeles, CA 90035.

ABSTRACT: The film emphasizes avoidance as the best protection from rape. Almost every conceivable situation in which urban women are alone and vulnerable is depicted, and a variety of prevention methods are portrayed.

CRITIQUE: Full of valuable tips for the elderly. However, it depicts frightening episodes. Narration by a woman is effective.

FORMAT: 20 min, 16 mm, color, sound.

*Crime on the Streets,* 1979, Aims Instructional Media, P.O. Box 1010, Hollywood, CA 90028.

ABSTRACT: This film dramatically portrays situations in which common sense could prevent rape (see Appendix T). Through excellent acting, it emphasizes that one cannot judge a criminal by appearances.

CRITIQUE: Suitable for general audiences—with the exception of senior citizens. The film may be very frightening to that group.

FORMAT: 18 min, 16 mm, color. Rental: $25.00; purchase: $245.00.

*Double Jeopardy,* 1979, MIT Teleprograms, Inc., 3710 Commercial Avenue, Northbrook, IL 60062, (800) 323-5343.

ABSTRACT: Depicts the problems that sexually abused children confront when they give testimony about their abuse in the criminal justice system. The children are realistically portrayed as experiencing double jeopardy: first the abuse and then the criminal prosecution process. The film presents alternate procedures that prevent further trauma for the victim and are both therapeutic for the child and helpful to the investigative/prosecution process.

CRITIQUE: Excellent for audiences of police personnel, attorneys, judges, legislators, rape crisis center staff/volunteers, social workers, nurses, and the general public.

FORMAT: 40 min, 16 mm, color. Discussion guide of film text included.

*Fighting Back,* 1974, Audiovisual Center, Indiana University, Bloomington, IN

ABSTRACT: This film was shot in the Women Against Rape Center in New York. Women discuss their experiences with rape, the socialization of women that fosters failure to resist assault, and the fears that women have about inflicting injury in an attempt to save their lives. It emphasizes the importance of women raising their consciousness about their socialization and gaining an awareness of their fears and strengths.

CRITIQUE: Very good for general audiences—with the exception of senior citizens.

FORMAT: 16 mm.

*If It Happens to You: Rape,* 1976, Distribution Center, Education Development Center, 39 Chapel Street, Newton, MA 02160.

ABSTRACT: This documentary drama portrays the care and counseling of a rape victim in an emergency department (ED). It focuses less on the rape exam than on the sensitive interviewing and support provided to the victim through the medical care, police interview, and follow-up care arrangements. Professionals (nurse, physician, police, counselor) are portrayed as helpful to the victim. The film has been shown on PBS television as part of the series "Something Personal."

CRITIQUE: The film is excellent for the education of professionals responsible for investigating and providing victim care, particularly those who see the victim in the immediate aftermath of rape. It emphasizes the sensitive reaction of professionals in easing a victim's self-blaming responses to a rape experience.

FORMAT: 14 min, color, sound, 16 mm. Rental: $15.00; purchase: $95.00.

*Incest: The Hidden Crime,* 1979, The Media Guild, 118 S. Acacia Avenue, Box 881, Solana Beach, CA 92075, (714) 755-9191.

ABSTRACT: The film presents a real family (an airline pilot, his wife, and their daughter) discussing the development and impact of incest in their lives. It unfolds what happened, how each family member felt about the event, and what happened once secrecy about the incest was broken. The film's dual goal is increased awareness among viewers and crime prevention. Sexual matters are discussed openly. Through this documentary the producers aim to convey that children need not face a life scarred by guilt, self-doubt, and fear.

CRITIQUE: Suitable for high school, college, adult, and general public audiences. The emotional upset of most child victims is not accurately presented because the child in this film has acquired some emotional distance from the abuse and has had the benefit of counseling. The long-term effects of child sexual abuse are not addressed. The abuser in the film, the father, does not appear upset over his offense, and the family dynamics of abuse are minimally explored. Guided discussion of the film is recommended.

FORMAT: 20 min, 16 mm, color film or videocassette. Rental: $22.00; purchase: $265 for film, $220.00 for videocassette.

*Incest: The Victim Nobody Believes,* 1979, Motorola Teleprograms, Inc., 4825 N. Scott Street, Suite 23, Schiller Park, IL 60176, (800) 323-5343.

ABSTRACT: Depicts adult women discussing their childhood sexual abuse victimization. The film portrays the impact of the crime on their psychosocial well-being and where they are now in their lives. The setting is informal, and the women openly share their feelings.

CRITIQUE: This film is appropriate for professional audiences and community education, particularly for groups that have not been previously exposed to child sexual abuse victims. It is useful as an awareness or consciousness-raising film.

FORMAT: 20 min, 16 mm, color, sound. Rental: $25.00.

*Investigation of Rape,* 1977, Motorola Teleprograms, Inc., 4825 N. Scott Street, Suite 23, Schiller Park, IL 60176, (800) 323-5343.

ABSTRACT: The film presents a complete rape investigation, beginning with the legal investigation and following with the rape examination for evidence collection and establishment of a chain of evidence. Crisis intervention techniques that portray humane and sensitive care of victims are depicted. Hospital personnel and police officers are shown with the victim.

CRITIQUE: Presents a complete portrayal of the complex forces, emotions, and procedures that merge and must be addressed by victims following a rape experience. The film is excellent for professional audiences. An outstanding instructor's manual accompanies the film.

FORMAT: 22 min, 16 mm, color, sound.

*Invitations to Burglary,* 1978, Aptos Film Productions, Inc., 729 Seward Street, Suite 203, Hollywood, CA 90038.

ABSTRACT: Emphasizing citizen responsibility in preventing crime, this film demonstrates how citizens can take preventive action against burglary. Narrated by Raymond Burr, the film depicts procedures and security devices for preventing crimes.

CRITIQUE: Since many rapes occur during a burglary, this film is excellent for community audiences interested in rape prevention. Such audiences are taught to remove invitations to criminal acts that are obvious to burglars. Practical and realistic advice is offered for crime prevention.

FORMAT: 22 min, 16 mm, color, sound. Purchase: $250.00.

*Killing Us Softly: Advertising's Image of Women,* 1979, Cambridge Documentary Films, P.O. Box 385, Cambridge, MA 02139.

ABSTRACT: Using advertising from various media, Jean Kilbourne brings the audience to an awareness of distortions and manipulations by advertisers that add up to a powerful form of cultural conditioning that negatively affects women. Issues addressed in this film include objectification of women; exploitation of sexuality; caricaturing of femininity and masculinity; victimization of children; tyranny of "ideal" beauty; limiting of role and career options for women; and gratification of violence against women.

CRITIQUE: The film is an excellent resource for students; women's groups; rape crisis centers; courses on contemporary issues, women's studies, abuse, and violence. It stimulates open communication and discussion; examines the effect of stereotypes on a woman's self-image; demonstrates the link between a woman's low self-image and self-destructiveness; and explores possibilities for change on issues affecting women's health.

FORMAT: 30 min, 16 mm, color, sound. Rental: $38.00 (1 day), $56.00 (2 days); purchase: $365.00. Free previews available to libraries only.

*No Lies,* 1979, Direct Cinema Ltd. Library, P.O. Box 135, Franklin Lakes, NJ 07147.

ABSTRACT: Portrays the emotional and psychologic impact of rape on a victim and how one woman coped with a sexual assault. The film begins with a filmmaker questioning a friend about her rape experience. Shown is the lack of understanding, the doubt, and the blame that victims often encounter from the general public—all of which adds to the victim's stress reaction.

CRITIQUE: This film's realistic portrayal often has a deep emotional impact on audiences and thus offers an excellent starting point for a course of instruction that actively involves the learner. Because of the impact that this film creates, it needs to be followed with guided discussion; the advisability of preparing the audience in advance of viewing should also be considered by the presenter.

FORMAT: 16 min, color, sound. Rental: $25.00; purchase: $285.00. Comes with excellent study guides for different audiences (college courses, women's groups) with questions that can be interchanged for various audiences to stimulate discussion.

*Nobody's Victim II,* 1978, Ramsgate Films, 704 Santa Monica Boulevard, Santa Monica, CA 90401.

ABSTRACT: The film is designed in three parts: (1) ways of avoiding danger in public (on streets, on public transportation, in cars) and in the home; (2) ways to handle unavoidable confrontation; and (3) ways of diverting the hostility of a rapist. Crime is presented as a reality of life. Women are encouraged to behave with confidence and alertness rather than to focus on their anger about crime. New facts, such as which criminals are most dangerous, are presented.

CRITIQUE: Appropriate for community education audiences interested in rape prevention, particularly groups of independent and self-reliant women.

FORMAT: 24 min, 16 mm, color, sound. Rental: $35.00; purchase: $350.00.

*No Exceptions,* 1977, Filmfair Communications, 10900 Ventura Boulevard, P.O. Box 1728, Studio City, CA 91604.

ABSTRACT: Presents rape prevention techniques, self-defense strategies, and the reporting of a rape experience.

CRITIQUE: The producers take the position that if a victim hurts a rapist but fails to escape she is risking death. This controversial position is not supported in the research literature. No other film takes such a stand. The content is not suitable for the elderly because it cannot be easily heard. Beyond this limitation, the film is suitable for community education if the presenter addresses the controversy about victim resistance.

FORMAT: 24 min, 15 mm, color, sound. Rental: $35.00; purchase: $350.00.

*Rape: A New Perspective,* 1979, Motorola Teleprograms, Inc., 4825 N. Scott Street, Suite 23, Schiller Park, IL 60176, (800) 323-5343.

ABSTRACT: This film depicts the way in which cross-examination of a rape victim challenges the truth of her assertion that she was raped. The producers use the analogy of cross-examining a robbery victim to get the point of "victim guilt" across to the audience. Portrayed are ways in which victims are forced to defend their life-style and habits, manner of dress, social activities, and selection of friends.

CRITIQUE: Suitable for a wide range of audiences, particularly for community groups since these persons serve as jurors in rape cases and for persons likely to be involved in counseling victims who elect to prosecute their assailants. The film is excellent for stimulating group discussion.

FORMAT: 7 min, 16 mm, color, sound. Rental: $25.00; purchase: $125.00.

*Rape: A Preventive Inquiry,* 1975, Motorola Teleprograms, Inc., 4825 N. Scott Street, Suite 23, Schiller Park, IL 60176, (800) 323-5343.

ABSTRACT: Draws on the experience of women as victims and as persons capable of preventing rape. The San Francisco Police Department assists with the presentation of rape from the perspective of the victim, of the rapist, and of the police. Emphasis is placed on (1) awareness of one's environment, (2) remaining calm, using one's wit and intuition; and (3) reporting rape to the police.

CRITIQUE: The film is effective in conveying rape prevention information and what to do if rape cannot be avoided. Because elderly persons may be frightened by the film, discussion of the content with the audience before and after the showing is important.

FORMAT: 17½ min, 16 mm, color, sound. Rental: $50.00; purchase: $295.00.

*Rape Culture,* 1979, Cambridge Documentary Films, Inc., P.O. Box 385, Cambridge, MA 02139.

ABSTRACT: This documentary searches the social forces in our culture that actively contribute to the crime of rape and the issues victims confront as a result of the crime. It examines popular media (films, advertising, and records) and interviews with victims, rapists, crisis workers, and experts in the field of victimology.

CRITIQUE: The film is suitable for community groups, high schools, colleges, and other organizations that provide rape education programs to teenagers and young adults. It is also useful for classes addressing contemporary issues and the media.

FORMAT: 35 min, 16 mm, color, sound. Rental: $40.00 (2 days).

*Rape Prevention: No Pat Answers,* 1975, Douglas County Rape Victim Support Project, P.O. Box 20877, University Station, Lawrence, KS 66045.

ABSTRACT: covers a wide range of prevention behaviors. It addresses a woman's fear of being aggressive, assertive ways to respond in protecting oneself, and aggressive resistance. Myths about rape are refuted. The offender's pattern of testing victim vulnerability is depicted, and helpful ideas for preventing child rape are presented. The film ends with a group of women discussing their feelings about rape and rape prevention.

CRITIQUE: This is currently *one of the best* rape prevention films on the market and is widely used by rape crisis centers. It is suitable for teenagers and the elderly, community groups, women's groups, community organizations, and students.

FORMAT: 20 min, 16 mm, color, sound. Rental: $10.00; purchase: $160.00.

*Rape: The Savage Crime,* 1979, Audio Visual Narrative Arts, Inc., Box 9, Pleasantville, NJ 10570.

ABSTRACT: Part 1 reviews the ways in which society has responded to rape over the centuries. The content offers some description of the rapist and explains the myths and misinformation that surround reporting and prosecuting the crime. Part 2 explores cultural conditioning that contributes to a woman's vulnerability to rape. Examined are ways in which the police/legal/medical systems view rape and how women react to rape. A rationale for the responses of systems and victims is provided.

CRITIQUE: The film is intended for a wide range of audiences. The content is not dramatic or shocking—like that of some films that require audience desensitization. Audiences suitable for viewing the film include community groups, women's groups and organizations, students, and classes in contemporary issues.

FORMAT: 30 min, color, sound, filmstrip. Rental: $7.50; purchase: $57.50.

*Rape: Victim or Victor,* 1976, MTI Teleprograms, Inc., 4825 N. Scott Street, Suite 23, Schiller Park, IL 60176, (800) 323-5343.

ABSTRACT: Uses a series of vignettes to show that there are no rules to guarantee women they are assault free. The film portrays situations in which greater awareness and prevention strategies can minimize the chances of becoming a victim. In the case of an assault, the film emphasizes the need for regaining composure and becoming aware of the right moment to escape.

CRITIQUE: Directed toward hospital social service departments, schools and libraries, women's groups, PTA groups, community organizations, students, rape crisis centers, crime prevention officers, students, and others. Used by rape crisis centers, this film is *highly recommended.*

FORMAT: 20 min, 16 mm, color film, sound, or ¾″ U-matic videocassette. A discussion leader's guide is also available. Rental: $40.00 (1 week); purchase: $275.00.

*Sexual Child Abuse: Four Case Studies,* 1979, Motorola Teleprograms, Inc., 4825 N. Scott Street, Suite 23, Schiller Park, IL 60176, (800) 323-5343.

ABSTRACT: This film comes in two parts. Presented in depth are (1) the lives of four women who were victims of child sexual abuse and (2) their experience in therapy as they worked through their feelings. The women reveal the impact of the trauma, where they are now with their lives, and what the therapist can do to help adult women who experienced sexual victimization as children.

CRITIQUE: Suitable for professional audiences, particularly persons who work with adult women who were victims of child sexual abuse. The film is appropriate for counselors in crisis centers, community mental health centers, hospital out-patient clinics, and psychiatric–mental health nurses. The film is also useful as a training tool in educational programs.

FORMAT: Part A, 27 min (2 women presented), Part B, 23 min (2 women presented). Rental: $110 for both films; purchase: $650 for film or $595 for videocassette. Parts A or B ordered separately. Rental: $55.00 for Part A or B; purchase: $410 for color film, $375 for videocassette.

*Someone Else's Crisis,* 1979, Motorola Teleprograms, Inc., 4825 N. Scott Street, Suite 23, Schiller Park, IL 60176.

ABSTRACT: Consists of five vignettes depicting crisis situations: (1) an armed robbery, (2) a violent rape, (3) a burglary in a residence, (4) a purse-snatching robbery, and (5) a child who has lost his dog. The presentation is explicit to help the audience empathize with the victim's emotional state. The police officer's role in providing emotional support prior to investigating the crime is emphasized.

CRITIQUE: With its emphasis on empathic response to the victim, this is an excellent film for teaching awareness of victim response to assault and crisis. It is suitable for a wide range of audiences.

FORMAT: 25 min, 16 mm, color, sound. Instructor's manual included. Rental: $50.00; purchase: $375.00.

*The Last Taboo: Sexual Child Abuse,* 1979, Motorola Teleprograms, Inc., 4825 N. Scott Street, Suite 23, Schiller Park, IL 60176, (800) 323-5343.

ABSTRACT: This film presents four adult women working through their feelings about child sexual abuse in their lives. Shown is role of professionals interacting with the women to help them work through their feelings.

CRITIQUE: Usually has a high degree of emotional impact on the audience. This film is recommended as a training film for professionals who work with child sexual abuse victims. It is also an excellent tool for educating nurses about therapeutic work with adult women who were child victims. The film is interconnected with another film, *Sexual Child Abuse: Four Case Studies.* Together the two programs form a complete offering that reflects the therapeutic work done with these women.

FORMAT: 28 min, 16 mm, color, sound. Rental: $65.00; purchase: $435.00 (film), $395 (videocassette).

*The Rape Examination,* 1978, Abbott Laboratories, Abbott Motion Pictures Professional Relations, D-383 Abbott Park, North Chicago, IL 60064. Contact the agency Film Library.

ABSTRACT: The film presents an explicit portrayal of the step-by-step medical procedure in treating a rape victim and collecting evidence of the assault for prosecution of an assailant. It begins with the victim's entrance into treatment in the emergency department. Professionals involved are very empathic and understanding while providing care to the victim. The gynecologic exam and the correct procedures for evidence collection (for most regions of the nation) are well presented.

CRITIQUE: This is *one of the best* teaching films available for use in the education of professionals responsible for victim care in an emergency department. The film presenter needs to identify any procedures presented that may differ from what is required in his or her own community. This film complements the content of Chapter 6 of this text.

FORMAT: 20 min, 16 mm, color, sound. Excellent monograph accompanies film for use in studying and reinforcing learning (additional copies can be ordered for $.50 per copy). Rental: $7.50.

*The Reality of Rape,* 1979, Motorola Teleprograms, Inc., 4825 N. Scott Street, Suite 23, Schiller Park, IL 60176, (800) 323-5343.

ABSTRACT: This film begins with a young woman hitchhiking, a high-risk behavior that puts women in a vulnerable position for rape. It depicts the way in which a rapist gains psychologic control over a victim and how fear, horror, and shock can paralyze a victim into submission and passivity. Portrayal of the rape as a violent act is more realistic than that of many films. Two police officers are shown interviewing the victim; one is supportive and empathic, but the other is less so.

CRITIQUE: Excellent as a teaching film, a training film, and a community or public information tool. Guided discussion after viewing is recommended.

FORMAT: 10 min, 16 mm, color, sound. Rental: $25.00; purchase: $175.00.

*Treating the Sexual Assault Victim,* 1979, Film and Video Service, P.O. Box 299, Wheaton, IL 60187.

ABSTRACT: This film consists of two color filmstrips accompanied by audiocassettes that can be advanced manually or automatically. Part 1 focuses on interpersonal communication, assessment, and crisis intervention skills. Part 2 presents the physical exam, collection of evidence, and medical treatment of the victim.

CRITIQUE: The filmstrips were developed for use in nursing schools and in-service training programs for staff in hospital settings. Emphasis is placed on assessment, interviewing, crisis intervention and counseling, medical treatment, and evidence collection. This resource is suitable for professional audiences.

FORMAT: 15 min, color, filmstrip. Preview: $10.00.

*Vulnerable to Attack,* 1979, Charles S. MacCrone Productions, 379 Sandalwood Drive, Aptos, CA 95003.

ABSTRACT: Informs women about preventing crime, ways to respond if approached, and ways to physically defend oneself against assault. Rape is presented as a violent rather than a sexual crime. The film is narrated by Greg Morris of "Mission Impossible," which may be an attractive feature for some audiences.

CRITIQUE: This film is excellent for women's groups, students, and public speaking engagements on rape prevention. It is not recommended for elderly persons because the prevention strategies require agility, the pace of the film is fast, and there are a few scenes that may be frightening.

FORMAT: 28 min, 16 mm, color, sound. Purchase: $395.00.

*When Will People Help?: The Social Psychology of Bystander Intervention,* 1976, Harcourt Brace Jovanovich, 757 Third Avenue, New York, NY 10017.

ABSTRACT: Explores why bystanders elect not to intervene in violent crimes. Attention is given to facts from social psychology studies that discuss why people are more likely to respond to emergencies when they are not in a crowd. The film demonstrates how field experiments and laboratory studies arrived at an explanation of bystander nonintervention; and it recommends ways of involving people in coming to the aid of victims. The 1965 case of Kitty Genovese is used as an example. The witness to the crime is presented as a victim too.

CRITIQUE: The film is excellent for neighborhood groups because it teaches citizens the importance of effectively looking out for one another. It is an outstanding educational resource for community workers such as nurses, police officers, and victim/witness assistants.

FORMAT: 25 min, 16 mm, color, sound. Rental: $44.00 (per week); purchase: $440.00.

*Who Do You Tell?*, 1979, MTI Teleprograms, Inc., 4825 N. Scott Street, Suite 23, Schiller Park, IL 60176, (800) 323-5343.

ABSTRACT: This film combines live interviews with children and cartoons in order to illustrate how children can handle problems that will not go away (such as sexual abuse) and may become more and more frightening for the young child. Not limited to sexual abuse, the film addresses other stressful situations and encourages the child to reach out to persons available for help. Support systems for the child are identified (e.g., community services and adults in the community).

CRITIQUE: Directed toward children 8 to 11 years old. Nurses working with children in this age group will find the film useful in preventive education and in efforts at case identification. This film is useful for community education projects, particularly within school systems because its format is acceptable to most schools.

FORMAT: 10 min, 16 mm, color, sound. Included are teaching guides, discussion questions, classroom activities, and suggested projects. Rental: $25.00; purchase: $120.00.

*Additional resources and film information can be obtained by writing to:*

The National Center for the Prevention and Control of Rape
5600 Fishers Lane
Rockville, MD 20852

National Organization for Victim Assistance
918 16th Street, N.W., Suite 503
Washington, DC 20006
(202) 466-NOVA

Criminal Justice and the Elderly
National Council of Senior Citizens
1511 K Street, N.W., Suite 540
Washington, DC 20005
(202) 638-4848

*Publication:* Guide to training materials in crime prevention and victim assistance for the elderly, ed. 2, Dec. 1979-Jan. 1981. Cost: $2.00.

## APPENDIX V

# Resolution on victimology*

WHEREAS, The number of reported cases of abused victims of all ages is increasing; and

WHEREAS, Abuse victims present themselves in all settings where registered nurses practice; and

WHEREAS, Comprehensive nursing care of abused victims requires a definite knowledge base in family dynamics, human sexuality, and victimology; and

WHEREAS, Registered nurses providing primary, secondary, and tertiary intervention generally are not prepared in victim health care; and

WHEREAS, This knowledge can only be assured with an adequate cadre of clinicians and faculty prepared in victimology; and therefore be it

RESOLVED, That the Council of Specialists in Psychiatric and Mental Health Nursing encourage graduate programs in psychiatric and mental health nursing **to assure adequate numbers of faculty to teach victimology and victimologist researchers to expand the scientific base for psychiatric and mental health nursing practice with victims;** and be it further

RESOLVED, That the Council of Specialists in Psychiatric and Mental Health Nursing encourage clinicians who care for abused victims to write and report their information concerning clinical practice.

---

*Approved by the membership of the Council of Specialists in Psychiatric and Mental Health Nursing at their annual business meeting, June 9, 1980.

# Index